Nuclear Cardiology

Editors

SHARMILA DORBALA
PIOTR SLOMKA

CARDIOLOGY CLINICS

www.cardiology.theclinics.com

May 2023 • Volume 41 • Number 2

ELSEVIER

1600 John F. Kennedy Boulevard • Suite 1800 • Philadelphia, Pennsylvania, 19103-2899

http://www.theclinics.com

CARDIOLOGY CLINICS Volume 41, Number 2
May 2023 ISSN 0733-8651, ISBN-13: 978-0-323-96167-7

Editor: Joanna Gascoine
Developmental Editor: Karen Justine S. Dino

Cardiology Clinics (ISSN 0733-8651) is published quarterly by Elsevier Inc., 360 Park Avenue South, New York, NY 10010-1710. Months of issue are February, May, August, and November. Business and Editorial Offices: 1600 John F. Kennedy Blvd., Ste. 1800, Philadelphia, PA 19103-2899. Customer Service Office: 3251 Riverport Lane, Maryland Heights, MO 63043. Periodicals postage paid at New York, NY and additional mailing offices. Subscription prices are $377.00 per year for US individuals, $743.00 per year for US institutions, $100.00 per year for US students and residents, $468.00 per year for Canadian individuals, $932.00 per year for Canadian institutions, $490.00 per year for international individuals, $932.00 per year for international institutions, $100.00 per year for Canadian students/residents and $220.00 per year for international students/residents. To receive student/resident rate, orders must be accompanied by name of affiliated institution, data of term, and the *signature* of program/residency coordinator on institution letterhead. Orders will be billed at individual rate until proof of status is received. Foreign air speed delivery is included in all *Clinics* subscription prices. All prices are subject to change without notice. **POSTMASTER:** Send address changes to *Cardiology Clinics*, Elsevier Health Sciences Division, Subscription Customer Service, 3251 Riverport Lane, Maryland Heights, MO 63043. **Customer Service: 1-800-654-2452 (U.S. and Canada); 314-447-8871 (outside U.S. and Canada). Fax: 314-447-8029. E-mail: journalscustomerservice-usa@elsevier.com (for print support); journalsonlinesupport-usa@elsevier.com (for online support).**

Reprints. For copies of 100 or more, of articles in this publication, please contact the Commercial Reprints Department, Elsevier Inc., 360 Park Avenue South, New York, NY 10010-1710. Tel.: 212-633-3874; Fax: 212-633-3820; E-mail: reprints@elsevier.com.

Cardiology Clinics is also published in Spanish by McGraw-Hill Interamericana Editores S. A., P.O. Box 5-237, 06500, Mexico D. F., Mexico; in Portuguese by Reichmann and Alfonso Editores Rio de Janeiro, Brazil; and in Greek by Dimitrios P. Lagos, 8 Pondon Street, GR115-28 Ilissia, Greece.

Cardiology Clinics is covered in *MEDLINE/PubMed (Index Medicus)*, *Excerpta Medica, The Cumulative Index to Nursing and Allied Health Literature* (CINAHL).

Contributors

EDITORIAL BOARD

JAMIL A. ABOULHOSN, MD, FACC, FSCAI, Director, Ahmanson/UCLA Adult Congenital Heart Center, Streisand/American Heart Association Endowed Chair, Divisions of Cardiology and Pediatric Cardiology, David Geffen School of Medicine at UCLA, Los Angeles, California, USA

DAVID M. SHAVELLE, MD, FACC, FSCAI, Associate Professor, Keck School of Medicine of USC, Director, General Cardiovascular Fellowship Program, Director, Cardiac

Catheterization Laboratory, LAC + USC Medical Center, Division of Cardiovascular Medicine, University of Southern California, Los Angeles, California, USA; MemorialCare Heart and Vascular Institute, Long Beach Medical Center, Long Beach, California, USA

AUDREY H. WU, MD, MPH, Associate Professor, Advanced Heart Failure and Transplant Program, Division of Cardiovascular Medicine, Department of Medicine, University of Michigan, Ann Arbor, Michigan, USA

EDITORS

SHARMILA DORBALA, MD, MPH, MASNC, FACC, Division of Cardiovascular Imaging, Department of Radiology, Cardiovascular Division, Division of Nuclear Medicine and Molecular Imaging, Cardiac Amyloidosis Program, Division of Cardiology, Department of Medicine, Director of Nuclear Cardiology, Brigham and Women's Hospital, Professor of

Radiology, Harvard Medical School, Boston, Massachusetts, USA

PIOTR SLOMKA, PhD, MASNC, FACC, Research Scientist, Artificial Intelligence in Medicine Program, Cedars-Sinai Medical Center, Los Angeles, California, USA

AUTHORS

SHADY ABOHASHEM, MD, Instructor, Department of Radiology, Massachusetts General Hospital, Cardiovascular Imaging Research Center, Boston, Massachusetts, USA

WANDA ACAMPA, MD, PhD, Department of Advanced Biomedical Sciences, University Federico II, Naples, Italy

ROBERTA ASSANTE, MD, PhD, Department of Advanced Biomedical Sciences, University Federico II, Naples, Italy

FRANCESCO BARTOLI, MD, Department of Translational Research and Advanced

Technologies in Medicine and Surgery, Regional Center of Nuclear Medicine, University of Pisa, Pisa, Italy

ROBERTO BONI, MD, Nuclear Medicine Department, ASST Papa Giovanni, Bergamo, Italy

ELISABETH BROUWER, MD, PhD, Department of Rheumatology and Clinical Immunology, University Medical Center Groningen, University of Groningen, the Netherlands

ALBERTO CUOCOLO, MD, Department of Advanced Biomedical Sciences, University Federico II, Naples, Italy

ADRIANA D'ANTONIO, MD, Department of Advanced Biomedical Sciences, University Federico II, Naples, Italy

VERONICA DELLA TOMMASINA, MD, Cardiology Unit, Ospedale Versilia – USL Toscana Nord-Ovest, Italy

MARCELO F. DI CARLI, MD, Executive Director, Cardiovascular Imaging Program, Departments of Medicine and Radiology, Division of Nuclear Medicine and Molecular Imaging, Cardiovascular Division, Brigham and Women's Hospital, Seltzer Family Professor of Radiology and Medicine, Harvard Medical School, Boston, Massachusetts, USA

SANJAY DIVAKARAN, MD, Division of Cardiovascular Medicine and Cardiovascular Imaging Program, Brigham and Women's Hospital, Harvard Medical School, Boston, Massachusetts, USA

SHARMILA DORBALA, MD, MPH, MASNC, FACC, Division of Cardiovascular Imaging, Department of Radiology, Cardiovascular Division, Division of Nuclear Medicine and Molecular Imaging, Cardiac Amyloidosis Program, Division of Cardiology, Department of Medicine, Director of Nuclear Cardiology, Brigham and Women's Hospital, Professor of Radiology, Harvard Medical School, Boston, Massachusetts, USA

W. LANE DUVALL, MD, Division of Cardiology, Director of Nuclear Cardiology, Hartford Hospital, Hartford, Connecticut, USA

PAOLA A. ERBA, MD, PhD, Department of Medicine and Surgery, University of Milan Bicocca and Nuclear Medicine Unit ASST Ospedale Papa Giovanni XXIII Bergamo (Italy), Bergamo, Italy

PAOLA FERRO, MD, Nuclear Medicine Department, ASST Papa Giovanni, Bergamo, Italy

OLIVIER GHEYSENS, MD, PhD, Department of Nuclear Medicine, Cliniques Universitaires Saint-Luc and Institute of Clinical and Experimental Research (IREC), Université Catholique de Louvain (UCLouvain), Brussels, Belgium

ALESSIA GIMELLI, MD, Fondazione Toscana Gabriele Monasterio, Imaging Department, Pisa, Italy

ANDOR W.J.M. GLAUDEMANS, MD, PhD, Department of Nuclear Medicine and Molecular Imaging, Medical Imaging Center, University Medical Center Groningen, University of Groningen, the Netherlands

SIMRAN S. GREWAL, DO, Fellow, Division of Cardiology, Department of Medicine, Cardiovascular Imaging Research Center, Massachusetts General Hospital, Boston, Massachusetts, USA

WILLIAM F. JIEMY, PhD, Department of Rheumatology and Clinical Immunology, University Medical Center Groningen, University of Groningen, the Netherlands

YOSHITO KADOYA, MD, Clinical and Research Fellow, Division of Cardiology, University of Ottawa Heart Institute, Ottawa, Ontario, Canada

JACEK KWIECINSKI, MD, PhD, Department of Interventional Cardiology and Angiology, KKiAI, Institute of Cardiology, Warsaw, Poland

SUVASINI LAKSHMANAN, MD, University of Iowa Hospitals and Clinics, Iowa, USA

FRANCESCA LAZZERI, MD, Department of Translational Research and Advanced Technologies in Medicine and Surgery, University of Pisa, Pisa, Italy

RICCARDO LIGA, MD, PhD, Dipartimento di Patologia Chirurgica, Medica, Molecolare e dell'Area Critica, University of Pisa, University Hospital of Pisa, Pisa, Italy

TERESA MANNARINO, MD, PhD, Department of Advanced Biomedical Sciences, University Federico II, Naples, Italy

SEAN R. MCMAHON, MD, Division of Cardiology, Associate Director,

Echocardiography Laboratory, Hartford Hospital, Hartford, Connecticut, USA

ROBERT J.H. MILLER, MD, FRCPC, FACC, Clinical Associate Professor, Department of Cardiac Sciences, University of Calgary, Calgary, Alberta, Canada

DOUWE J. MULDER, MD, PhD, Division of Vascular Medicine, Department of Internal Medicine, University of Groningen, University Medical Center Groningen, the Netherlands

PIETER NIENHUIS, BSc, Department of Nuclear Medicine and Molecular Imaging, Medical Imaging Center, University Medical Center Groningen, University of Groningen, the Netherlands

MICHAEL T. OSBORNE, MD, Assistant Professor, Division of Cardiology, Department of Medicine, Cardiovascular Imaging Research Center, Massachusetts General Hospital, Boston, Massachusetts, USA

ETEE K. PATEL, MD, Division of Cardiology, Hartford Hospital, Hartford, Connecticut, USA

COSTANZA PICCOLO, BSc, Unit of Immunology, Rheumatology, Allergy and Rare Diseases (UnIRAR), IRCCS San Raffaele Hospital, Vita-Salute San Raffaele University, Milan, Italy

TERRENCE D. RUDDY, MD, FRCPC, FACC, FSNMMI, Clinician-Scientist and Professor, Division of Cardiology, University of Ottawa Heart Institute, Ottawa, Ontario, Canada
MARIA SANDOVICI, MD, PhD, Department of Rheumatology and Clinical Immunology, University Medical Center Groningen, University of Groningen, the Netherlands

RIEMER H.J.A. SLART, MD, PhD, Department of Nuclear Medicine and Molecular Imaging, Medical Imaging Center, University Medical Center Groningen, University of Groningen, the Netherlands; Biomedical Photonic Imaging Group, Faculty of Science and Technology, University of Twente, Enschede, the Netherlands

BEREND G.C. SLIJKHUIS, MD, Division of Vascular Medicine, Department of Internal Medicine, University of Groningen, University Medical Center Groningen, the Netherlands

GARY R. SMALL, PhD, MB, Clinician-Investigator and Associate Professor, Division of Cardiology, University of Ottawa Heart Institute, Ottawa, Ontario, Canada

ANAHITA TAVOOSI, MD, Clinical and Research Fellow, Division of Cardiology, University of Ottawa Heart Institute, Ottawa, Ontario, Canada

AHMED TAWAKOL, MD, Associate Professor, Division of Cardiology, Department of Medicine, Cardiovascular Imaging Research Center, Massachusetts General Hospital, Boston, Massachusetts, USA

MERRILL THOMAS, MD, MSc, University of Missouri-Kansas City School of Medicine, Saint Luke's Mid America Heart Institute, Kansas City, Missouri, USA

RANDALL C. THOMPSON, MD, MASNC, University of Missouri-Kansas City School of Medicine, Saint Luke's Mid America Heart Institute, Kansas City, Missouri, USA

ALESSANDRO TOMELLERI, MD, Unit of Immunology, Rheumatology, Allergy and Rare Diseases (UnIRAR), IRCCS San Raffaele Hospital, Vita-Salute San Raffaele University, Milan, Italy

KORNELIS S.M. VAN DER GEEST, MD, PhD, Department of Rheumatology and Clinical Immunology, University Medical Center Groningen, University of Groningen, the Netherlands

ANAM WAHEED, MD, Division of Cardiovascular Imaging, Department of Radiology, Cardiovascular Division, Brigham and Women's Hospital, Boston, Massachusetts, USA

ROGER GLENN WELLS, PhD, Medical Physicist and Associate Professor, Division of Cardiology, University of Ottawa Heart Institute, Ottawa, Ontario, Canada

EMILIA ZAMPELLA, MD, PhD, Department of Advanced Biomedical Sciences, University Federico II, Naples, Italy

Contents

The clinical presentation of coronary artery disease (CAD) has changed during the last 20 years with less ischemia on stress testing and more nonobstructive CAD on coronary angiography. Single-photon emission computed tomography (SPECT) myocardial perfusion imaging should include the measurement of myocardial flow reserve and assessment of coronary calcium for the diagnosis of nonobstructive CAD and coronary microvascular disease. SPECT/CT systems provide reliable attenuation correction for better specificity and low-dose CT for coronary calcium evaluation. SPECT MFR measurement is accurate, well validated, and repeatable.

PET allows the assessment of cardiovascular pathophysiology across a wide range of cardiovascular conditions. By imaging processes directly involved in disease progression and adverse events, such as inflammation and developing calcifications (microcalcifications), PET can not only enhance our understanding of cardiovascular disease, but also, as shown for 18F-sodium fluoride, has the potential to predict hard endpoints. In this review, the recent advances in disease activity assessment with cardiovascular PET, which provide hope that this promising technology could be leveraged in the clinical setting, shall be discussed.

Myocardial perfusion imaging by nuclear cardiology is widely validated for the diagnosis, risk stratification, and management of patients with suspected or known coronary artery disease. Numerous radiopharmaceuticals are available for single-photon emission computed tomography and PET modalities. Each tracer shows advantages and limitations that should be taken into account in performing an imaging examination. This review aimed to summarize the state-of-the-art radiotracers used for myocardial perfusion imaging and blood flow quantification, highlighting the new technologic advances and promising possible applications.

Artificial intelligence (AI) encompasses a variety of computer algorithms that have a wide range of potential clinical applications in nuclear cardiology. This article will introduce core terminology and concepts for AI including classifications of AI as well as training and testing regimens. We will then highlight the potential role for

AI to improve image registration and image quality. Next, we will discuss methods for AI-driven image attenuation correction. Finally, we will review advancements in machine learning and deep-learning applications for disease diagnosis and risk stratification, including efforts to improve clinical translation of this valuable technology with explainable AI models.

Nuclear cardiac imaging techniques may quantitatively investigate major disease mechanisms of different cardiac pathologies.

This review provides an overview of the techniques used in nuclear cardiology for the assessment of suspected or known cardiac sarcoidosis, how radionuclide imaging assists with regard to diagnosis, risk stratification, and monitoring response to therapy, and work that is on the horizon with novel tracers.

Cardiac single photon emission computed tomography using ^{99m}Tc-bone avid tracers allows for an accurate noninvasive diagnosis of transthyretin (ATTR) cardiac amyloidosis, a historically underdiagnosed disease. This imaging is recommended in select populations who demonstrate clinical and imaging features of infiltrative cardiomyopathy. It is imperative to concomitantly assess for light chain (AL) cardiac amyloidosis independent of radionuclide scintigraphy for timely management of AL amyloidosis, a deadly disease requiring urgent therapy. Clinical judgement is also key and in some select scenarios an endomyocardial biopsy may be needed even after a noninvasive evaluation.

Infective endocarditis (IE) is associated with high morbidity and mortality. Early diagnosis is crucial for adequate patient management. Due to difficulties in the diagnosis, a multidisciplinary discussion in addition to the integration of clinical signs, microbiology data, and imaging data is used. Imaging, including echocardiography, molecular imaging techniques, and coronary CT angiography (CTA) is central to detect infections involving heart valves and implanted cardiovascular devices, also allowing for early detection of septic emboli and metastatic. This article describes the main clinical application of white blood cell SPECT/CT and [^{18}F]FDG-PET/CT and CTA in IE and infections associated with cardiovascular implantable electronic devices.

Systemic vasculitides comprise a group of autoimmune diseases affecting blood vessels. [18F]-fluoro-2-deoxy-d-glucose positron emission tomography/computed tomography (FDG-PET/CT) plays an important role in the diagnosis and therapeutic monitoring of vasculitides affecting large-sized and medium-sized vessels. FDG-PET/CT also provides complementary information to other vascular imaging tools. The resolution and sensitivity of newer generation scanners continues to increase, hereby improving the ability of FDG-PET/CT to accurately assess the full disease extent in patients with vasculitis. Novel tracers targeting specific immune cells will allow for more detailed detection of vascular infiltrates.

Radionuclide Imaging of Heart-Brain Connections   **267**

Shady Abohashem, Simran S. Grewal, Ahmed Tawakol, and Michael T. Osborne

The heart and brain have a complex interplay wherein disease or injury to either organ may adversely affect the other. The mechanisms underlying this connection remain incompletely characterized. However, nuclear molecular imaging is uniquely suited to investigate these pathways by facilitating the simultaneous assessment of both organs using targeted radiotracers. Research within this paradigm has demonstrated important roles for inflammation, autonomic nervous system and neurohormonal activity, metabolism, and perfusion in the heart-brain connection. Further mechanistic clarification may facilitate greater clinical awareness and the development of targeted therapies to alleviate the burden of disease in both organs.

CARDIOLOGY CLINICS

CARDIOLOGY CLINICS

SERIES OF RELATED INTEREST

Heart Failure Clinics
Available at: https://www.heartfailure.theclinics.com/
Cardiac Electrophysiology Clinics
Available at: https://www.cardiacep.theclinics.com/
Interventional Cardiology Clinics
Available at: https://www.interventional.theclinics.com/

Preface
Nuclear Cardiology in 2023

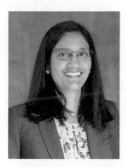

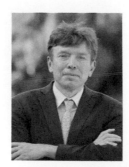

Sharmila Dorbala, MD, MPH, MASNC, FACC   Piotr Slomka, PhD, MASNC, FACC

Editors

Nuclear Cardiology techniques have become essential for the evaluation and management of various cardiovascular diseases. Recent advancements in imaging technologies, such as hybrid PET/CT and PET/MR scanners, new image reconstruction software, and repurposing of existing radionuclide tracers, have enabled personalized therapies. In this issue of *Cardiology Clinics* on Nuclear Cardiology, experts discuss technological advancements and radiotracer developments that have revolutionized the field and enabled comprehensive evaluation and image-guided management of cardiovascular diseases.

The authors cover the use of single-photon emission computed tomography (SPECT) myocardial perfusion imaging (MPI) radiotracers and their use for risk stratification. They discuss the emerging technological SPECT-MPI advancements that make low-radiation dose and myocardial blood flow quantification possible. The value of coronary artery calcification to the MPI is also highlighted. In addition, the authors discuss various molecular imaging tracers, including ^{99m}Tc-pyrophosphate and ^{18}F-sodium fluoride, which have been repurposed for cardiac imaging. These hot-spot tracers measure disease activity and aid in the personalized evaluation and management of cardiac amyloidosis, coronary disease, and aortic valve disease. Furthermore, the authors discuss the rapidly emerging role of ^{18}F-Fluorodeoxyglucose–PET/CT in the management of patients with various inflammatory cardiovascular diseases, including cardiac sarcoidosis, vasculitis, and infective endocarditis. This includes

its use for prosthetic valve and cardiac implantable electronic device evaluations. These advancements in nuclear cardiology offer a comprehensive evaluation of cardiovascular diseases, including the heart-brain connection. This systems-based approach can improve our understanding of how cardiovascular disease impacts an individual's overall well-being and health.

We thank Dr Audrey H. Wu for the opportunity to edit this issue on Nuclear Cardiology. It has been a great pleasure to work with each of the authors; we thank them for their insightful contributions. Our special thanks to Karen Justine S. Dino Solomon and her team for their support and guidance throughout this issue.

Sharmila Dorbala, MD, MPH, MASNC, FACC
Division of Nuclear Medicine and
Molecular Imaging
Department of Radiology
Brigham and Women's Hospital
Harvard Medical School
70 Francis Street Shapiro
5th Floor, Room 128
Boston, MA 02115, USA

Piotr Slomka, PhD, MASNC, FACC
Cedars-Sinai Medical Center
North Tower A047, 8700 Beverly Boulevard
Los Angeles, CA 90048, USA

E-mail addresses:
sdorbala@bwh.harvard.edu (S. Dorbala)
piotr.slomka@cshs.org (P. Slomka)

Cardiol Clin 41 (2023) xiii
https://doi.org/10.1016/j.ccl.2023.03.001
0733-8651/23/

Advances in Single-Photon Emission Computed Tomography
Hardware, Software, and Myocardial Flow Reserve

Terrence D. Ruddy, MD, FRCPC, FSNMMI*, Yoshito Kadoya, MD,
Anahita Tavoosi, MD, Gary R. Small, PhD, MB, Roger Glenn Wells, PhD

KEYWORDS

- Myocardial perfusion imaging • Solid-state CZT SPECT • SPECT/CT • Myocardial flow reserve
- Coronary artery calcium

KEY POINTS

- Temporal changing of coronary artery disease (CAD) presentation with less ischemia on stress testing and more nonobstructive CAD on coronary angiography, consistent with more patients with ischemia with nonobstructive CAD (INOCA).
- Need for single-photon emission computed tomography (SPECT) myocardial perfusion imaging (MPI) to include MFR measurement and coronary calcium assessment for diagnosis of INOCA and coronary microvascular disease.
- Higher counts with solid-state cadmium-zinc-telluride SPECT camera systems or focusing collimation permit lower radiation dose or shorter imaging times for MPI with similar image quality and diagnostic accuracy.
- Hybrid SPECT/CT systems provide reliable attenuation and scatter correction of MPI images for better specificity and diagnostic accuracy and low dose CT for coronary calcium evaluation.
- SPECT MFR measurement is accurate, validated with very good diagnostic accuracy compared with coronary angiography and PET myocardial blood flow, and repeatable.

INTRODUCTION

Single-photon emission computed tomography (SPECT) technology for myocardial perfusion imaging (MPI) has improved remarkably during the last 15 years.[1,2] New solid-state cardiac camera systems using cadmium-zinc-telluride (CZT) detectors combined with novel collimator designs have been introduced D-SPECT (Spectrum Dynamics, Caesarea, Israel), NM Discovery 530/570c (General Electric Healthcare, Haifa, Israel). Cardiofocal collimators can be added to dual-head Anger cameras as an upgrade or part of a new camera system using specialized software (Siemens, SmartZoom, Erlangen, Germany). Fanbeam collimation has been combined with solid-state photodiode detectors and Cs(I) crystals (Digirad Cardius 3 XPO, Digirad Corporation, Poway, CA, USA). These camera innovations improve effective image resolution and increase count sensitivity (**Fig. 1**). The greater count sensitivity permits lower radiation doses or shorter imaging times with similar image quality and diagnostic accuracy. Dynamic list mode imaging with stationary gantry CZT camera designs and higher count rates facilitate measurement of myocardial blood flow

Division of Cardiology, University of Ottawa Heart Institute, 40 Ruskin Street, Ottawa, Ontario K1Y 4W7, Canada
* Corresponding author.
E-mail address: truddy@ottawaheart.ca

Cardiol Clin 41 (2023) 117–127
https://doi.org/10.1016/j.ccl.2023.01.001
0733-8651/23/© 2023 Elsevier Inc. All rights reserved.

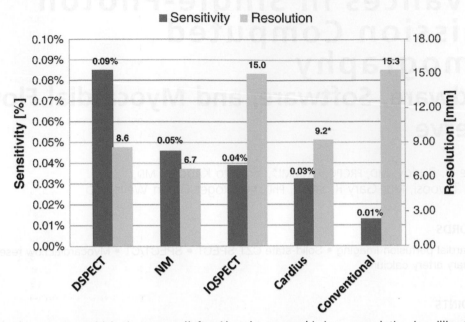

Fig. 1. Absolute count sensitivity in percent (*left axis*) and tomographic image resolution in millimeters (*right axis*) of the new cardiac SPECT systems as compared with the conventional dual head system. DSPECT, spectrum dynamics DSPECT system; IQSPECT, Symbia system with dual head astigmatic collimators from Siemens; NM, GE Alcyone 530c/570c system; Cardius Digirad X ACT with fan beam (FB27) collimator and n-speed reconstruction. Conventional = conventional dual-headed SPECT with low-energy high-resolution collimators. * Digirad XACT smallest orbit radius is approximately 20 cm and testing was conducted at that distance, as compared to standard 15 cm for NEMA NU-1 2001. (*From* Slomka PJ, Pan T, Berman DS, Germano G. Advances in SPECT and PET Hardware. Prog Cardiovasc Dis. 2015 May-Jun;57(6):566-78.)

(MBF) and myocardial flow reserve (MFR). Computed tomography (CT) is available on several SPECT/CT systems for CT-based attenuation correction and coronary calcium evaluation. These advances in SPECT hardware combined with improved reconstruction software have led to major improvements in SPECT MPI: lower dose, faster studies, MBF measurement, attenuation correction with CT, and assessment of coronary calcium.

The role of SPECT MPI in the management of coronary artery disease (CAD) is evolving with ongoing temporal changes in presentation and nature of CAD.[3] For decades, stress SPECT MPI has been crucial to decision-making for patients with suspected or known CAD. Demonstration of ischemia in a symptomatic patient would frequently lead to coronary angiography and revascularization. However, the frequency of ischemia in symptomatic patients evaluated for CAD with stress MPI has declined,[4] and the prevalence of nonobstructive CAD in patients with angina undergoing coronary angiography has increased to about 40% to 50%.[5,6] Ischemia in patients with nonobstructive CAD (INOCA) may result in symptoms of dyspnea and angina or myocardial infarction and has an adverse prognosis.[5] This shift in the spectrum of CAD may be due to increasing obesity and diabetes, which may contribute to coronary microvascular disease (CMD) and more diffuse atherosclerosis.[7] Fortunately, INOCA may be identified with modern SPECT/CT MPI technology. The presence of coronary calcium identifies CAD, which may be obstructive or nonobstructive. The presence or absence of perfusion defects suggests obstructive or nonobstructive CAD. Reduced MFR (and no perfusion defects) may indicate reduced flow due to diffuse nonobstructive CAD or CMD. Appreciating the changes in CAD phenotype and implementing current SPECT technology will permit SPECT MPI to meet the current and future clinical needs for diagnosis, guiding treatment, and determining prognosis.

SINGLE-PHOTON EMISSION COMPUTED TOMOGRAPHY HARDWARE ADVANCES
Solid-State Cadmium-Zinc-Telluride Single-Photon Emission Computed Tomography Systems

The detector material used in the 2 commercially available cardiac-dedicated CZT SPECT systems (Spectrum Dynamics D-SPECT, GE Discovery NM 530/570c) provides an improved energy response compared with less expensive NaI(Tl) crystal detectors. The digital detector coupled with the CZT crystal includes an application-specific integrated circuit, heat sink, and digital board (**Fig. 2**) and no photomultiplier tubes. The reduced size of the CZT detector permits novel gantry and camera system designs (**Fig. 3**).

The D-SPECT has 6 or 9 vertical columns of pixelated CZT detector arrays, each 4 cm × 16 cm, and positioned in a 90° gantry. Each column has a high-sensitivity parallel-hole tungsten collimator and can be closely positioned to the patient improving spatial resolution. The collimator holes are square and larger than those of conventional collimators to further improve sensitivity. The Discovery NM 530/570c has a curved gantry with 19 16 cm × 16 cm pixelated CZT detectors, each interfaced with a single-hole pinhole collimator. Data are acquired simultaneously by all detectors with the gantry stationary. Improved sensitivity is related to the multiple detectors, larger collimator holes than standard collimators, and a field of view focused on the heart. With both systems, resolution is maintained using CZT detectors and software utilizing resolution recovery algorithms.

Solid-state CZT SPECT cameras have better sensitivity (5 to 8 times) and spatial resolution (2

times higher) compared with standard Anger cameras (see **Fig. 1**) and permit lower radiation doses and/or shorter imaging times.[1] Reducing acquisition time decreases motion artifacts and increases patient comfort. Diagnostic accuracy for obstructive CAD is similar for low-dose MPI.[8,9] Two-position imaging (prone and supine or semireclined and upright) is facilitated with improved count sensitivity and can help identify attenuation and respiratory artifacts.[10–12] A meta-analysis of the diagnostic accuracy of CZT SPECT MPI for obstructive CAD, including 20 studies and 2350 patients, reported a sensitivity of 84% and a specificity of 72%[13] (**Fig. 4**). Several prognostic studies have demonstrated similar risk prediction of cardiac events with CZT SPECT MPI compared with Anger camera studies.[14–16] The largest and most recent study compared quantitative versus visual analysis of CZT SPECT MPI in 19,495 patients and found increasing risk of cardiac events with worsening of visual assessment (normal scan 2% annual event rate).[16] In patients with normal scans, quantitative assessment further stratified risk and added prognostic value.

Adding CT with a hybrid SPECT/CT system or separate CT acquisition can enhance MPI by adding attenuation correction (AC) and evaluation of coronary calcium. Although the Discovery NM570c was available about 10 years ago as a hybrid system with a diagnostic CT, the increased cost limited its clinical use. More recently, new solid-state general-purpose SPECT/CT systems Veriton-CT (Spectrum Dynamics, Caesarea, Israel), Starguide (GE Healthcare, Haifa, Israel), and Discovery NM/CT 870 CZT (GE Healthcare, Haifa, Israel) have been introduced, and they can be used for MPI. The Veriton-CT has a ring gantry of 12 CZT variable-radius detector columns, each 4 cm × 32 cm, and up to a 128-slice CT. This gantry design permits accurate 3-dimensional patient contouring and greater count sensitivity. The GE Starguide has a multidetector 360° ring-shaped adaptive gantry with 12 CZT detectors and interfaced with a conventional CT. Each detector has 7 modules of 16 × 16 2.46 mm^2 collimated pixels and a tungsten collimator. The Discovery NM/CT 870 CZT has improved energy and image resolution with better image quality due to the CZT detectors. However, the Discovery NM/CT 870 CZT system has standard collimators and count sensitivity like usual Anger camera systems.

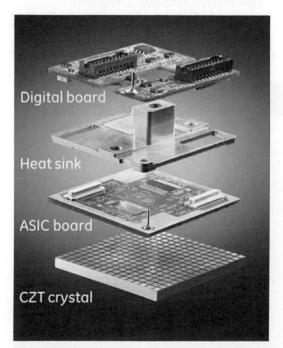

Fig. 2. Solid-state detector coupled with a CZT crystal. ASIC, application-specific integrated circuit. (*From* Slomka PJ, Pan T, Berman DS, Germano G. Advances in SPECT and PET Hardware. Prog Cardiovasc Dis. 2015 May-Jun;57(6):566-78.)

Focusing Collimation

Focusing or converging/diverging collimators can increase the sensitivity of conventional dual head Anger cameras by magnifying the region of interest.

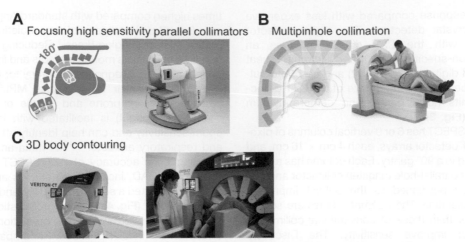

A Focusing high sensitivity parallel collimators

B Multipinhole collimation

C 3D body contouring

Fig. 3. Solid-state camera systems and collimator designs. (*A*). Focusing high sensitivity parallel collimators. Each of the 6 or 9 detector columns has 1 square hole collimator and can rotate 45° to focus on the heart. With the D-SPECT system, patients are positioned on a chair and can be imaged in both upright and semisupine positions. D-SPECT & VERITON. Used with permission from Spectrum Dynamics Medical. (*B*). Multipinhole collimation. Each of the 19 detector arrays are coupled to a pinhole collimator and are stationary. With the Discovery NM 530c system, patients can be imaged in the supine and prone positions. Used with permission of GE HealthCare Technologies Inc. (*C*). Three-dimensional contouring collimation. With the general purpose Veriton, 12 detector blocks with swivel motion can optimize sensitivity. D-SPECT & VERITON. Used with permission from Spectrum Dynamics Medical.

The center of the field of view is magnified with the converging collimation in the axial and trans-axial directions, and the periphery is minimized with the diverging collimation (**Fig. 5**). Image counts can be further increased by using a cardio-centric orbit to optimize the heart-to-collimator distance. Cardio-focal collimators (Siemens, SmartZoom) can be part of a new camera system or an inexpensive upgrade replacing existing collimators.

Single-Photon Emission Computed Tomography/Computed Tomography Systems

Hybrid SPECT/CT systems are now available and provide reliable attenuation and scatter correction

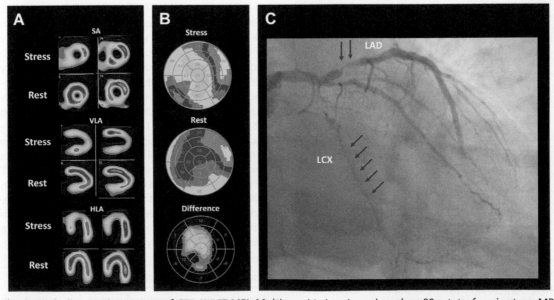

Fig. 4. High diagnostic accuracy of CZT SPECT MPI. Multivessel ischemia on low-dose 99m-tetrofosmin stress MPI (*A, B*) in a symptomatic male obese patient and subsequent coronary angiography showing severe left anterior descending and circumflex CAD (*C*).

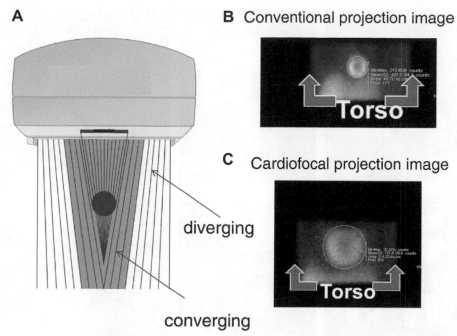

A

B Conventional projection image

C Cardiofocal projection image

diverging

converging

Fig. 5. Siemens IQ SPECT acquisition geometry with the diverging/converging (cardiofocal) collimator (*A*) allowing increased sensitivity in the heart region by selective focusing in the maximum zoom area. Projection images obtained with conventional (*B*) and cardiofocal (*C*) collimators. (*From* Slomka PJ, Pan T, Berman DS, Germano G. Advances in SPECT and PET Hardware. Prog Cardiovasc Dis. 2015 May-Jun;57(6):566-78.)

of MPI images for better specificity and diagnostic accuracy. The low-dose CT can be used for coronary calcium evaluation (**Fig. 6**).

SOFTWARE ADVANCES

Improved image reconstruction software is an essential component of solid-state camera systems and contributes to improved spatial resolution and count sensitivity. Image resolution is decreased with high-sensitivity collimation using larger collimator holes. Resolution is recovered through accurate modeling of the collimators and detectors. Image quality can be further improved with iterative reconstruction using constraints based on myocardial anatomic priors. These constraints assume a range for myocardial shape and thickness or can use CT data.

These new iterative reconstruction algorithms have been validated and can decrease scan times (or dose) by 50% while preserving image quality[17] and providing diagnostic quality concordant with full-time imaging with or without CT AC.[18]

Single-Photon Emission Computed Tomography Measurement of Myocardial Blood Reserve

MBF and MFR, measured with PET, add diagnostic and prognostic values to PET MPI in patients with suspected or known obstructive CAD.[19] However, PET MPI is less frequently performed than SPECT due to the higher costs of PET radiotracers and camera systems and the greater access to SPECT. Adding SPECT measurement of MFR to routine SPECT MPI would increase the availability and use of MFR with MPI.

Preclinical validation
The feasibility and accuracy of CZT SPECT measurement of MBF has been shown in a preclinical porcine model using ^{201}Tl, ^{99m}Tc-tetrofosmin, and ^{99m}Tc-sestamibi. The MBF values at rest and during dipyridamole stress with transient left anterior descending (LAD) coronary ischemia were accurate and correlated well (r = 0.75–0.90, P < .01 for all) with simultaneous microsphere measurements.[20] Timmins and colleagues[21] showed that accuracy and precision were maintained with dynamic SPECT measurement of MBF using one-fourth (^{99m}Tc tracers) and one-half dose (^{201}Tl).

Clinical validation with invasive coronary angiography and fractional flow reserve
Very good diagnostic accuracy of CZT SPECT measurement of MFR for the detection of obstructive CAD has been demonstrated with comparisons to invasive coronary angiography and FFR.[22–28] Ben Bouallègue and colleagues[22]

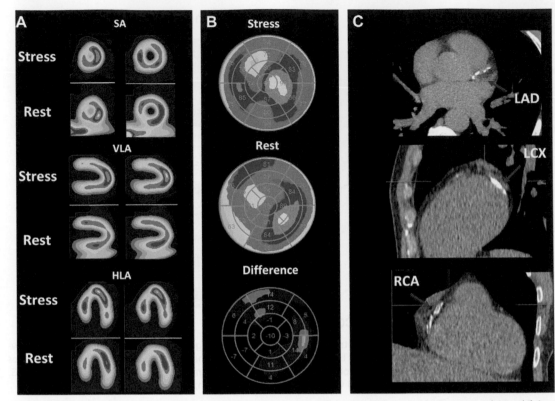

Fig. 6. Additional value of coronary artery calcium evaluation for MPI. Three-vessel coronary calcium (*C*) in an asymptomatic male patient with multiple risk factors and minimal ischemia on low-dose 99m-tetrofosmin stress MPI (*A, B*). Coronary angiography showed mild-to-moderate multivessel CAD.

evaluated regional MFR in 23 patients with known multivessel and reported diagnostic accuracy of 81% for the detection of obstructed arteries on visual analysis and 85% for arteries with abnormal FFR. Shiraishi and colleagues[23] evaluated the predictive value of a global MFR for the detection of left main or 3 vessel CAD in 55 patients. Using receiver operating characteristic (ROC) curve analysis, global MFR alone had a diagnostic accuracy of 80% for left main and 3-vessel CAD. Miyagawa and colleagues[24] showed that global MFR had a high diagnostic accuracy for predicting 3 vessel CAD and greater diagnostic accuracy than relative stress MPI in 69 patients. De Souza and colleagues[25] described the feasibility of a rapid acquisition protocol for measuring global and regional MFR in 41 patients. Rest and stress (supine and prone) static-gated imaging immediately followed dynamic imaging for a total imaging time less than 40 minutes. Regional MFR had a sensitivity of 63% and a specificity of 74% for the detection of an obstructed artery. Acampa and colleagues[26] showed the feasibility of measurement of MBF and MFR using a low-dose protocol in 173 patients with suspected or known CAD in 91 patients. Total perfusion defect, global stress MBF

and global MFR were predictive of obstructive CAD with univariate analysis but only global MFR was an independent predictor using multivariate analysis. Pang and colleagues[27] reported similar diagnostic accuracy of stress MBF and MFR for obstructive CAD using low doses in 57 patients with suspected or known CAD. Zavadovsky and colleagues[28] confirmed the predictive value of global stress MBF for the prediction of multivessel CAD (MVD) in 52 patients with stable CAD. Global stress MBF and MFR had a greater diagnostic accuracy for MVD than relative perfusion with semi-quantitative analysis, based on ROC analysis. Only stress MBF was an independent predictor of MVD on multivariate analysis.

Clinical validation with positron emission tomography comparisons

CZT SPECT measurement of MBF and MFR has been well validated with comparisons to PET.[29–33]

Nkoulou and colleagues[29] demonstrated the need for extraction fraction correction for SPECT measurements with a comparison of MBF and MFR measured with SPECT using ^{99m}Tc-tetrofosmin versus PET using ^{13}N-ammonia in 28 patients. SPECT and PET images were reconstructed with

AC and MBF calculated with a 1-tissue compartment model and no correction for extraction fraction. Although the correlation between SPECT and PET MBF was fair (0.62), SPECT severely underestimated PET MBF at high flows due to the much lower extraction of ^{99m}Tc-tetrofosmin compared with ^{13}N-ammonia. SPECT MFR predicted an abnormal PET MFR with a diagnostic accuracy of 75%.

Wells and colleagues[30] compared SPECT measurements of MBF and MFR to PET in 31 patients with known CAD. Accuracy and precision of global SPECT MBF improved with correction for motion and blood binding. SPECT global MBF and MFR differed from PET by 2% ± 32% (MBF) and 2% ± 28% (MFR). AC did not improve global

and regional MBF correlations with PET or detection of abnormal PET MFR. Optimized SPECT global MFR, with motion and blood binding correction and no attenuation correction, had an AUC of 0.95 using ROC analysis for the detection of abnormal PET MFR. Results were similar for regional analysis for SPECT MFR detection of abnormal PET MFR.

Agostini and colleagues[31] reported very good correlations between global and regional MBF and MFR measured with SPECT and ^{15}O-water PET in 30 stable patients with CAD with FFR of all 3 coronary arteries (WATERDAY study). Diagnostic accuracy of SPECT global stress MBF and MFR was high for the detection of reduced PET global stress MBF and MFR. SPECT and PET

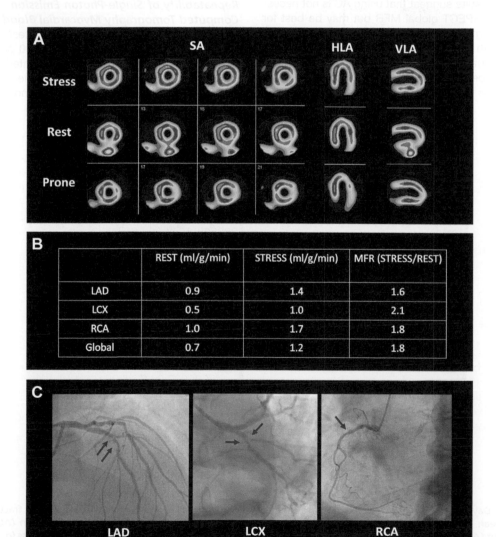

	REST (ml/g/min)	STRESS (ml/g/min)	MFR (STRESS/REST)
LAD	0.9	1.4	1.6
LCX	0.5	1.0	2.1
RCA	1.0	1.7	1.8
Global	0.7	1.2	1.8

Fig. 7. Incremental diagnostic value of MBF measurement for MPI. Mild ischemia of lateral wall on MPI (*A*) and reduced global stress flow and reserve (*B*) in a symptomatic male patient. Angiography showed severe left anterior descending and circumflex CAD (*C*).

regional MFR had high and similar diagnostic accuracy for the detection of an abnormal FFR.

Giubbini and colleagues[32] showed good correlations of global MFR measured using SPECT with (r = 0.52) and without AC (r = 0.50) compared with PET in 54 patients with suspected or known CAD. However, global rest and stress global MBF with SPECT and no AC were higher than PET and more like PET with attenuation correction. SPECT global MBF correlated better with PET with AC (r = 0.59) than without AC (r = 0.48). Diagnostic accuracy for the detection of reduced PET global MFR with SPECT MFR was very good and did not differ with AC or without AC. Thus, results for global MFR did not differ with and without AC but were more accurate for global MBF with AC. These results suggest that using AC is not necessary for SPECT global MFR but may be best for SPECT global MBF for physiological studies in sites with CT availability.

Acampa and colleagues[33] described fair correlations between SPECT and PET global stress MBF (r = 0.44) and MFR (r = 0.56) in 58 patients.

SPECT studies were low dose and without AC. Global rest MBF was similar with SPECT and PET but global stress MBF and MFR were higher with SPECT. SPECT global MFR had a very good diagnostic accuracy (80%) for the detection of reduced PET MFR. SPECT and PET regional MFR had a similar very good diagnostic accuracy for specific vessel obstructive CAD.

Panjer and colleagues[34] reported a meta-analysis and systematic review of the diagnostic accuracy of SPECT MFR for the detection of obstructive CAD defined as reduced PET MFR or reduced FFR. The pooled analysis of 9 studies with 421 patients showed a sensitivity of 79% and specificity of 85% (**Fig. 7**).

Repeatability of Single-Photon Emission Computed Tomography Myocardial Blood Flow

Wells and colleagues evaluated the test–retest repeatability of SPECT global MBF in 30 patients with repeat testing at a mean interval of 18 days.[35] The precision measured as the average coefficient of variation using Bland-Altman

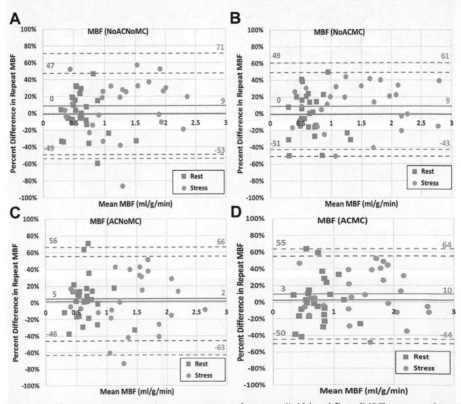

Fig. 8. Day-to-day differences in repeated measurements of myocardial blood flow (MBF) expressed as a fraction of the mean MBF. Images were analyzed without (*A* and *B*) and with (*C* and *D*) attenuation correction (AC) and without (*A* and *C*) and with (*B* and *D*) motion correction (MC). Results are shown for rest (*blue*) and stress (*orange*). The means are indicated with solid lines and the 95% confidence limits with dashed lines. Results are shown for user 1; results for user 2 were similar. (*From* Wells RG, Radonjic I, Clackdoyle D, Do J, Marvin B, Carey C, et al: Test-Retest precision of myocardial blood flow measurements with 99mTc-tetrofosmin and solid-state detector single photon emission computed tomography. Circ Cardiovasc Imaging 2020:13(2);e009769: with permission)

analysis was between 28% and 31% for MBF (**Fig. 8**) and 33% to 38% for MFR, calculated with and without correction for attenuation and motion. Interobserver repeatability was 11% to 15% for MBF and 13% to 22% for MFR. De Souza and colleagues[36] reported improved accuracy of SPECT MBF, compared with ^{13}N-ammonia PET, and repeatability with 2 serial SPECT studies using spline-fitted reconstruction algorithms compared with standard reconstruction.

Prognostic value of single-photon emission computed tomography myocardial blood flow

The prognostic value of SPECT MFR for predicting major adverse cardiac events has been shown in one recent study.[37] Liga and colleagues followed 129 patients with chest pain undergoing SPECT MPI and invasive coronary angiography for cardiac death, nonfatal myocardial infarction, and urgent revascularizations with a median follow-up of 65 months. Patients had early revascularization for clinical indications (64 patients). Events included nonfatal myocardial infarctions (7 patients) and late revascularization for urgent angina (13 patients). Relative perfusion semiquantitative scores and prevalence of obstructive CAD were similar in patients with and without events. However, events were associated with lower MFR and higher angiographic scores (incorporating severity, location, and extent of CAD). Multivariate analysis showed that low MFR and high angiographic scores were independent predictors of events.

FUTURE DIRECTIONS

SPECT MPI with solid-state camera systems has improved significantly with faster and lower dose studies and measurement of MFR. Attenuation correction and coronary calcium evaluation is possible with CT. Although several sites have realized much of this potential, many sites still need to upgrade hardware and software.

Although spatial resolution has been improved with solid-state cameras, patient and respiratory motion remains an issue for image quality. Data-driven correction methods for respiratory motion are feasible using list mode data.[38] Myocardium-to-blood-pool contrast can be improved with end-respiratory gating and further enhanced with dual respiratory/cardiac gating.[39] Using a center of mass approach, patient motion can be detected and then rejected to reconstruct images with less artifacts.[40] These software approaches for motion correction could be applied to dynamic list mode data used for measurement of MFR and improve accuracy and repeatability. Advanced 4D reconstruction algorithms that integrate data from all the dynamic frames[41,42] could reduce image noise and improve the variability of SPECT MBF measurements.[36]

Artificial intelligence techniques with machine or deep learning are being developed for rapid and accurate interpretation of SPECT MPI studies and may improve diagnosis and risk stratification in patients with suspected or known CAD.[43,44]

SUMMARY

Advanced technology with solid-state SPECT cameras combined with new reconstruction software results in improved photon sensitivity and image resolution compared with conventional Anger cameras. Increased sensitivity can also be achieved by retrofitting conventional dual head cameras with inexpensive cardiofocal collimators. SPECT MPI studies can now be acquired with half (or less) the usual radiation dose or acquisition time and have similar diagnostic value as full-dose or time conventional MPI studies. Several new SPECT systems are equipped with CT for attenuation correction and coronary calcium assessment.

Measurement of MFR with dynamic list mode imaging is feasible with stationary solid-state cameras due to the greater count sensitivity and improved temporal resolution. SPECT MBF and MFR measurements are accurate and have good day-to-day repeatability and interobserver variability. The presence of severe multivessel CAD can be identified by reduced global stress MBF and MFR. Reduced regional stress MBF and MFR have high diagnostic accuracy for obstructive CAD of specific vessels.

These technological innovations will allow SPECT MPI to grow and expand to meet the changing needs of the future.

CLINICS CARE POINTS

- Symptomatic patients with angina are now less likely to have obstructive coronary artery disease (CAD) and often have diffuse nonobstructive CAD or microvascular disease (or a combination).

- Diffuse nonobstructive CAD may be identified by the presence of coronary calcium, reduced myocardial flow reserve (MFR) and no relative perfusion defect.

- Reduced MFR is seen with coronary microvascular disease in patients with no coronary calcium or relative perfusion defects.

- MFR measurement is possible with positron emission (PET) or single photon emission computed (SPECT) tomography.
- Nuclear cardiology laboratories need to evolve from providing only relative perfusion imaging to adding evaluation of coronary calcium and MFR.

DISCLOSURE

Drs T.D. Ruddy and R.G. Wells have received research grants from GE HealthCare.

REFERENCES

1. Slomka PJ, Pan T, Berman DS, et al. Advances in SPECT and PET hardware. Prog Cardiovasc Dis 2015;57:566–78.
2. Slomka PJ, Miller RJH, Hu LH, et al. Solid-state detector SPECT myocardial perfusion imaging. J Nucl Med 2019;60:1194–204.
3. Di Carli MF. Changing epidemiology of CAD: why should we pay attention? J Nucl Cardiol 2021;28: 386–8.
4. Jouni H, Askew JW, Crusan DJ, et al. Temporal trends of single-photon emission computed tomography myocardial perfusion imaging in patients with coronary artery disease: a 22-year experience from a tertiary academic medical center. Circ Cardiovasc Imaging 2017;10:e005628.
5. Jespersen L, Hvelplund A, Abildstrøm SZ, et al. Stable angina pectoris with no obstructive coronary artery disease is associated with increased risks of major adverse cardiovascular events. Eur Heart J 2012;33:734–44.
6. Maddox TM, Stanislawski MA, Grunwald GK, et al. Nonobstructive coronary artery disease and risk of myocardial infarction. JAMA 2014;312:1754–63.
7. Virani SS, Alonso A, Benjamin EJ, et al. American heart association council on epidemiology and prevention statistics committee and stroke statistics subcommittee. heart disease and stroke statistics-2020 update: a report from the american heart association. Circulation 2020;141:e139–596.
8. Gimelli A, Bottai M, Genovesi D, et al. High diagnostic accuracy of low-dose gated-SPECT with solid-state ultrafast detectors: preliminary clinical results. Eur J Nucl Med Mol Imaging 2012;39: 83–90.
9. Sharir T, Pinskiy M, Pardes A, et al. Comparison of the diagnostic accuracies of very low stress-dose with standard-dose myocardial perfusion imaging: automated quantification of one-day, stress-first SPECT using a CZT camera. J Nucl Cardiol 2016; 23:11–20.
10. Nakazato R, Tamarappoo BK, Kang X, et al. Quantitative upright-supine high-speed SPECT myocardial perfusion imaging for detection of coronary artery disease: correlation with invasive coronary angiography. J Nucl Med 2010;51:1724–31.
11. Duvall WL, Slomka PJ, Gerlach JR, et al. High-efficiency SPECT MPI: comparison of automated quantification, visual interpretation, and coronary angiography. J Nucl Cardiol 2013;20:763–73.
12. Nakazato R, Slomka PJ, Fish M, et al. Quantitative high-efficiency cadmium-zinc-telluride SPECT with dedicated parallel-hole collimation system in obese patients: results of a multi-center study. J Nucl Cardiol 2015;22:266–75.
13. Zhang YQ, Jiang YF, Hong L, et al. Diagnostic value of cadmium-zinc-telluride myocardial perfusion imaging versus coronary angiography in coronary artery disease: a PRISMA-compliant meta-analysis. Medicine (Baltim) 2019;98:e14716.
14. Oldan JD, Shaw LK, Hofmann P, et al. Prognostic value of the cadmium-zinc-telluride camera: a comparison with a conventional (Anger) camera. J Nucl Cardiol 2016;23:1280–7.
15. Engbers EM, Timmer JR, Mouden M, et al. Prognostic value of myocardial perfusion imaging with a cadmium-zinc-telluride SPECT Camera in patients suspected of having coronary artery disease. J Nucl Med 2017;58:1459–63.
16. Otaki Y, Betancur J, Sharir T, et al. 5-year prognostic value of quantitative versus visual MPI in subtle perfusion defects: results from REFINE SPECT. JACC Cardiovasc Imaging 2020;13:774–85.
17. Borges-Neto S, Pagnanelli RA, Shaw LK, et al. Clinical results of a novel wide beam reconstruction method for shortening scan time of Tc-99m cardiac SPECT perfusion studies. J Nucl Cardiol 2007;14: 555–65.
18. Ali I, Ruddy TD, Almgrahi A, et al. Half-time SPECT myocardial perfusion imaging with attenuation correction. J Nucl Med 2009;50:554–62.
19. Murthy VL, Bateman TM, Beanlands RS, et al. Clinical quantification of myocardial blood flow using PET: joint position paper of the SNMMI cardiovascular council and the ASNC. J Nucl Med 2018;59:273–93.
20. Wells RG, Timmins R, Klein R, et al. Dynamic SPECT measurement of absolute myocardial blood flow in a porcine model. J Nucl Med 2014;55:1685–91.
21. Timmins R, Klein R, Petryk J, et al. Reduced dose measurement of absolute myocardial blood flow using dynamic SPECT imaging in a porcine model. Med Phys 2015;42:5075–83.
22. Ben Bouallègue F, Roubille F, Lattuca B, et al. SPECT myocardial perfusion reserve in patients with multivessel coronary disease: correlation with angiographic findings and invasive fractional flow reserve measurements. J Nucl Med 2015;56: 1712–7.

23. Shiraishi S, Sakamoto F, Tsuda N, et al. Prediction of left main or 3-vessel disease using myocardial perfusion reserve on dynamic thallium-201 single-photon emission computed tomography with a semi-conductor gamma camera. Circ J 2015;79:623–31.

24. Miyagawa M, Nishiyama Y, Uetani T, et al. Estimation of myocardial flow reserve utilizing an ultrafast cardiac SPECT: comparison with coronary angiography, fractional flow reserve, and the SYNTAX score. Int J Cardiol 2017;244:347–53.

25. de Souza ACDAH, Gonçalves BKD, Tedeschi AL, et al. Quantification of myocardial flow reserve using a gamma camera with solid-state cadmium-zinc-telluride detectors: relation to angiographic coronary artery disease. J Nucl Cardiol 2021;28:876–84.

26. Acampa W, Assante R, Mannarino T, et al. Low-dose dynamic myocardial perfusion imaging by CZT-SPECT in the identification of obstructive coronary artery disease. Eur J Nucl Med Mol Imaging 2020; 47:1705–12.

27. Pang Z, Wang J, Li S, et al. Diagnostic analysis of new quantitative parameters of low-dose dynamic myocardial perfusion imaging with CZT SPECT in the detection of suspected or known coronary artery disease. Int J Cardiovasc Imaging 2021;37:367–78.

28. Zavadovsky KV, Mochula AV, Maltseva AN, et al. The diagnostic value of SPECT CZT quantitative myocardial blood flow in high-risk patients. J Nucl Cardiol 2022;29:1051–63.

29. Nkoulou R, Fuchs TA, Pazhenkottil AP, et al. Absolute myocardial blood flow and flow reserve assessed by gated SPECT with cadmium-zinc-telluride detectors using 99mTc-tetrofosmin: head-to-head comparison with 13N-ammonia PET. J Nucl Med 2016;57:1887–92.

30. Wells RG, Marvin B, Poirier M, et al. Optimization of SPECT measurement of myocardial blood flow with corrections for attenuation, motion, and blood binding compared with PET. J Nucl Med 2017;58: 2013–9.

31. Agostini D, Roule V, Nganoa C, et al. First validation of myocardial flow reserve assessed by dynamic 99mTc-sestamibi CZT-SPECT camera: head to head comparison with 15O-water PET and fractional flow reserve in patients with suspected coronary artery disease. The WATERDAY study. Eur J Nucl Med Mol Imaging 2018;45:1079–90.

32. Giubbini R, Bertoli M, Durmo R, et al. Comparison between N13NH3-PET and 99mTc-tetrofosmin-CZT-SPECT in the evaluation of absolute myocardial blood flow and flow reserve. J Nucl Cardiol 2021; 28:1906–18.

33. Acampa W, Zampella E, Assante R, et al. Quantification of myocardial perfusion reserve by CZT-SPECT: a head-to-head comparison with 82rubidium PET. J Nucl Cardiol 2021;28:2827–39.

34. Panjer M, Dobrolinska M, Wagenaar NRL, et al. Diagnostic accuracy of dynamic CZT-SPECT in coronary artery disease. A systematic review and meta-analysis. J Nucl Cardiol 2022;29:1686–97. Epub ahead of print. PMID: 34350553.

35. Wells RG, Radonjic I, Clackdoyle D, et al. Test-retest precision of myocardial blood flow measurements with 99mTc-tetrofosmin and solid-state detector single photon emission computed tomography. Circ Cardiovasc Imaging 2020;13:e009769.

36. de Souza ACDAH, Harms HJ, Martell L, et al. Accuracy and reproducibility of myocardial blood flow quantification by single photon emission computed tomography imaging in patients with known or suspected coronary artery disease. Circ Cardiovasc Imaging 2022;15:e013987.

37. Liga R, Neglia D, Kusch A, et al. Prognostic role of dynamic CZT imaging in CAD patients: interaction between absolute flow and CAD burden. JACC Cardiovasc Imaging 2022;15:540–2.

38. Daou D, Sabbah R, Coaguila C, et al. Feasibility of data-driven cardiac respiratory motion correction of myocardial perfusion CZT SPECT: a pilot study. J Nucl Cardiol 2017;24:1598–607.

39. Chan C, Harris M, Le M, et al. End-expiration respiratory gating for a high-resolution stationary cardiac SPECT system. Phys Med Biol 2014;59:6267–87.

40. Kennedy JA, William Strauss H. Motion detection and amelioration in a dedicated cardiac solid-state CZT SPECT device. Med Biol Eng Comput 2017; 55:663–71.

41. Shrestha U, Sciammarella M, Alhassen F, et al. Measurement of absolute myocardial blood flow in humans using dynamic cardiac SPECT and 99mTc-tetrofosmin: method and validation. J Nucl Cardiol 2017;24:268–77.

42. Reutter BW, Gullberg GT, Huesman RH. Direct least-squares estimation of spatiotemporal distributions from dynamic SPECT projections using a spatial segmentation and temporal B-splines. IEEE Trans Med Imaging 2000;19:434–50.

43. Slomka PJ, Miller RJ, Isgum I, et al. Application and translation of artificial intelligence to cardiovascular imaging in nuclear medicine and noncontrast CT. Semin Nucl Med 2020;50:357–66.

44. Miller RJH, Huang C, Liang JX, et al. Artificial intelligence for disease diagnosis and risk prediction in nuclear cardiology. J Nucl Cardiol 2022;29:1754–62.

Novel PET Applications and Radiotracers for Imaging Cardiovascular Pathophysiology

Jacek Kwiecinski, MD, PhD

KEYWORDS

- PET • ^{18}F-sodium fluoride • Vulnerable plaque • Aortic stenosis • Coronary artery disease

KEY POINTS

- Assessment of disease activity with PET radiotracers elucidates the pathophysiology, and can serve for risk stratification and prognostication of disease progression of a wide range of cardiovascular conditions.
- Although the activity of several different PET tracers has been investigated, the literature is most advanced for ^{18}F-sodium fluoride, which is also the only PET tracer with available prognostic information in atherosclerotic plaque and aortic stenosis imaging.
- Further studies are necessary to validate the utility of PET tracers in imaging cardiovascular pathophysiology and ultimately to facilitate clinical adoption of this promising technology.

INTRODUCTION

Although the evaluation of the presence and extent of myocardial ischemia is the hallmark of nuclear cardiology, recent advances in PET have allowed the assessment of cardiovascular pathophysiology beyond myocardial perfusion imaging.[1] These novel applications are most apparent in atherosclerotic plaque imaging and valvular heart disease.[2]

In coronary artery disease, the assessment of the processes which drive plaque progression and rupture with PET complement multimodal assessments of anatomic, morphologic, and hemodynamic disease severity. The three processes that have been the primary imaging targets are inflammation, active calcification (microcalcifications) and, most recently, developing thrombus.[1]

IMAGING ATHEROSCLEROTIC PLAQUE INFLAMMATION

The initial efforts focused primarily on imaging coronary plaque inflammation with ^{18}F-fluorodeoxyglucose PET (FDG PET), which provides a reliable and reproducible measure of vascular inflammation as it indicates increased metabolic activity of macrophages, and probably also reflects contributions from local hypoxia and efficiency of tracer delivery by the microcirculation.[3,4] Unfortunately, coronary ^{18}F-FDG imaging is hampered by problems related to tracer uptake in the myocardium. Despite stringent dietary recommendations, suppression of myocardial activity is typically achieved in 57% to 85% of patients.[4–6] Often suboptimal suppression results in a patchy distribution of myocardial uptake that can obscure activity in one or more coronary vessels.[6]

Given the limitations of [18]FDG coronary imaging, it was proposed that tracers with established roles in cancer imaging (^{68}Ga-DOTATATE, 11C-PK11195, and ^{18}F-fluoromethylcholine) might be more-specific for vascular inflammation and better-suited to atherosclerotic plaque imaging than FDG.[7–9] Especially, ^{68}Ga-DOTATATE which binds to the somatostatin subtype-2 receptor on the surface of activated macrophages, is particularly promising. ^{68}Ga-DOTATATE PET offers

Department of Interventional Cardiology and Angiology, KKiAI, Institute of Cardiology, Alpejska 42, Warsaw 04-628, Poland
E-mail address: jkwiecinski@ikard.pl

Cardiol Clin 41 (2023) 129–139
https://doi.org/10.1016/j.ccl.2023.01.002

measurement of both generalized atherosclerotic disease activity and detailed information about local plaque functional phenotype distinguishing culprit from non-culprit coronary lesions.[9]

IMAGING ATHEROSCLEROTIC PLAQUE THROMBOSIS

Aside from the detection of vascular inflammation, subclinical plaque thrombosis has recently gained considerable interest. The glycoprotein IIb/IIIa (GPIIb/IIIa) receptor on activated platelets is a key player in thrombus formation and an attractive target for molecular imaging. The ^{18}F-labeled fiban-class ligand (^{18}F-GP1) is a novel radiotracer that binds with high affinity to the GPIIb/IIIa receptor on activated platelets.[10] Early results of a prospective study involving 51 patients with recent myocardial infarction showed that ^{18}F-GP1 binds to activated platelets and in vivo thrombus with high specificity. Indeed, ^{18}F-GP1 identified intracoronary thrombus beyond the resolution of computed tomography (CT) and accurately identified the culprit vessels. Furthermore, ^{18}F-GP1 can depict activated platelets within the coronary arteries, aiding in the identification of thrombus formation in both the left atrium and left ventricle, and potentially facilitating the distinction between type 1 and type 2 myocardial infarction[11] **(Fig. 1)**.

IMAGING ACTIVE CALCIFICATION PROCESSES WITHIN THE CARDIOVASCULAR SYSTEM

Although the activity of several different PET tracers has now been investigated in the coronary arteries, the literature is most advanced for ^{18}F-sodium fluoride (^{18}F-NaF), which is also the only PET tracer with available prognostic information.[12] Although ^{18}F-NaF has been developed for bone imaging (as it is directly incorporated into the exposed bone crystal [hydroxyapatite] via an exchange mechanism with hydroxyl groups), on whole-body PET scans, it became apparent that the activity of ^{18}F-NaF is often detectable within the atherosclerotic plaque.[13–20] These initial observations have led to dedicated cardiovascular studies focusing specifically on imaging calcifications within the atherosclerotic plaques and cardiac valves.

DEDICATED CARDIOVASCULAR ^{18}F-NaF IMAGING

In an observational study examining the role of active valvular calcifications in patients with aortic stenosis, Dweck and colleagues[21] demonstrated that ^{18}F-NaF activity is increased in patients with both aortic sclerosis and stenosis, displaying a progressive rise in uptake with increasing disease severity. Although this study

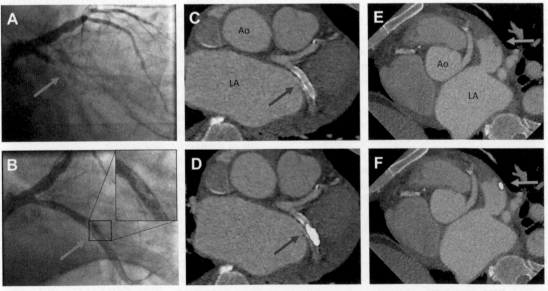

Fig. 1. Imaging plaque thrombosis. Typing a myocardial infarction. Invasive coronary angiography shows a proximally occluded left circumflex artery (*A; arrow*) and a persistent filling defect following recanalization (*B; arrow*). ^{18}F-GP1 PET/CT shows uptake colocalized to the stented coronary segment indicating thrombus behind the stent (*D; arrow*). ^{18}F-GP1 PET/CT scan shows uptake colocalized to a filling defect indicating an additional thrombus in the left atrial appendage (*F; arrow*). Corresponding CTA images in panels (*C and E*) respectively. (Reprinted with permission from Elsevier. The Lancet, August 2021, 398 (10299), page e9.)

established the feasibility of evaluating ^{18}F-NaF activity in patients with aortic stenosis, the dataset also served as the basis for a post hoc analysis of ^{18}F-NaF coronary uptake.[22] Dweck and colleagues have demonstrated that this technique is both feasible and repeatable and that it can provide key insights into coronary artery plaque biology. Among 119 study participants, ^{18}F-NaF activity was higher in patients with atherosclerosis compared with control subjects, displaying a progressive rise with an increasing atherosclerotic burden. Furthermore, the study suggested that ^{18}F-NaF uptake can be used to discriminate between patients with active and inactive coronary calcification. Those with active calcification (38%) were more likely to have clinically significant coronary artery disease (CAD), a higher incidence of previous major adverse cardiovascular events, lower serum high-density lipoprotein cholesterol concentrations, and higher Framingham risk scores. This initial study led to further investigations including the study of patients with recent myocardial infarction.

In a prospective clinical trial by Joshi and colleagues,[6] patients with myocardial infarction (n = 40) and stable angina (n = 40) underwent ^{18}F-NaF PET. Using invasive coronary angiography as the gold standard for determining the culprit plaque, the area of greatest ^{18}F-NaF uptake in the coronary arteries localized the culprit in 37 of 40 patients. Moreover, in patients with stable coronary artery disease, ^{18}F-NaF uptake identified coronary plaques with high-risk features on intravascular ultrasound. The authors concluded that ^{18}F-NaF PET holds major promise as a means of identifying high-risk and ruptured plaque, and potentially informing the future management and treatment of patients with stable and unstable coronary artery disease (**Fig. 2**). Despite the compelling findings of the study, the relatively modest ^{18}F-NaF uptake difference in culprit versus non-culprit plaques (~34% higher target-to-background ratio [TBR]) reported in the analysis could hamper clinical implementation. Fortunately, over the past decade, several technical refinements focused on mitigating the detrimental effects of motion and providing a more global measure of ^{18}F-NaF activity have been proposed.

OPTIMIZING ^{18}F-NaF CORONARY IMAGING

With the encouraging data suggesting that ^{18}F-NaF PET can potentially detect unstable coronary artery disease, further study focused on critical clinical as well as technical aspects of ^{18}F-NaF PET. Over the past years, the latter efforts have

enhanced this promising imaging modality by establishing tools for motion correction, optimized acquisition, and reconstruction protocols.[23] We have learned that by applying corrections for cardiac contractions, tidal breathing and gross patient motion, the reproducibility of ^{18}F-NaF coronary uptake measurements can be improved significantly.[24–29] For optimal image quality, it is vital to acquire data with time-of-flight information and preferably with a greater than 1-hour delay from tracer injection.[30,31]

In the initial ^{18}F-NaF PET studies, image analysis was typically performed using a maximum activity approach where the reader delineated volumes of interest only around areas with visually increased tracer activity and recorded the maximal activity (typically as maximum TBR). This method has several limitations.[32] Aside from the small difference between culprit and non-culprit lesions, the per plaque maximum TBR approach relies on labor-intensive and subjective visual detection of lesions and does not truly reflect disease activity across the entire coronary vasculature. This shortcoming has been addressed with a novel measure of coronary ^{18}F-NaF uptake—the coronary microcalcification activity (CMA).[33,34] This method allows evaluation of coronary ^{18}F-NaF activity on a per-vessel and per-patient basis, providing more global assessments of disease activity in the coronary arteries (**Fig. 3**).

By leveraging CT angiography-derived whole-vessel three-dimensional volumes of interest, ^{18}F-NaF PET tracer activity can be expressed as the global CMA mimicking an approach successfully implemented in oncology and cardiac sarcoidosis.[35,36] CMA represents both the volume and intensity of coronary ^{18}F-NaF activity, similar to the Agatston method for CT calcium scoring.[37] Rather than being limited to reporting the highest TBR or the number of plaques with increased tracer activity, CMA reflects the whole-coronary ^{18}F-NaF uptake burden. As a result, in patients and vessels with multiple foci of uptake, CMA provides a continuous measure of disease activity across the coronary vasculature. The proposed approach moves away from a single hot spot approach to a patient-level total ^{18}F-NaF activity burden assessment, and hence, does not rely on a single-pixel-value as traditional uptake measures (TBR or standard uptake values). Importantly, in a study evaluating the repeatability and reproducibility of CMA, this novel measure showed excellent intra- and interobserver repeatability and interscan reproducibility and narrow limits of agreements within and between scans.[34]

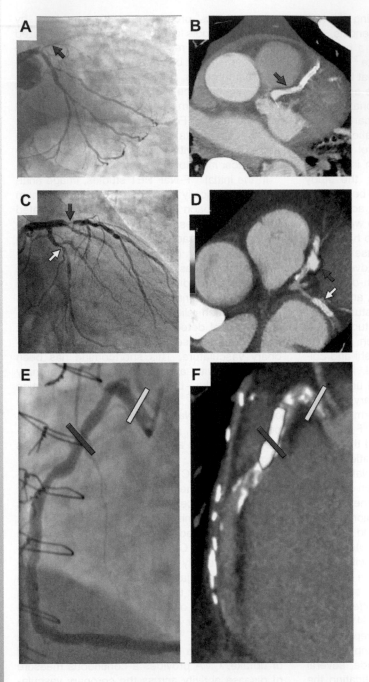

Fig. 2. Focal ¹⁸F-NaF in patients with myocardial infarction and stable angina. Patient with acute myocardial infarction with (*A*) proximal occlusion (*red arrow*) of the left anterior descending artery on invasive coronary angiography and (*B*) intense focal ¹⁸F-NaF uptake (*yellow–red*) at the site of the culprit plaque (*red arrow*) on PET. Patient with anterior myocardial infarction with (*C*) culprit (*red arrow*; left anterior descending artery) and bystander non-culprit (*white arrow*; circumflex artery) lesions on invasive coronary angiography that were both stented during the index admission. Only the culprit lesion had increased ¹⁸F-NaF uptake on PET (*D*). In a patient with stable angina with previous coronary artery bypass grafting, invasive coronary angiography (*E*) showed non-obstructive disease in the right coronary artery. Corresponding PET scan (*F*) showed a region of increased ¹⁸F-NaF in the mid-right coronary artery and a region without increased uptake in the proximal vessel. This figure was originally published in the Lancet under the Creative Commons Attribution 4.0 International License (http://creativecommons.org/licenses/by/4.0/). (Reprinted with permission from Elsevier. The Lancet, February 2014, 383 (9918), Pages 705-713.)

¹⁸F-NaF POSITRON EMISSION TOMOGRAPHY CORONARY STUDIES

while the cardiac imaging community has been awaiting data highlighting the outcome implications of coronary ¹⁸F-NaF uptake, multiple studies have provided compelling data regarding the association between unfavorable plaque morphology and plaque activity on PET. Whether imaged non-invasively with coronary CT angiography or intracoronary imaging (including intravascular ultrasound and optical coherence tomography), plaques displaying adverse features have been shown to present with more pronounced ¹⁸F-NaF activity than stable lesions.[38,39] Of interest compared to maximum TBR values, CMA showed a stronger association with established anatomical quantitative risk indices derived from CT angiography including the low attenuation plaque volume.[40,41]

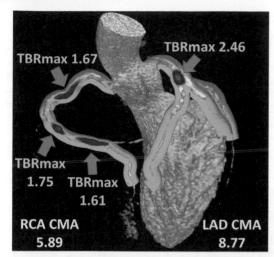

Fig. 3. Three-dimensional rendering of coronary CT angiography with superimposed tubular whole-vessel volumes of interest (*light green*) employed for evaluation of 18F-sodium fluoride uptake (*blue and red*). Despite the relatively lower target-to-background ratio maximum (TBRmax) due to multiple foci of increased 18F-NaF activity, the CMA in the right coronary artery (RCA) is only moderately lower than in the left anterior descending (LAD) coronary artery which presented with a very high TBRmax. (*From Kwiecinski J, Cadet S, Daghem M, et al. Whole-vessel coronary 18F-sodium fluoride PET for assessment of the global coronary microcalcification burden. Eur J Nucl Med Mol Imaging. 2020;47(7):1736-1745.*)

Additionally, three independent studies have linked 18F-NaF uptake to coronary inflammation in patients with stable disease. In observational studies, the pericoronary adipose tissue density—which acts as a surrogate measure of plaque inflammation and can be derived from standard coronary CT angiography datasets—was shown to be closely associated with 18F-NaF[42–44] uptake. These correlations persisted following adjustments for risk factors, coronary calcium scores, and stenosis highlighting at a noninvasive imaging level the association between osteogenesis and inflammation in atherosclerosis which has been widely reported on the molecular level.[45]

Several independent studies have now demonstrated that baseline 18F-NaF uptake predicts the progression of coronary plaque during follow-up.[46–48] 18F-NaF PET was recently used in a study which investigated both coronary artery disease activity and progression in patients with and without prior coronary artery bypass (CABG) surgery.[49] It was demonstrated that both disease activity and disease progression are higher in bypassed native vessels and that this is independent of the overall plaque burden. The study supported the hypothesis that CABG surgery accelerates disease activity and progression in the native coronary vasculature.

18F-NaF UPTAKE AS A PREDICTOR OF MYOCARDIAL INFARCTION

Several observational studies have served as a basis for a post hoc analysis which established the prognostic implications of 18F-NaF coronary uptake. In a two-center multimodality imaging study in 293 patients with advanced established coronary artery disease, CMA emerged as the most powerful independent predictor of myocardial infarction outperforming all other established predictors, including the burden of comorbidities, cardiovascular risk scores, coronary artery calcium scoring, and the presence, severity, and extent of obstructive coronary artery disease (**Fig. 4**).[50] Importantly, while patients with high coronary 18F-NaF activity had an eight-fold risk of myocardial infarction, there were no subsequent myocardial infarctions in patients who had no coronary 18F-NaF uptake (CMA = 0). Concordant findings regarding the prognostic utility of 18F-NaF have been also reported in a smaller observational study.[51]

In parallel to the data supporting the prognostic implications of 18F-NaF coronary uptake, CT-derived plaque morphology and compositions have also emerged as robust predictors of outcomes.[40,41] Given the robust evidence supporting the prognostic implications of the low attenuation plaque burden—assessed with quantitative plaque analysis derived from contrast-enhanced coronary CT angiography—recently we have assessed the prognostic utility of these measurements along with 18F-NaF coronary PET.[52] As multiple coronary CT angiography-derived measures are correlated, and these also show a close association with 18F-NaF coronary uptake, we have used machine learning to overcome the challenges posed by the collinearity of these variables. Our machine learning model incorporating the information from these two modalities alongside clinical factors outperformed the individual components analyzed separately with a high c-statistic of 0.85 reinforcing the necessity of considering multimodality imaging data for optimal risk stratification.[52]

IMAGING 18F-NaF ATHEROSCLEROTIC PLAQUE UPTAKE BEYOND THE CORONARY ARTERIES

Given the fact that calcification plays a central role across a wide spectrum of cardiovascular

Patients with advanced established coronary artery disease

⬇

Coronary disease activity on ¹⁸F-NaF PET: the only predictor of fatal or non-fatal MI
(independent of calcium score, coronary artery lumen stenosis, risk scores & co-morbidities)

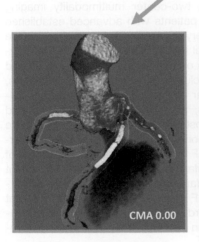 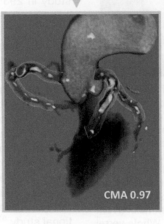 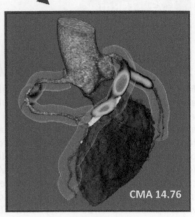

CMA 0.00   CMA 0.97   CMA 14.76

No Activity   **Low Activity**   **High Activity**
(CMA=0)   (CMA 0.01 to 1.56)   (CMA > 1.56)
No MI on follow up   Intermediate risk   8-fold risk of future MI
Continue medical therapy   Close Observation   Intensify Therapy

Fig. 4. ¹⁸F-sodium fluoride PET as a marker of disease activity in the coronary arteries is a predictor of fatal or non-fatal myocardial infarction (MI) in patients with established coronary artery disease. ¹⁸F-NaF PET can be used to measure disease activity across the coronary vasculature and to stratify patients into those with no, low and high disease activity. (*From* Kwiecinski J, Tzolos E, Adamson PD, et al. Coronary 18F-Sodium Fluoride Uptake Predicts Outcomes in Patients With Coronary Artery Disease. J Am Coll Cardiol. 2020;75(24):3061-3074.)

conditions affecting the vasculature and cardiac valves, and given the promising findings of initial ¹⁸F-NaF coronary imaging, multiple studies have explored the utility of these imaging modalities beyond coronary artery disease. Similar to coronary vasculature throughout arteries of the human body, increased ¹⁸F-NaF uptake is associated with adverse events and disease progression. This includes carotid arteries, the aorta, penile, and lower limb arteries.[53–56]

Similar to coronary artery disease, early ¹⁸F-NaF studies have suggested a link between carotid plaque activity and cerebrovascular accidents.[54] This relationship has been studied both in patients imaged shortly following ischemic stroke and stable individuals who underwent carotid endarterectomy shortly after PET. The latter subcohort enabled in-depth histological validation of the PET findings demonstrating that plaques with increased tracer activity have increased calcification activity (tissue non-specific alkaline phosphatase, osteocalcin activity) as well as greater macrophage infiltration and evidence of cell death (apoptosis, cleaved-caspase-3 expression and the presence of a necrotic core).

Recently, ¹⁸F-NaF activity within the ascending aorta has been shown to act as an independent predictor of ischemic stroke.[57,58] Among 461 patients with advanced stable coronary artery disease or aortic stenosis, 23 experienced ischemic stroke over the 6.1 ± 2.3 years of follow-up, and the thoracic aortic ¹⁸F-NaF activity was associated with a 10-fold increased future risk of ischemic stroke. From the clinical perspective, the study indicated that thoracic ¹⁸F-NaF PET can provide a simultaneous assessment of both thoracic aorta and coronary ¹⁸F-NaF activity on a single scan. As a result, by identifying individuals at high risk of both stroke and myocardial infarction, ¹⁸F-NaF PET imaging might allow for optimizing intensive or advanced preventive therapies in patients at the highest risk of these two potentially debilitating adverse events.

Concordant findings have been reported in peripheral vascular disease.[56] In lower limb arterial atherosclerosis, baseline calcification activity (evidenced with ^{18}F-NaF PET) can identify patients who will progress to symptomatic restenosis within a year. Moreover, according to the study, symptomatic anatomic restenosis is associated with persistent calcification activity following percutaneous transluminal angioplasty. This suggests that the atherosclerotic activity of the vascular wall determines downstream restenosis

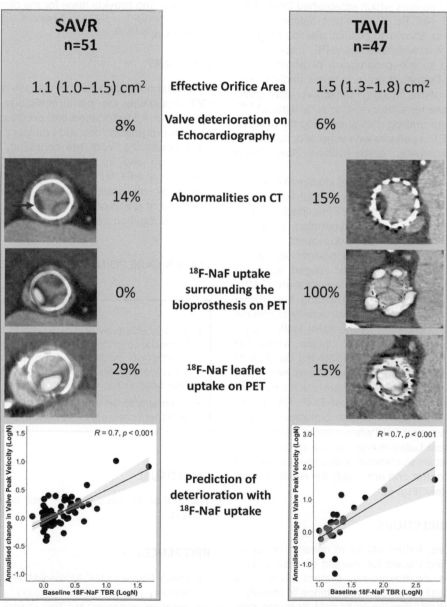

Fig. 5. Comparison of imaging findings and valve deterioration in TAVR versus surgical aortic valve replacement (SAVR). Echocardiographic, CT, and ^{18}F-sodium fluoride (^{18}F-NaF) findings in 47 patients with TAVR with 51 patients with SAVR who underwent the same research imaging protocol. Hypoattenuating leaflet thickening (*red arrow*). (*From* Kwiecinski J, Tzolos E, Cartlidge TRG, et al. Native Aortic Valve Disease Progression and Bioprosthetic Valve Degeneration in Patients With Transcatheter Aortic Valve Implantation. Circulation. 2021;144(17):1396-1408.)

and that this could potentially be a target for patient selection and therapeutic manipulation.

IMAGING AORTIC VALVE STENOSIS WITH ^{18}F-NaF POSITRON EMISSION TOMOGRAPHY

Beyond atherosclerosis, recently substantial advancements in ^{18}F-NaF PET have been made in aortic stenosis imaging. These include translating technical advancements into valvular imaging and clinical studies which established the clinical utility of ^{18}F-NaF PET.[59–62] In fact, before baseline ^{18}F-NaF was shown to predict disease progression of atherosclerosis, baseline PET tracer uptake was linked to the progression of aortic stenosis.[46–48,63] Despite these prognostic implications, the uptake of this imaging modality in native aortic valve disease remains limited to clinical trials.[64–66] Recently, compelling data supporting the utility of ^{18}F-NaF PET in patients with surgical or transcatheter bioprosthetic aortic valves have been published.[67,68]

In prospective observational studies of over 100 bioprosthetic valve recipients without known bioprosthesis failure, ^{18}F-NaF PET identified subclinical bioprosthetic valve degeneration, providing powerful prediction of subsequent valvular dysfunction and highlighting patients at risk of valve failure.[67,68] In patients imaged following transcatheter aortic valve implantation (TAVI), ^{18}F-NaF has facilitated establishing that within the native aortic valve disease activity continues despite immobilization of the valve leaflets after TAVI. Interestingly, ^{18}F-NaF uptake within the native aortic valve increased with the duration of implantation and, on histological analysis, there was evidence of activation of pro-calcific markers in explanted native valves post-TAVI. The observations that the valve remains biologically active several years after TAVI when mechanical stresses are no longer being exerted on the valve leaflets, confirm that aortic stenosis is an actively regulated disease process and not simply the result of valve wear and tear (**Fig. 5**).

FUTURE DIRECTIONS

In the future, further efforts to develop or repurpose existing tracers for imaging disease activity within the cardiovascular system should be made. It shall be of great importance to identify a patient cohort who would benefit from the proposed developments thus providing a rationale for the clinical use of this novel technology. Although for ^{18}F-NaF, the path toward clinical implementation seems shortest, we still await more data. Undoubtedly employing ^{18}F-NaF PET

in the context of clinical trials, exploring the potential of novel therapies will become a stronghold of this technology as multiple examples of such applications in both valvular and coronary artery disease are already ongoing.

Given the complexity of ^{18}F-NaF PET, further efforts to simplify data acquisition, reconstruction, and analysis shall be necessary for more widespread implementation of this promising technology. Fortunately, such developments are already underway and provide hope for the dissemination of ^{18}F-NaF PET beyond academic institutions.[52,69,70]

SUMMARY

In conclusion, assessment of disease activity with PET elucidates the pathophysiology, and can serve for risk stratification and prognostication of disease progression of a wide range of cardiovascular conditions. With the constantly improving technology and accumulating data supporting the utility of PET for in-depth characterization of cardiovascular disease activity, we stand at a threshold of precision medicine where direct disease interrogation can facilitate clinical decision-making.

CLINICS CARE POINTS

- Disease activity assessments with PET have the potential to enhance the clinical maganagement of our patients by informing upon the activity of key biological processes driving disease progression and outcomes.

- It remains to be established how to incorporate these measures into clinical practice.

DISCLOSURE

The author declares that he has no conflict of interest.

REFERENCES

1. Dweck MR, Doris MK, Motwani M, et al. Imaging of coronary atherosclerosis - evolution towards new treatment strategies. Nat Rev Cardiol 2016;13(9): 533–48.
2. Tzolos E, Dweck MR. 18F-Sodium fluoride (18F-NaF) for imaging microcalcification activity in the cardiovascular system. Arterioscler Thromb Vasc Biol 2020;40(7):1620–6.

3. Rudd JH, Warburton EA, Fryer TD, et al. Imaging atherosclerotic plaque inflammation with [18F]-fluoro-deoxyglucose positron emission tomography. Circulation 2002;105:2708–11.

4. Rogers IS, Nasir K, Figueroa AL, et al. Feasibility of FDG imaging of the coronary arteries: comparison between acute coronary syndrome and stable angina. JACC Cardiovasc Imaging 2010;3:388–97.

5. Cheng VY, Slomka PJ, Le Meunier L, et al. Coronary arterial ^{18}F-FDG uptake by fusion of PET and coronary CT angiography at sites of percutaneous stenting for acute myocardial infarction and stable coronary artery disease. J Nucl Med 2012;53(4):575–83.

6. Joshi NV, Vesey AT, Williams MC, et al. 18F-fluoride positron emission tomography for identification of ruptured and high-risk coronary atherosclerotic plaques: a prospective clinical trial. Lancet 2014;383:705–13.

7. Gaemperli O, Shalhoub J, Owen DRJ, et al. Imaging intraplaque inflammation in carotid atherosclerosis with 11C-PK11195 positron emission tomography/computed tomography. Eur Heart J 2012;33(15):1902–10.

8. Bucerius J, Schmaljohann J, Bohm I, et al. Feasibility of 18F-fluoromethylcholine PET/CT for imaging of vessel wall alterations in humans – first results. Eur J Nucl Med Mol Imaging 2008;35:815–20.

9. Tarkin JM, Joshi FR, Evans NR, et al. Detection of atherosclerotic Inflammation by 68Ga-DOTATATE PET compared to [18F]FDG PET imaging. J Am Coll Cardiol 2017;69(14):1774–91.

10. Tzolos E, Bing R, Andrews J, et al. In vivo coronary artery thrombus imaging with 18F-GP1 PET-CT. Eur Heart J 2021;42(Supplement_1). ehab724.0261.

11. Tzolos E, Bing R, Newby DE, et al. Categorising myocardial infarction with advanced cardiovascular imaging. Lancet 2021;398:e9.

12. Kwiecinski J, Slomka PJ, Dweck MR, et al. Vulnerable plaque imaging using 18F-sodium fluoride positron emission tomography. Br J Radiol 2020;93(1113):20190797.

13. Czernin J, Satyamurthy N, Schiepers C. Molecular mechanisms of bone 18F-NaF deposition. J Nucl Med 2010;51:1826–9.

14. Derlin T, Richter U, Bannas P, et al. Feasibility of 18F-sodium fluoride PET/CT for imaging of atherosclerotic plaque. J Nucl Med 2010;51:862–5.

15. Li Y, Berenji GR, Shaba WF, et al. Association of vascular fluoride uptake with vascular calcifi cation and coronary artery disease. Nucl Med Commun 2012;33:14–20.

16. Beheshti M, Saboury B, Mehta NN, et al. Detection and global quantification of cardiovascular molecular calcification by fluoro18-fluoride positron emission tomography/computed tomography—a novel concept. Hell J Nucl Med 2011;14:114–20.

17. Janssen T, Bannas P, Herrmann J, et al. Association of linear 18Fsodiumfluoride accumulation in femoral arteries as a measure of diffuse calcification with cardiovascular risk factors: a PET/CT study. J Nucl Cardiol 2013;20:569–77.

18. Irkle A, Vesey AT, Lewis DY, et al. Identifying active vascular microcalcification by (18)F-sodium fluoride positron emission tomography. Nat Commun 2015;6:7495.

19. Creager MD, Hohl T, Hutcheson JD, et al. 18F-Fluoride signal amplification identifies microcalcifications associated with atherosclerotic plaque instability in positron emission tomography/computed tomography images. Circ Cardiovasc Imaging 2019;12(1):e007835.

20. McKenney-Drake ML, Territo PR, Salavati A, et al. 18F-NaF PET imaging of early coronary artery calcification. J Am Coll Cardiol 2016;9:627–8.

21. Dweck MR, Jones C, Joshi NV, et al. Assessment of valvular calcification and inflammation by positron emission tomography in patients with aortic stenosis. Circulation 2012;125(1):76–86.

22. Dweck MR, Chow MW, Joshi NV, et al. Coronary arterial 18F-sodium fluoride uptake: a novel marker of plaque biology. J Am Coll Cardiol 2012;59:1539–48.

23. Kwiecinski J, Lassen ML, Slomka PJ. Advances in quantitative analysis of 18f-sodium fluoride coronary imaging. Mol Imaging 2021;2021:8849429.

24. Lassen ML, Kwiecinski J, Dey D, et al. Triple-gated motion and blood pool clearance corrections improve reproducibility of coronary 18F-NaF PET. Eur J Nucl Med Mol Imaging 2019;46:2610–20.

25. Kwiecinski J, Adamson PD, Lassen ML, et al. Feasibility of coronary 18F-sodium fluoride PET assessment with the utilization of previously acquired CT angiography. Circ Cardiovasc Imaging 2018;11(12):e008325.

26. Lassen ML, Kwiecinski J, Slomka PJ. Gating approaches in cardiac PET imaging. Pet Clin 2019;14(2):271–9.

27. Lassen M.L., Kwiecinski J., Cadet S., et al., Data-driven gross patient motion detection and compensation: implications for coronary 18 F-NaF PET imaging, J Nucl Med, 2018, 2019;60(6):830-836.

28. Tzolos E, Lassen ML, Pan T, et al. Respiration-averaged CT versus standard CT attenuation map for correction of 18F-sodium fluoride uptake in coronary atherosclerotic lesions on hybrid PET/CT. J Nucl Cardiol 2022;29:430–9.

29. Lassen ML, Tzolos E, Pan T, et al. Anatomical validation of automatic respiratory motion correction for coronary 18F-sodium fluoride positron emission tomography by expert measurements from four-dimensional computed tomography. Med Phys 2022;49(11):7085–94.

30. Kwiecinski J, Berman DS, Lee SE, et al. Three-hour delayed imaging improves assessment of coronary

18F-sodium fluoride PET. J Nucl Med 2019;60(4): 530–5.

31. Doris MK, Otaki Y, Krishnan SK, et al. Optimization of reconstruction and quantification of motion-corrected coronary PET-CT. J Nucl Cardiol 2020; 27(2):494–504.

32. Bellinge JW, Francis RJ, Majeed K, et al. In search of the vulnerable patient or the vulnerable plaque: (18) F-sodium fluoride positron emission tomography for cardiovascular risk stratification. J Nucl Cardiol 2018;25:1774–83.

33. Kwiecinski J, Cadet S, Daghem M, et al. Whole-vessel coronary 18F-sodium fluoride PET for assessment of the global coronary microcalcification burden. Eur J Nucl Med Mol Imaging 2020;47: 1736–45.

34. Tzolos E, Kwiecinski J, Lassen ML, et al. Observer repeatability and interscan reproducibility of 18F-sodium fluoride coronary microcalcification activity. J Nucl Cardiol 2022;29(1):126–35.

35. Steven ML, Yusuf E, Timothy A, et al. Tumor treatment response based on visual and quantitative changes in global tumor glycolysis using pet-fdg imaging: the visual response score and the change in total lesion glycolysis. Clin Positron Imaging 1999; 2(3):159–71.

36. Ahmadian A, Brogan A, Berman J, et al. Quantitative interpretation of FDG PET/CT with myocardial perfusion imaging increases diagnostic information in the evaluation of cardiac sarcoidosis. J Nucl Cardiol 2014;21:925–39.

37. Agatston AS, Janowitz WR, Hildner FJ, et al. Quantification of coronary artery calcium using ultrafast computed tomography. J Am Coll Cardiol 1990;15: 827–32.

38. Kwiecinski J, Dey D, Cadet S, et al. Predictors of 18F-sodium fluoride uptake in patients with stable coronary artery disease and adverse plaque features on computed tomography angiography. Eur Heart J Cardiovasc Imaging 2020;21:58–66.

39. Lee JM, Bang J-I, Koo B-K, et al. Clinical relevance of 18 F-sodium fluoride positron-emission tomography in noninvasive identification of high-risk plaque in patients with coronary artery disease. Circulation 2017;10 [pii:e006704].

40. Lin A, Manral N, McElhinney P, et al. Deep learning from coronary computed tomography angiography for atherosclerotic plaque and stenosis quantification and cardiac risk prediction: an international multicentre study. Lancet Digital Health 2022;4(4):256–65.

41. Williams MC, Kwiecinski J, Doris M, et al. Low-attenuation noncalcified plaque on coronary computed tomography angiography predicts myocardial infarction: results from the multicenter SCOT-HEART trial. Circulation 2020;141(18):1452–62.

42. Wen W, Mingxin G, Yun M, et al. Associations between coronary/aortic 18F-sodium fluoride uptake and pro-atherosclerosis factors in patients with multivessel coronary artery disease. J Nucl Cardiol 2022;29(6):3352–65.

43. Kwiecinski J, Dey D, Cadet S, et al. Peri-coronary adipose tissue density is associated with (18)F- sodium fluoride coronary uptake in stable patients with high-risk plaques. JACC Cardiovasc Imaging 2019;12:2000–10.

44. Kitagawa T, Nakamoto Y, Fujii Y, et al. Relationship between coronary arterial 18F-sodium fluoride uptake and epicardial adipose tissue analyzed using computed tomography. Eur J Nucl Med Mol Imaging 2020;47:1746–56.

45. Aikawa E, Nahrendorf M, Figueiredo JL, et al. Osteogenesis associates with inflammation in early-stage atherosclerosis evaluated by molecular imaging in vivo. Circulation 2007;116:2841–50.

46. Doris MK, Meah MN, Moss AJ, et al. Coronary 18F-fluoride uptake and progression of coronary artery calcification. Circ Cardiovasc Imaging 2020;13(12): e011438.

47. Bellinge JW, Francis RJ, Lee SC, et al. 18F-sodium fluoride positron emission tomography activity predicts the development of new coronary artery calcifications. Arterioscler Thromb Vasc Biol 2021;41(1): 534–41.

48. Ishiwata Y, Kaneta T, Nawata S, et al. Quantification of temporal changes in calcium score in active atherosclerotic plaque in major vessels by 18F-sodium fluoride PET/CT. Eur J Nucl Med Mol Imaging 2017;44(9):1529–37.

49. Kwiecinski J, Tzolos E, Fletcher AJ, et al. Bypass grafting and native coronary artery disease activity. JACC Cardiovasc Imaging 2022;15(5):875–87.

50. Kwiecinski J, Tzolos E, Adamson PD, et al. 18F-sodium fluoride coronary uptake predicts outcome in patients with coronary artery disease. J Am Coll Cardiol 2020;75:3061–74.

51. Kitagawa T, Yamamoto H, Nakamoto Y, et al. Predictive value of 18F-sodium fluoride positron emission tomography in detecting high-risk coronary artery disease in combination with computed tomography. J Am Heart Assoc 2018;7(20):e010224.

52. Kwiecinski J, Tzolos E, Meah M, et al. Machine-learning with 18F-sodium fluoride PET and quantitative plaque analysis on CT angiography for the future risk of myocardial infarction. J Nucl Med 2022;63(1): 158–65.

53. Nakahara T, Narula J, Tijssen JG, et al. 18F-fluoride positron emission tomographic imaging of penile arteries and erectile dysfunction. J Am Coll Cardiol 2019;73(12):1386–94.

54. Vesey AT, Jenkins WS, Irkle A, et al. 18F-fluoride and 18F-fluorodeoxyglucose positron emission tomography after transient ischemic attack or minor ischemic stroke: case-control study. Circ Cardiovasc Imaging 2017;10(3):e004976.

55. Forsythe RO, Dweck MR, McBride OMB, et al. F-18-Somp(3) study. J Am Coll Cardiol 2018;71(5):513–23.

56. Chowdhury MM, Tarkin JM, Albaghdadi MS, et al. Vascular positron emission tomography and restenosis in symptomatic peripheral arterial disease: a prospective clinical study. JACC Cardiovasc Imaging 2020;13(4):1008–17.

57. Fletcher AJ, Tew YY, Tzolos E, et al. Thoracic aortic 18F-sodium fluoride activity and ischemic stroke in patient with established cardiovascular disease. JACC Cardiovasc Imaging 2022;15:1274–88.

58. Fletcher AJ, Lembo M, Kwiecinski J, et al. Quantifying microcalcification activity in the thoracic aorta. J Nucl Cardiol 2022;29:1372–85.

59. Massera D, Doris MK, Cadet S, et al. Analytical quantification of aortic valve 18F-sodiumfluoride PET uptake. J Nucl Cardiol 2020;27:962–72.

60. Lassen ML, Tzolos E, Massera D, et al. Aortic valve imaging using 18F-sodium fluoride: impact of triple motion correction. EJNMMI Phys 2022;9(1):4.

61. Nakamoto Y, Kitagawa T, Sasaki K, et al. Clinical implications of 18F-sodium fluoride uptake in subclinical aortic valve calcification: its relation to coronary atherosclerosis and its predictive value. J Nucl Cardiol 2021;28(4):1522–31.

62. Tzolos E, Kwiecinski J, Berman D, et al. Latest advances in multimodality imaging of aortic stenosis. J Nucl Med 2022;63(3):353–8.

63. Dweck MR, Jenkins WSA, Vesey AT, et al. 18F-sodium fluoride uptake is a marker of active calcification and disease progression in patients with aortic stenosis. Circ Cardiovasc Imaging 2014;7(2):371–8.

64. ClinicalTrials.gov. National Library of Medicine (U.S.). Study investigating the effect of drugs used to treat osteoporosis on the progression of calcific aortic stenosis. (SALTIRE II). Available at: https://ClinicalTrials.gov/show/NCT02132026. Accessed June 4, 2022.

65. ClinicalTrials.gov. National Library of Medicine (U.S.). Bicuspid aortic valve stenosis and the effect of vitamin K2 on calciummetabolism on 18F-NaF PET/MRI. (BASIK2). Available at: https://ClinicalTrials.gov/show/NCT02917525. Accessed June 4, 2022.

66. Peeters FECM, Doris MK, Cartlidge TRG, et al. Sex differences in valve-calcification activity and calcification progression in aortic stenosis. JACC Cardiovasc Imaging 2020;13(9):2045–6.

67. Kwiecinski J, Tzolos E, Cartlidge TRG, et al. Native aortic valve disease progression and bioprosthetic valve degeneration in patients with transcatheter aortic valve implantation. Circulation 2021;144:1396–408.

68. Cartlidge TRG, Doris MK, Sellers SL, et al. Detection and prediction of bioprosthetic aortic valve degeneration. J Am Coll Cardiol 2019;73:1107–19.

69. Singh A, Kwiecinski J, Cadet S, et al. Automated nonlinear registration of coronary PET to CT angiography using pseudo-CT generated from PET with generative adversarial networks. J Nucl Cardiol 2022. https://doi.org/10.1007/s12350-022-03010-8.

70. Piri R, Edenbrandt L, Larsson M, et al. "Global" cardiac atherosclerotic burden assessed by artificial intelligence-based versus manual segmentation in 18F-sodium fluoride PET/CT scans: head-to-head comparison. J Nucl Cardiol 2021. https://doi.org/10.1007/s12350-021-02758-9.

Radionuclide Tracers for Myocardial Perfusion Imaging and Blood Flow Quantification

Teresa Mannarino, MD, PhD, Roberta Assante, MD, PhD,
Adriana D'Antonio, MD, Emilia Zampella, MD, PhD, Alberto Cuocolo, MD,
Wanda Acampa, MD, PhD*

KEYWORDS

• Myocardial perfusion imaging • Myocardial blood flow • Myocardial perfusion reserve

KEY POINTS

- Ideal tracers for myocardial perfusion imaging should have a high first-pass extraction fraction, linearly correlated to coronary blood flow and adequate myocardial retention.
- [99m]Technetium (^{99m}Tc)-labeled compounds were not traditionally considered ideal tracers for myocardial blood flow (MBF).
- The implementation of novel single-photon emission tomography instrumentation has contributed to explore the clinical potential of flow quantification with ^{99m}Tc-tracers.
- Quantification of MBF by the new cadmium zinc telluride (CZT) camera is not only technically possible but also promising for different clinical applications.

INTRODUCTION

Myocardial perfusion imaging (MPI) is a well-established noninvasive tool for the diagnosis and risk stratification of patients with suspected or known coronary artery disease (CAD). Different published guidelines discuss the most appropriate noninvasive or invasive testing for the diagnosis or management of patients with CAD.[1,2] Both single-photon emission tomography (SPECT) and positron emission tomography (PET) are routinely used for the evaluation of myocardial perfusion and left ventricular (LV) function, identifying possible areas of myocardial ischemia related to obstructive CAD. At the same time, radionuclide imaging allows the quantification of myocardial blood flow (MBF), which could be useful in the diagnostic workout of specific categories of patients such as those with multivessel or microvascular disease. In the past several years, the diagnostic and prognostic value of MPI has significantly improved, due to two relevant factors: (1) technical improvements in SPECT camera, for acquisition protocols, imaging processing, and data analysis and (2) more availability of PET radiotracers and PET/computed tomography (CT) cameras. PET imaging is considered the gold standard for the evaluation of myocardial perfusion compared with SPECT imaging due to the possibility to obtain attenuation correction, higher spatial resolution, and ability to evaluate absolute quantification of MBF. Moreover, in the last decade, the developments and wide availability of PET radiotracers have further increased their clinical use. However, SPECT imaging represents the most common method used for cardiac perfusion evaluation due to the lower costs and widespread availability of cameras. In addition, the introduction of cardiac-dedicated SPECT with solid-state-detectors has improved spatial

Department of Advanced Biomedical Sciences, University Federico II, Via Sergio Pansini 5, Naples 80131, Italy
* Corresponding author.
E-mail address: acampa@unina.it

Cardiol Clin 41 (2023) 141–150
https://doi.org/10.1016/j.ccl.2023.01.003

resolution with a reduced imaging times and lower radiation dose, and the possibility to obtain dynamic data, similar to PET. Several radiotracers are available for both SPECT and PET studies. The main characteristic of these radio-labeled compounds is their capability to be extracted from the coronary arteries in relation to blood flow and concentrated inside the perfused myocardial tissue.[3] This review attempts to provide an update on the SPECT and PET tracers for clinical MPI and their utility in the quantification of MBF, highlighting the new possibilities over the last few years.

POSITRON EMISSION TOMOGRAPHY AND SINGLE-PHOTON EMISSION COMPUTED TOMOGRAPHY TRACERS FOR MYOCARDIAL PERFUSION IMAGING

Exercise or pharmacologic stress MPI represents a powerful tool to detect regional myocardial ischemia and infarction. Ideal perfusion tracers have the capability to be avidly taken up by the tissue and permanently or irreversibly retained. Therefore, the ideal tracer should have a high first-pass extraction fraction, linear correlation to coronary blood flow, and adequate myocardial retention. Moreover, it should be bound to an isotope with acceptable dosimetric characteristics, half-life, and a good energy window to provide images of good quality. **Table 1** summarizes the physical and kinetic properties of the most commonly used radiotracers for MPI. **Fig. 1** shows PET and SPECT radiotracer kinetics related to MBF.

Cardiac PET for MPI has been considered the most accurate modality to study patients with suspected or known CAD and several published data in literature have assessed its diagnostic and prognostic value.[4,5] The use of hybrid PET/CT allows to obtain in a single session both PET and CT images, combining the analysis of functional and anatomic parameters, such as coronary atherosclerotic burden, besides the great advantage of providing a more accurate attenuation correction for PET images. In particular, three PET myocardial perfusion tracers are currently available for clinical use: oxygen-15 (^{15}O) water, ^{13}N ammonia, and ^{82}Rubidium. ^{15}O-water has limited use in MPI because of the extremely short half-life (2.1 min) with the need for an on-site cyclotron for its production, close to the gantry, the high cost, and the low availability. Moreover, due to its physical characteristics and poor myocardial retention (as it is freely diffusible), myocardial perfusion image quality with ^{15}O-water is suboptimal with a low myocardial-to-background count

ratio. But due to its high first-pass extraction in relation to blood flow, ^{15}O-water provides ideal quantitation of MBF. ^{13}N-ammonia has a physical half-life of 9.96 min and a high first-pass extraction (70% to 80%), it has a good retention in myocardial cells and a rapid clearance from the blood pool, so good quality perfusion images can be provided. Several published studies in patients with suspected or known CAD have been conducted using PET imaging by ^{13}N-ammonia, and it has shown high diagnostic and prognostic value.[6,7] ^{82}Rubidium (^{82}Rb), the most common PET radiotracer for clinical use, is a potassium analog that enters cells using Na$^+$/K$^+$ cotransporter. It has the great advantage to be produced by a generator (^{82}Sr/^{82}Rb), so, despite the high costs, it is more accessible. It has an ultra-short half-life of 75.5 s, therefore the use of pharmacologic vasodilation is the only option for imaging at peak hyperemic stress, performed while the patient is lying on the bed. On the other hand, its use allows a very low radiation dose exposure. This aspect is relevant considering that with the growing incidence of cardiovascular disease, increasing the use of nuclear cardiology can increase patient exposure to radiation.[8] The use of ^{82}Rb PET has been widely validated and several studies have shown a high diagnostic value in identifying obstructive CAD and a good prognostic value. Several studies[9,10] have shown the equivalence of these above-mentioned tracers in flow quantification, thus ^{13}N-ammonia and ^{82}Rubidium are currently used in different centers according to logistic availability and local expertise. The kinetic properties and characteristics of the PET and SPECT perfusion tracers have been extensively described previously.[11]

The most commonly used tracers for SPECT imaging are ^{99m}Technetium (^{99m}Tc) complexes, which have been introduced in myocardial SPECT imaging since the 1990s. The introduction of ^{99m}Tc-sestamibi (methoxyisobutyl isoitrile) and ^{99m}Tc-tetrofosmin (1,2-bis[bis(2-ethoxyethyl) phosphino] ethane) has deeply changed the history of MPI. The favorable characteristics of ^{99m}Tc, such as the relatively higher energy photons, half-life (6h), good myocardial retention, and lower costs have led to the wide diffusion of these tracers in nuclear cardiology. ^{99m}Tc-sestamibi and ^{99m}Tc-tetrofosmin have very similar characteristics. They are lipophilic cations and pass inside the myocytes following the transmembrane potential, thus can be considered as markers of cell integrity. The first-pass extraction fraction is approximately 54% for tetrofosmin and 68% for sestamibi.[12] ^{99m}Tc-labeled tracers allow for gated MPI, leading to the measurement of LV ejection fraction and volumes in combination with

Table 1
PET and single-photon emission computed tomography tracers used for clinical myocardial perfusion imaging

Tracer	Modality	Half-Life	Energy	Production	First-Pass Myocardial Extraction	Kinetics	Dose Range (MBq)
[15]O-water	PET	2.1 min	511 KeV	On-site cyclotron	100%	Diffusion	350 to 750
[13]N-ammonia	PET	10 min	511 KeV	On-site cyclotron	80%	Diffusion/active transport	350 to 750
[82]Rubidium	PET	72 s	511 KeV	Generator	70%	Na+/K+ cotransporter	750 to 1500
[18]F-flurpiridaz	PET	2 h	511 KeV	On-site/regional cyclotron	94%	Mitochondrial complex 1	100 to 250
[99m]Tc-sestamibi	SPECT	6 h	140 KeV	Generator	68%	Diffusion	250 to 1100
[99m]Tc-tetrofosmin	SPECT	6 h	140 KeV	Generator	54%	Diffusion	250 to 1100

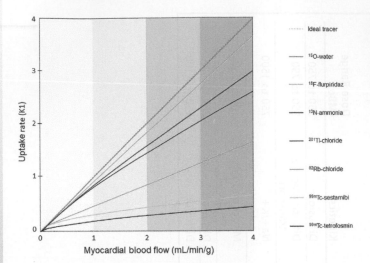

Fig. 1. Radiotracer kinetics related to MBF. The uptake rate (K1) is obtained by extraction fraction × MBF.

Legend:
- Ideal tracer
- ^{15}O-water
- ^{18}F-flurpiridaz
- ^{13}N-ammonia
- ^{201}Tl-chloride
- ^{82}Rb-chloride
- ^{99m}Tc-sestamibi
- ^{99m}Tc-tetrofosmin

myocardial perfusion evaluation.[13] However, different studies have tried to attempt the possibility to perform dynamic studies using conventional 2-detector NaI SPECT to quantify MBF, with limited success.[14,15]

The introduction of new machines equipped with high-resolution semiconductor CZT detectors has improved spatial, temporal, and energy resolution as compared with traditional gamma cameras, providing better image quality using ^{99m}Tc-radiotracers in a shorter acquisition time with a reduction of radiation exposure to the patient, without affecting diagnostic accuracy.[16,17] In a meta-analysis including 40 studies, a good diagnostic performance has been shown for the two gamma camera systems, with slightly higher accuracy for CZT-SPECT, due to the improved technological characteristics.[16] Therefore, these results encourage the clinical use of the CZT-SPECT camera in detecting CAD as a valid replacement for traditional systems.

MYOCARDIAL BLOOD FLOW QUANTIFICATION UPDATE

PET MPI has been considered for many years the gold standard for the evaluation of myocardial perfusion and is routinely used for MBF quantification, considering the availability of tracers such as ^{15}O-water showing linear correlation with MBF, also in hyperemic conditions. For MBF quantification, tracer kinetic modeling is used to simplify the physiological process of tracer uptake in mathematical terms. Tracer kinetic models used for analysis are based on one or two tissue compartments with multiple kinetic parameters, according to the mechanism of tracer uptake from capillaries into

myocytes. However, although MBF quantification by PET imaging is validated and shows high diagnostic and prognostic value, the cost of PET procedures is high and the availability of PET cameras for cardiology applications is lower compared with SPECT. ^{99m}Tc-labeled compounds were not traditionally considered as ideal tracers for MBF quantification, due to their suboptimal extraction characteristics at maximal hyperemia. However, the introduction of novel cardio-dedicated CZT cameras has opened new possible clinical scenarios to use the available ^{99m}Tc-perfusion radiotracers.[18,19] The implementation of novel SPECT instrumentation has contributed to explore the clinical potential of flow quantification with dynamic image acquisition. Indeed, the feasibility of quantification of MBF using dynamic list-mode acquisition has been reported.[20] Dynamic images are performed by a list mode acquisition and then data are reformatted and reconstructed into 60 to 70 frames. The acquisition must be started from the time of tracer injection, using an automatic injector which allows to obtain high reproducibility and controlled injected activity.[21] A factor analysis is used to generate left and right ventricular blood pool time–activity curves from the reconstructed multiframe datasets.[20] These curves serve as input functions in kinetic analysis. Regional and global time–activity curves are generated and a two-compartment kinetic model, with input functions, is derived using factor analysis. K1 parameter values (^{99m}Tc-sestamibi uptake) are calculated for the stress and rest images, and K2 values (^{99m}Tc-compound washout) are settled to zero. The myocardial perfusion reserve (MPR) index is then calculated as the ratio of the stress and rest K1 values

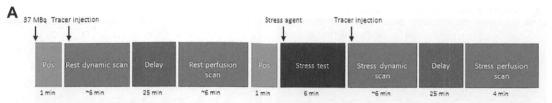

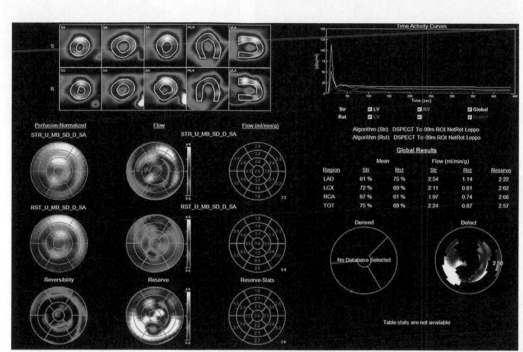

Fig. 2. Dynamic CZT study: (*A*) acquisition protocol and (*B*) dynamic processing of data.

(MPR index = K1 stress/K1 rest). For MBF quantification, a net retention model proposed by Jeffrey Leppo and Katsuya Yoshida[22,23] can be used. A dynamic study protocol by D-SPECT and MBF analysis is depicted in **Fig. 2**. Published data have shown that MBF quantification by CZT camera using ^{99m}Tc-sestamibi is feasible and showed high diagnostic accuracy in identifying obstructive CAD.[20,21] Specifically, it has been shown that MPR is lower in patients with perfusion defects and regions supplied by obstructed coronary arteries.[20] Moreover, a cutoff of < 2.1 has been indicated as the best value for the identification of obstructive CAD.[21] It should be considered that using ^{99m}Tc-compounds as a perfusion agent for the measurement of the MPR index, the retention estimates at high flow rates may be underestimated because of the nonlinear relationship between radiotracer extraction and MBF. However, different studies compared MBF and MPR measurements obtained by dynamic CZT-SPECT to the values obtained by ^{15}O-water, ^{13}N-ammonia, and [82]Rubidium PET imaging[24–26] showing good correlations between the

two different methods. In particular, Agostini and colleagues comparing ^{99m}Tc-sestamibi CZT to ^{15}O-water PET showed that hyperemic and rest MBF values were significantly higher from dynamic CZT-SPECT MPI than from ^{15}O-water PET, but they resulted in similar MPR. Moreover, they showed a high concordance between MPR-CZT and fractional flow reserve in vessel territories.[24] Similarly, Yamamoto and colleagues[25] comparing ^{13}N-ammonia PET and CZT-SPECT showed that MBF was overestimated by D-SPECT at high values, due to the differences between the two different tracers and unfavorable kinetic of ^{99m}Tc-sestamibi. However, MBF and MPR results correlated well between the two modalities. Similarly, Acampa and colleagues[26] showed that hyperemic MBF and MPR values obtained by CZT-SPECT are higher than those measured by [82]Rb-PET imaging, but with a moderate correlation between the two methods. Global MPR by CZT-SPECT had good accuracy in the identification of reduced MPR by PET. The two methods also showed similar results in the identification of

A Stress-rest myocardial perfusion imaging

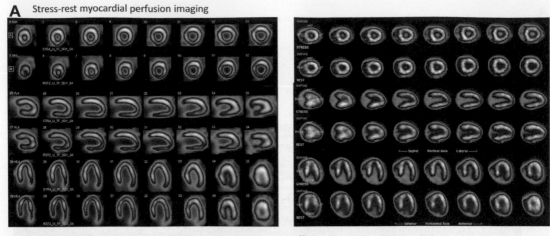

99mTc Sestamibi CZT   82Rubidium PET

B Absolute quantification of myocardial blood flow

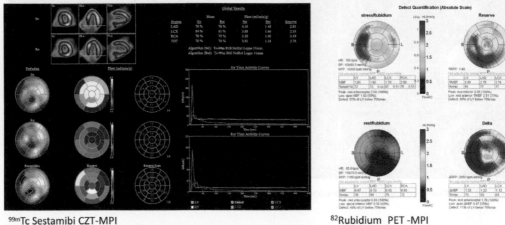

99mTc Sestamibi CZT-MPI   82Rubidium PET -MPI

Fig. 3. Direct comparison between CZT and PET in a patient with suspected CAD: (*A*) myocardial perfusion imaging reconstruction and (*B*) myocardial perfusion reserve quantification.

obstructive CAD in corresponding coronary arteries. **Fig. 3**A and B shows an example of a comparison between CZT and PET studies in a patient with suspected CAD. Thus, the technological improvement provided by CZT cameras partially overcomes the limitations related to the physical characteristics of the available 99mTc-radiotracers. It should be considered that the different PET perfusion tracers have different properties explaining the different results observed in PET studies compared with 99mTc-tracers in SPECT studies. In particular, 82Rb has lower extraction (40% to 70%) compared with 13N-ammonia and 15O-water, despite the advantages of a higher retention rate and optimal image quality. It should be outlined that sestamibi has a slightly higher first-pass extraction as compared with tetrofosmin, supporting the theoretical idea that sestamibi should be preferred in case of dynamic

acquisitions. However, few studies using tetrofosmin as a radiotracer showed good results in comparison to PET tracers,[27–29] further data providing a direct comparison between the two 99mTc-tracers and according to pharmacological stress used should be provided. All these results suggest that quantification of MBF by the new CZT camera is not only technically possible but also advantageous and promising for future applications. **Table 2** shows a summary of the main studies focused on the diagnostic accuracy of dynamic CZT SPECT in the evaluation of MBF.[30–35]

FUTURE PERSPECTIVES

Research activity has focused on the use of 18F as an isotope for its favorable characteristics.18F-flurpiridaz represents a new PET tracer with a high myocardial extraction fraction and longer half-life

Table 2
Summary of published studies evaluating the diagnostic value of CZT single-photon emission computed tomography

Study Year	Camera	Number of Patients	Radiotracer	Compartment Model	Software for MBF Quantification	Gold Standard
Bouallègue et al,[30] 2015	DNM530c	23	Tetrofosmin	1-compartment	In-house software	FFR by ICA
Nkoulou et al,[27] 2016	DNM570c	28	Tetrofosmin	1-compartment	PMOD	^{13}N-ammonia PET
Miyagawa et al,[31] 2017	DNM530c	69	Tetrofosmin/sestamibi	1-compartment	In-house software	FFR by ICA
Wells et al,[28] 2017	DNM530c	29	Tetrofosmin	1-compartment	FlowQuant	[82]Rb/^{13}N-ammonia PET
Agostini et al,[24] 2018	D-SPECT	30	Sestamibi	Net retention	Corridor 4DM	^{15}O-water PET/FFR by ICA
Han et al,[32] 2018	DNM530c	34	Sestamibi	1-compartment	Corridor 4DM	FFR by ICA
de Souza et al,[33] 2019	DNM530c	41	Sestamibi	Net retention	Corridor 4DM	ICA
Giubbini et al,[29] 2019	DNM530c	54	Tetrofosmin	Net retention	Corridor 4DM	^{13}N-ammonia PET
Acampa et al,[21] 2020	D-SPECT	173	Sestamibi	Net retention	Corridor 4DM	ICA
Acampa et al,[26] 2020	D-SPECT	25	Sestamibi	Net retention	Corridor 4DM	[82]Rb PET
Zavadovsky et al,[34] 2020	DNM570c	52	Sestamibi	Net retention	Corridor 4DM	ICA
Zavadovsky et al,[35] 2021	DNM570c	23	Sestamibi	Net retention	Corridor 4DM	FFR by ICA
Yamamoto et al,[25] 2022	D-SPECT	14	Sestamibi	2-compartment	Corridor 4DM	^{13}N-ammonia PET

Abbreviations: FFR, fractional flow reserve; ICA, invasive coronary angiography.

than rubidium and ammonia. A recently completed phase III trial has shown that ^{18}F-flurpiridaz provides excellent image quality.[36] ^{18}F-flurpiridaz binds to mitochondrial complex 1 in the heart and has higher myocardial extraction than other available SPECT and PET tracers. The binding to ^{18}F guarantees the advantages of the fluoride complexes, such as the manageable half-life and the possibility to be produced in a regional cyclotron with unit dose delivery to sites (as with thallium and ^{18}F-FDG). Moreover, it could be useful in patients where an exercise stress test is indicated. In the Phase-III Clinical Trial[36] ^{18}F-flurpiridaz showed superior sensitivity and specificity in identifying obstructive CAD, compared with SPECT. In addition, data about the evaluation of regional MBF and MPR in patients with CAD as compared with healthy subjects have shown a significant difference in stress MBF and MPR between normal and known CAD territories.[37] ^{18}F-flurpiridaz is a strong candidate to be a clinically approved radiotracers for MPI in the near future. Although ^{99m}Tc-tetrofosmin and ^{99m}Tc-sestamibi are widely available with new potential applications using the new cameras, these compounds are still far from having all the desirable characteristics of an ideal tracer. Thus, in the last decades, various attempts to identify a new ideal tracer to use in MPI have been reported. ^{125}I-ZIROT (7-(Z)-[(125)I]iodorotenone) has shown higher myocardial extraction (84%) and retention characteristics than sestamibi in rats and in isolated perfused rabbit hearts. Its analog labeled with ^{123}I showed better regional myocardial flow than sestamibi in dog models.[38] ^{99m}Tc-N-DBODC5 (N,N-bis(ethoxyethyl)dithiocarbamates) is a lipophilic cationic tracer that has shown safety, good biodistribution, and high image quality in preliminary studies; it has been compared with sestamibi in a clinical study by Ma and colleagues[39] for the detection of CAD. Moreover, some authors[40] also evaluated the pharmacokinetics and biodistribution in 10 healthy humans of [99m]Tc N-MPO (2-mercaptopyridine N-oxide), finding that the high heart uptake of this compound, combined with a fast liver clearance, may suggest a possible utilization as a myocardial tracer. However, further studies about the properties of these new tracers for dynamic acquisition and MBF quantification in humans are still lacking.

SUMMARY

Several radiotracers are available for PET and SPECT MPI. The absence of a single tracer with all the characteristics of the ideal compound makes it necessary to choose one tracer over the other based on clinical need, the information we want to obtain, and local availability. The introduction of novel cardio-dedicated CZT cameras has opened the possibility of using the available [99m]Tc- radiotracers for flow quantification. In addition, technical advances in promising molecules as well as new applications of already-known radiopharmaceuticals will further advance MPI.

CLINICS CARE POINTS

- Different studies have demonstrated that MBF and MPR values obtained by CZT-SPECT show good correlation with those obtained by PET modality.
- MBF quantification by CZT camera using ^{99m}Tc-sestamibi is routinely feasible and showed high diagnostic accuracy in identifying obstructive CAD.
- The development of new ^{99m}Tc-labeled tracers for SPECT applications with optimal tracer kinetics may further improve the daily clinical practice.

DISCLOSURES

T. Mannarino, R. Assante, A. D'Antonio, and A. Cuocolo declare that they have nothing to disclose. W. Acampa is a consultant for Spectrum Dynamics.

REFERENCES

1. Acampa W, Gaemperli O, Gimelli A, et al. Document Reviewers. Role of risk stratification by SPECT, PET, and hybrid imaging in guiding management of stable patients with ischaemic heart disease: expert panel of the EANM cardiovascular committee and EACVI. Eur Heart J Cardiovasc Imaging 2015 Dec;16(12):1289–98.
2. Knuuti J, Wijns W, Saraste A, et al. ESC Scientific Document Group, 2019 ESC Guidelines for the diagnosis and management of chronic coronary syndromes: the Task Force for the diagnosis and management of chronic coronary syndromes of the European Society of Cardiology (ESC). Eur Heart J 2020;41(3):407–77.
3. Acampa W, Di Benedetto C, Cuocolo A. An overview of radiotracers in nuclear cardiology. J Nucl Cardiol 2000;7(6):701–7.
4. Ruddy TD, Tavoosi A, Taqueti VR. Role of nuclear cardiology in diagnosis and risk stratification of coronary microvascular disease. J Nucl Cardiol 2022. https://doi.org/10.1007/s12350-022-03051-z.

5. Zampella E, Acampa W, Assante R, et al. Combined evaluation of regional coronary artery calcium and myocardial perfusion by [82]Rb PET/CT in predicting lesion-related outcome. Eur J Nucl Med Mol Imaging 2020;47(7):1698–704.

6. von Felten E, Benz DC, Benetos G, et al. Prognostic value of regional myocardial flow reserve derived from ^{13}N-ammonia positron emission tomography in patients with suspected coronary artery disease. Eur J Nucl Med Mol Imaging 2021;49(1):311–20.

7. Fathala A, Aboulkheir M, Shoukri MM, et al. Diagnostic accuracy of ^{13}N-ammonia myocardial perfusion imaging with PET-CT in the detection of coronary artery disease. Cardiovasc Diagn Ther 2019;9(1):35–42.

8. Lindner O, Pascual TN, Mercuri M, et al. INCAPS Investigators Group. Nuclear cardiology practice and associated radiation doses in Europe: results of the IAEA Nuclear Cardiology Protocols Study (INCAPS) for the 27 European countries. Eur J Nucl Med Mol Imaging 2016;43(4):718–28.

9. Prior JO, Allenbach G, Valenta I, et al. Quantification of myocardial blood flow with 82Rb positron emission tomography: clinical validation with 15O-water. Eur J Nucl Med Mol Imaging 2012;39(6):1037–47.

10. Renaud JM, DaSilva JN, Beanlands RS, et al. Characterizing the normal range of myocardial blood flow with [82]rubidium and ^{13}N-ammonia PET imaging. J Nucl Cardiol 2013;20(4):578–91.

11. deKemp RA, Renaud JM, Klein R, et al. Radionuclide tracers for myocardial perfusion imaging and blood flow quantification. Cardiol Clin 2016;34(1):37–46.

12. Glover DK, Ruiz M, Yang JY, et al. Myocardial 99mTcTetrofosmin uptake during adenosine-induced vasodilatation with either a critical or mild coronary stenosis. Circulation 1997;96(7):2332–8.

13. Acampa W, Evangelista L, Petretta M, et al. Usefulness of stress cardiac single-photon emission computed tomographic imaging late after percutaneous coronary intervention for assessing cardiac events and time to such events. Am J Cardiol 2007;100(3):436–41.

14. Ito Y, Katoh C, Noriyasu K, et al. Estimation of myocardial blood flow and myocardial flow reserve by 99mTc-sestamibi imaging: comparison with the results of [15O]H2O PET. Eur J Nucl Med Mol Imaging 2003;30(2):281–7.

15. Daniele S, Nappi C, Acampa W, et al. Incremental prognostic value of coronary flow reserve assessed with single-photon emission computed tomography. J Nucl Cardiol 2011 Aug;18(4):612–9.

16. Cantoni V, Green R, Acampa W, et al. Diagnostic performance of myocardial perfusion imaging with conventional and CZT single-photon emission computed tomography in detecting coronary artery disease: a meta-analysis. J Nucl Cardiol 2021 Apr;28(2):698–715.

17. Acampa W, Buechel RR, Gimelli A. Low dose in nuclear cardiology: state of the art in the era of new cadmium-zinc-telluride cameras. Eur Heart J Cardiovasc Imaging 2016;17(6):591–5.

18. Duvall WL, Croft LB, Ginsberg ES, et al. Reduced isotope dose and imaging time with a high-efficiency CZT SPECT camera. J Nucl Cardiol 2011;18(5):847–57.

19. Meyer C, Weinmann P. Validation of early image acquisitions following Tc-99 m sestamibi injection using a semiconductors camera of cadmium-zinc-telluride. J Nucl Cardiol 2017;24(4):1149–56.

20. Ben-Haim S, Murthy VL, Breault C, et al. Quantification of myocardial perfusion reserve using dynamic SPECT imaging in humans: a feasibility study. J Nucl Med 2013;54(6):873–9.

21. Acampa W, Assante R, Mannarino T, et al. Low-dose dynamic myocardial perfusion imaging by CZT-SPECT in the identification of obstructive coronary artery disease. Eur J Nucl Med Mol Imaging 2020;47(7):1705–12.

22. Leppo JA, Meerdink DJ. Comparison of the myocardial uptake of a technetium-labeled isonitrile analogue and thallium. Circ Res 1989;65:632–9.

23. Yoshida K, Mullani N, Gould KL. Coronary flow and flow reserve by PET simplified for clinical applications using rubidium-82 or nitrogen-13-ammonia. J Nucl Med 1996;37:1701–12.

24. Agostini D, Roule V, Nganoa C, et al. First validation of myocardial flow reserve assessed by dynamic 99mTc-sestamibi CZT-SPECT camera: head to head comparison with 15O-water PET and fractional flow reserve in patients with suspected coronary artery disease. The WATERDAY study. Eur J Nucl Med Mol Imaging 2018;45(7):1079–90.

25. Yamamoto A, Nagao M, Ando K, et al. First validation of myocardial flow reserve derived from dynamic 99mTc-Sestamibi CZT-SPECT camera compared with 13N-ammonia PET. Int Heart J 2022;63(2):202–9.

26. Acampa W, Zampella E, Assante R, et al. Quantification of myocardial perfusion reserve by CZT-SPECT: a head to head comparison with 82Rubidium PET imaging. J Nucl Cardiol 2021;28(6):2827–39.

27. Nkoulou R, Fuchs TA, Pazhenkottil AP, et al. Absolute myocardial blood flow and flow reserve assessed by gated SPECT with cadmium-zinc-telluride detectors using 99mTc-tetrofosmin: head-to-head comparison with 13N-ammonia PET. J Nucl Med 2016;57(12):1887–92.

28. Wells RG, Marvin B, Poirier M, et al. Optimization of SPECT measurement of myocardial blood flow with corrections for attenuation, motion, and blood binding compared with PET. J Nucl Med 2017;58(12):2013–9.

29. Giubbini R, Bertoli M, Durmo R, et al. Comparison between N13NH3-PET and 99mTc-Tetrofosmin-CZT SPECT in the evaluation of absolute myocardial blood flow and flow reserve. J Nucl Cardiol 2019. https://doi.org/10.1007/s12350-019-01939x.

30. Ben Bouallègue F, Roubille F, Lattuca B, et al. SPECT myocardial perfusion reserve in patients with multivessel coronary disease: correlation with angiographic findings and invasive fractional flow reserve measurements. J Nucl Med 2015;56(11): 1712–7.

31. Miyagawa M, Nishiyama Y, Uetani T, et al. Estimation of myocardial flow reserve utilizing an ultrafast cardiac SPECT: comparison with coronary angiography, fractional flow reserve, and the SYNTAX score. Int J Cardiol 2017;244:347–53.

32. Han S, Kim Y-H, Ahn J-M, et al. Feasibility of dynamic stress 201Tl/rest 99mTc-tetrofosmin single photon emission computed tomography for quantification of myocardial perfusion reserve in patients with stable coronary artery disease. Eur J Nucl Med Mol Imaging 2018;45(12):2173–80.

33. do A H de Souza AC, Gonçalves BKD, Tedeschi AL, et al. Quantification of myocardial flow reserve using a gamma camera with solid-state cadmium-zinc-telluride detectors: relation to angiographic coronary artery disease. J Nucl Cardiol 2021;28:876–84.

34. Zavadovsky KV, Mochula AV, Maltseva AN, et al. The diagnostic value of SPECT CZT quantitative myocardial blood flow in high-risk patients. J Nucl Cardiol 2020. https://doi.org/10.1007/s12350-020-02395-8.

35. Zavadovsky KV, Mochula AV, Boshchenko AA, et al. Absolute myocardial blood flows derived by dynamic CZT scan vs invasive fractional flow reserve: correlation and accuracy. J Nucl Cardiol 2021; 28(1):249–59.

36. Maddahi J, Lazewatsky J, Udelson JE, et al. Phase-III clinical trial of fluorine-18 flurpiridaz positron emission tomography for evaluation of coronary artery disease. J Am Coll Cardiol 2020;76(4):391–401.

37. Packard RR, Huang SC, Dahlbom M, et al. Absolute quantitation of myocardial blood flow in human subjects with or without myocardial ischemia using dynamic flurpiridaz F 18 PET. J Nucl Med 2014;55(9): 1438–44.

38. Broisat A, Ruiz M, Goodman NC, et al. Myocardial uptake of 7'-(Z)-[(123)I]iodorotenone during vasodilator stress in dogs with critical coronary stenoses. Circ Cardiovasc Imaging 2011;4(6):685–92.

39. Ma H, Li S, Wu Z, et al. Comparison of 99mTc-N-DBODC5 and 99mTc-MIBI of myocardial perfusion imaging for diagnosis of coronary artery disease. BioMed Res Int 2013;2013:145427.

40. Gao S, Zhao G, Wen Q, et al. Pharmacokinetics and biodistribution of 99mTc N-MPO in healthy human volunteers. Clin Nucl Med 2014;39(1):e14–9.

Artificial Intelligence in Nuclear Cardiology

Robert J.H. Miller, MD

KEYWORDS

- Artificial intelligence • Machine learning • Deep learning • Nuclear cardiology

KEY POINTS

- Artificial intelligence (AI) refers to algorithms that perform tasks normally characteristic of human intelligence.
- AI techniques have been developed to improve image quality, reduce misregistration, or simulate attenuation correction imaging.
- Machine learning can improve the identification of obstructive coronary artery disease or risk prediction by combining clinical, stress, and imaging variables.
- Deep learning provides accurate prediction of disease diagnosis directly from image data.
- Methods to explain AI predictions to physicians, termed explainable AI, are a critical step toward clinical implementation.

INTRODUCTION

Artificial intelligence (AI) is a rapidly expanding field, which refers to any computer algorithm that performs tasks normally characteristic of human intelligence.[1] These algorithms could potentially be applied to many facets of nuclear cardiology including image reconstruction through clinical reporting. In particular, the vast array of clinical, stress, and imaging information associated with a typical myocardial perfusion scan is ideal for AI approaches that objectively integrate this data to improve disease diagnosis and risk prediction. Although AI applications can be initially daunting to many clinicians, understanding of key terminology and processes can dramatically improve understanding and the potential clinical impact of these algorithms. Enlightened by a review of key terminology, this article will review recent AI approaches for image reconstruction, which could be used to improve image quality or reduce radiation exposure as well as methods to automate image registration. Next, AI-driven attenuation correction (AC) of myocardial perfusion images and automated segmentation of coronary artery calcium (CAC) from AC imaging will be summarized. We will also discuss algorithms that leverage clinical, stress, and imaging information to accurately predict the presence of disease or cardiovascular risk. We will contrast this with deep learning (DL) approaches to provide similar predictions directly from images. Finally, we will review methods that are being developed to improve clinical implementation of these technologies including explainable AI.

ARTIFICIAL INTELLIGENCE TERMINOLOGY, TRAINING, AND TESTING
Artificial Intelligence Terminology

Although there is an increasing and broad interest in AI, the terminology remains a barrier to understanding for many clinicians and researchers. AI can be applied broadly to describe any computer algorithm, which performs a task normally characteristic of human intelligence such as understanding language, recognizing images, and learning patterns from past events to predict future events.[1] Machine learning (ML) algorithms are an example of AI, which typically use precoded data to perform a task, without being explicitly programmed about the importance of the various features.[2] ML algorithms can be developed to classify patients into specific categories (termed

Department of Cardiac Sciences, University of Calgary, GAA08, 3230 Hospital Drive Northwest, Calgary, Alberta T2N 2T9, Canada
E-mail address: robert.miller@albertahealthservices.ca

Cardiol Clin 41 (2023) 151–161
https://doi.org/10.1016/j.ccl.2023.01.004

supervised learning), for example, identifying patients with obstructive coronary artery disease (CAD). In unsupervised learning, ML algorithms are tasked with learning the inherent structure of the data without being specifically instructed which groups are present or which features are relevant. Unsupervised ML has been applied to identify different phenotypes of patients with heart failure with preserved ejection fraction[3] but could also be applied to nuclear cardiology. ML algorithms are well suited to integrate the vast amount of information from nuclear cardiology studies while considering nonlinearity as well as collinearity and interactions among variables.

DL is a subset of ML, which refers to algorithms using a multilayered learning approach. A graphical representation of some commonly used models in nuclear cardiology is shown in **Fig. 1**. Convolutional neural networks (CNNs) are one DL approach, which is frequently applied to image data.[1,4] CNNs differ from the classic artificial neural network in that the neurons from adjacent layers are only connected to other neurons in the near vicinity. CNNs are well suited for image interpretation and segmentation because the model architecture maintains information regarding the spatial structure of the image (ie, features from far away regions are not likely to influence each other). It is also possible to combine the CNN layers with some fully connected layers—usually as the late layers of the network—to allow connections between any features (nodes) of the layers. This approach has been used in cardiovascular image classification for example.[4–6]

An autoencoder is a specific DL architecture, which is tasked with copying the input layer to the output layer but with inner hidden layers that have fewer dimensions than either the input or output layers. Because the inner hidden layers have fewer dimensions, the algorithm only extracts the most critical information.[7] This approach has been used to denoise images in order to improve the image quality.[8] U-Net is a related model architecture, which incorporates skip connections, where information form one layer is carried forward across layers (or skips layers).[9] The skip connections allow the model to recover fine image details that may otherwise be lost in the contracting layers of the model. Although these are 3 commonly used DL algorithms, model architectures are rapidly evolving enabling new or improved clinical applications.

Artificial Intelligence Training

The process of identifying features and determining their relative importance for predicting the outcome of interest is referred to as training. Training datasets should be large, heterogenous, and ideally representative of the population in which the algorithm will eventually be applied. Model parameters are derived during the training process and are not set in any way. Hyperparameters are variables that control the learning process, for example, learning rate or number of iterations. Methods used to optimize the hyperparameters of the model are termed "tuning." Importantly, the data used for training and tuning the model should not be used in any way during model testing.

Artificial Intelligence Testing

Testing, which is also sometimes referred to as validation, is the process in which an AI model is applied to a new data set to evaluate its performance. This process may be performed once or several times. Additionally, this process may be applied to a random set of the study population or patients separated by a specific grouping factor. Two commonly used procedures are k-fold cross-validation and repeated external testing as depicted in **Fig. 2**. In k-fold cross-validation, the population is randomly divided into k-folds (or sets of data), with each fold sequentially held-out for testing.[10] Repeated testing decreases the variance in estimating model accuracy and is preferred to testing in a single random sample.[11] In external testing, the patients selected for training and tuning are from a different population than those eventually used for model testing.[12] External testing (frequently called external validation) provides an estimate of the model performance when it is applied in a new, unrelated population.[12] Occasionally when no external population is available for testing, temporal splits or rolling cross-validation are used to evaluate whether changes in patient characteristics over time significantly influence prediction performance.[13] Although it is important to assess model prediction performance (how accurately it classifies cases), it is also important to assess calibration (a measure of how closely predicted probability matches actual probability).[14] Failure in either prediction performance or calibration (identifying low-risk patients as high-risk patients) could have negative influences on downstream patient management.[15]

ARTIFICIAL INTELLIGENCE TO IMPROVE IMAGE QUALITY, REGISTRATION, AND ATTENUATION CORRECTION
Utilizing Artificial Intelligence to Improve Image Quality

AI algorithms have been applied extensively to image reconstruction to improve image quality. For

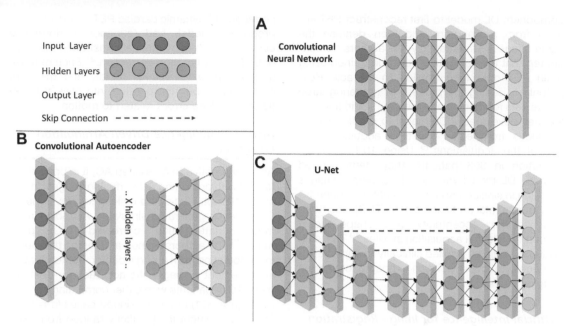

Fig. 1. Different deep-learning architectures. Neural networks are typically comprised of input and output layers with many hidden inner layers. Each neuron, or node, is connected to many neurons in the following layer, with all information moving forward through the network (feed-forward). In convolutional neural networks (A), neurons only feed-forward to local (spatially related) neurons in the next layer. Convolutional autoencoders (B) are connected to the next layer in a similar fashion to convolutional neural networks but are characterized by inner hidden layers with fewer dimensions than either the input or the output layer. This forces the network to identify only the most salient features. U-Net (C) is similar to a convolutional autoencoder but with skip connections, which help maintain fine image features that may be lost in the contracting layers of the model.

example, Ramon and colleagues demonstrated the feasibility of denoising low-dose single photon emission computed tomography (SPECT) images using DL.[16] The authors used stacked autoencoders trained to predict full-dose images from low-dose image reconstructions.[16] In simulations, images denoised with DL using one-sixteenth of the clinical dose achieved similar image quality to images using one-eighth dose denoised with standard methods.[16] Song and colleagues demonstrated that a CNN, trained in 95 patients and tested in 24 patients, improved spatial resolution compared with conventional postprocessing methods.[17] Wang and colleagues trained a 2-

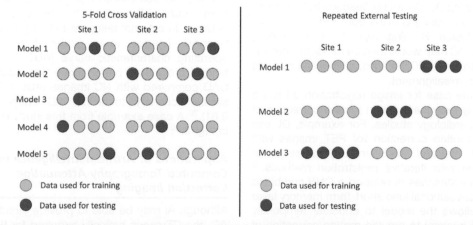

Fig. 2. Comparison of 5-fold cross-validation and repeated external testing. In k-fold cross-validation, the data set is randomly divided into k folds (or sets), in this case 5. Each set is sequentially held-out from model training to be used for testing. In repeated external testing, data sets are grouped according to factors such as site. Each site is held-out for testing the model developed using data from the remaining sites.

component DL model to first reconstruct PET images from a sinogram and then denoise the same images.[18] Interestingly, the authors demonstrated that their algorithm could be trained using brain PET data then applied to thoracic PET, potentially easing the process of gathering large image sets for training and testing.[18] Shiri and colleagues developed a DL model to predict full acquisitions from either half-time acquisitions or half of the acquisitions.[19] Using 10-fold cross-validation in 363 patients, they demonstrated that the DL model was able to generate images resulting in similar automatic quantitation of perfusion (stress total perfusion deficit [TPD]) and function (volume, eccentricity, and shape index) compared with full acquisition studies.[19] These algorithms could be applied clinically to improve image quality, reduce radiation exposure, or shorten imaging times.

Artificial Intelligence for Image Registration and Motion Correction

All PET and many SPECT myocardial perfusion scans are acquired with computed tomography (CT) for AC.[20] AC imaging improves the diagnostic accuracy of SPECT[21] but can be complicated by errors during image registration.[22] AI could potentially be used to reduce the frequency or extent of image misregistration. Ko and colleagues trained a CNN-based algorithm to predict the offset between images compared with manually coregistered SPECT/CT images using 402 cases.[23] The algorithm was tested using 100 cases and demonstrated residual misalignment between image pairs of 2.38 ± 2.00 mm during testing.[23] Another method to address image misregistration is to generate AC maps, directly from PET or SPECT images using DL. Shi and colleagues trained an algorithm to predict AC maps from SPECT myocardial perfusion imaging alone.[24] The resulting synthetic AC map would then be perfectly coregistered with the SPECT images, eliminating artifacts related to misalignment.

As is the case for image registration, AI has a potentially prominent role in motion correction of nuclear cardiology studies. For example, DL can provide motion correction for PET images with lower normalized root mean square error compared with iterative registration methods.[25] Guo and colleagues developed a CNN combined with a convolutional long short-term memory layer (which allows the model to consider temporally adjacent images) to provide motion correction of fluorodeoxyglucose PET images.[26] Similarly, Shi and colleagues applied a convolutional long short-term memory network to provide motion

correction of dynamic cardiac PET images.[27] Their proposed model had superior performance compared with conventional registration methods or CNN-based motion correction.[27] Each of these methods provides results rapidly and therefore could readily be incorporated into clinical workflows to reduce errors related to motion.

Artificial Intelligence-Driven Attenuation Correction

As an alternative to CT-based AC, it is possible to task AI with predicting AC perfusion images. In one such attempt, Hagio and colleagues developed a CNN, which generates simulated AC polar maps from nonattenuation corrected (NC) polar maps.[28] The authors trained and tested the model in a population from a single center, demonstrating improvement in diagnostic accuracy for obstructive CAD in patients with either correlating angiography (n = 351) or low-likelihood cases (n = 327). The improvement in specificity ranged from 26% (in higher quality studies) to 8% (when considering lower quality studies as well). Chen and colleagues DL network incorporated gender, body mass index, and images from 3 scatter windows together with NC images to predict AC images.[29] The authors demonstrated that their predicted AC images more closely matched the actual AC images compared with a traditional U-Net model, with normalized mean square error of 2.01% versus 2.23%.[29] More recently, Shanbhag and colleagues developed a generative adversarial network (GAN) model, which predicts AC SPECT images (DL-based AC [DeepAC]) from nonattenuation corrected (NC) images.[30] The goal of the GAN architecture is to iteratively train the generator network (in this case a modified U-Net model) until it generates images that are indistinguishable from actual AC images by the discriminator network. In external testing with 604 patients, the DeepAC images (area under the receiver-operating characteristic curve [AUC] 0.79) had higher prediction performance for obstructive CAD compared with NC images (AUC 0.70) and similar accuracy to actual AC images (AUC 0.81).[30] A case example from this study is shown in **Fig. 3.**[30]

Applications of Artificial Intelligence to Computed Tomography Attenuation Correction Imaging

Although AI may be able to provide direct image AC, the CT scans typically acquired for this purpose also contain valuable anatomic information. For example, CAC can be identified from low-dose CT attenuation scans in order to provide

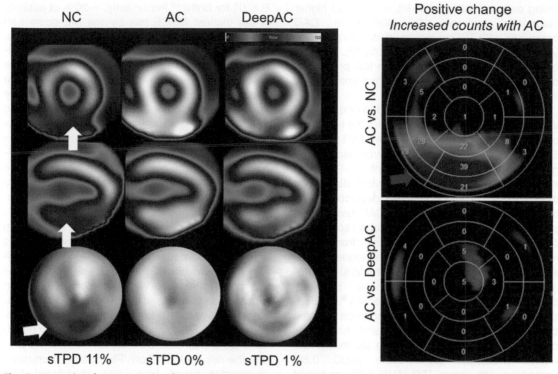

Fig. 3. Example of DeepAC. On short-axis images (*top*), vertical long axis (*middle*), and polar maps (*bottom*), there was a defect in the inferior wall on NC, images (*white arrows*) that essentially resolved with actual AC and DeepAC imaging. Standard quantification by stress TPD was abnormal for NC images only. There was positive change (increased counts with AC) in the inferior wall for AC versus NC (*red arrow*). There was no significant change seen between AC versus DeepAC images. The patient had no CAD on coronary CT angiography. This research was originally published in the Journal of Nuclear Medicine. (This research was originally published in JNM. Shanbhag AD, Miller RJH, Pieszko K, et al. Deep Learning-based Attenuation Correction Improves Diagnostic Accuracy of Cardiac SPECT [published online ahead of print, 2022 Sep 22]. J Nucl Med. 2022. jnumed.122.264429; DOI: https://doi.org/10.2967/jnumed.122.264429. © SNMMI.)

risk stratification.[31] Several AI models have been developed which can automate this segmentation process.[32–34] For example, Zeleznik and colleagues developed a DL model, which could quantify CAC from gated and ungated CT, demonstrating excellent agreement with expert reader quantification of CAC.[34] However, CT scans obtained for AC are acquired with lower radiation doses, resulting in noisier images, which make segmentation more difficult. Despite this challenge, DL-derived CAC scores can have good agreement with expert readers.[35,36] Additionally, Pieszko and colleagues recently demonstrated that CAC quantified by DL from CT attenuation scans obtained during PET imaging provides similar risk stratification as expert reader quantified CAC.[37] Similar results have been demonstrated with DL CAC scores for SPECT myocardial perfusion imaging (MPI) using external validation.[38] Importantly, the fully automated DL CAC results can be obtained in less than 1 second compared with ~5 minutes for expert reader

scores. These techniques could potentially be further refined to assess other features, such as epicardial adipose tissue volume and attenuation,[39] to allow physicians to more fully use anatomic information from CT.

ARTIFICIAL INTELLIGENCE TO IMPROVE PATIENT CLASSIFICATION
Artificial Intelligence for Disease Diagnosis

AI can efficiently and accurately classify patients, such as identifying patients with obstructive CAD. Arsanjani and colleagues demonstrated that an ML model, which integrated TPD, ischemic changes and left ventricular ejection fraction could identify patients with obstructive CAD more accurately than TPD alone (diagnostic accuracy 86% vs 81%; P < .01).[40] Eisenberg and colleagues developed an ML model, which included a larger number of clinical, stress, and imaging variables to identify patients with a low probability of obstructive CAD for rest scan cancellation.[41]

Using external testing, the ML model had higher diagnostic accuracy for obstructive CAD compared with TPD or reader visual interpretation (AUC 0.82 vs 0.74 and 0.68, $P < .05$). ML can also be used to identify patients with a low probability of abnormal perfusion for stress-first imaging using pretest features alone.[42]

Although ML models rely on coded or quantified variables, DL algorithms can predict the likelihood of obstructive CAD directly from MPI images. Spier and colleagues have also developed a DL algorithm, which achieved agreement of ∼90% with expert visual interpretation of myocardial perfusion.[43] Betancur and colleagues developed a DL model to diagnose obstructive CAD using 1638 patients from 9 centers.[5] With matched specificity, DL improved the per-vessel sensitivity from 64.4% (with TPD) to 69.8% ($P < .01$).[5] Subsequently, the authors showed that using upright and supine imaging data improved diagnostic accuracy compared with combined TPD analysis.[6] DL identification of CAD from SPECT polar maps has also been externally tested. Otaki and colleagues demonstrated that an explainable DL model had higher prediction performance (AUC 0.80) compared with stress TPD (AUC 0.73) or expert reader interpretation (AUC 0.71, $P < .001$ for both) in an external population of 555 patients.[44] However, when these DL models are trained using only patient who underwent invasive coronary angiography (a highly selected population), the estimated probability of CAD may overestimate actual risk. Methods for augmenting the training population with low-risk patients can improve model calibration, particularly for women, without affecting diagnostic accuracy.[45] DL-based approaches to diagnosis can be applied to diseases other than CAD. For example, Togo and colleagues developed a CNN to identify patients with cardiac sarcoidosis, which had improved diagnostic accuracy compared with standard quantification.[46] Recently, another CNN was developed to diagnose transthyretin cardiac amyloidosis from bone scintigraphy imaging.[47]

Artificial Intelligence for Risk Prediction

AI algorithms also have a potential role in refining risk prediction following MPI by rapidly, objectively, and accurately integrating large amounts of clinical, stress, and imaging data. In one such study, an ML model was developed using SPECT MPI data from a single center (n = 2619) for major adverse cardiovascular event (MACE) prediction using 10-fold cross-validation.[48] The ML model had higher AUC for MACE (0.81) compared with either stress TPD (0.73), or ischemic TPD (0.71,

$P < .01$ for both).[48] Importantly, ∼20% of patients in the highest MACE risk by the ML score had "normal" expert visual interpretation of perfusion. In a subsequent multicenter study, Hu and colleagues demonstrated that ML could improve the prediction of revascularization on a per patient and per-vessel basis compared with quantitative image analysis alone.[49] ML models have also been developed to identify patients with a low risk of MACE for rest scan cancellation.[50] In one such study, patients selected for rest scan cancellation with clinical methods had higher all-cause mortality (1.0%–1.3%) compared with patients selected by ML thresholds identifying a similar proportion of patients (0.2%–0.6%).[50] DL models have also been developed to predict MACE from rest and stress myocardial blood flow as well as myocardial flow reserve polar maps.[51] Using 5-fold cross-validation, the AUC was 0.90 for the DL model compared with 0.85 for a regression model incorporating clinical history, ventricular function, myocardial blood flow, and myocardial flow reserve. Singh and colleagues recently developed an explainable DL model, which could predict the risk of death from PET relative perfusion, myocardial blood flow, and myocardial flow reserve polar maps. In simulated prospective testing with 1135 patients, the DL model had a higher prediction performance (AUC 0.82) compared with myocardial flow reserve (AUC 0.70) or a comprehensive regression model (AUC 0.75).[52] A similar approach has also been used to predict death or myocardial infarction from SPECT perfusion, thickening, and motion polar maps.[53] In external testing with 9019 patients, the model had higher prediction performance (AUC 0.73) compared with a logistic regression model (AUC 0.70) or stress TPD (AUC 0.65).[53] These last studies demonstrate the potential for DL to integrate multiple image sources to improve the prediction performance.

Reducing Barriers to Clinical Implementation

Although the potential for improvements from AI techniques is clear, methods to implement them clinically still require further investigation. One example of attempts to improve clinical translation is studies investigating methods to decrease the number of variables requiring collection for ML models. Alonso and colleagues demonstrated that an ML model using only 6 variables provided superior risk prediction compared with a logistic regression model with 14 variables.[54] Rios and colleagues demonstrated that an ML model with 12 manually input and 11 imaging variables had similar prediction performance for MACE

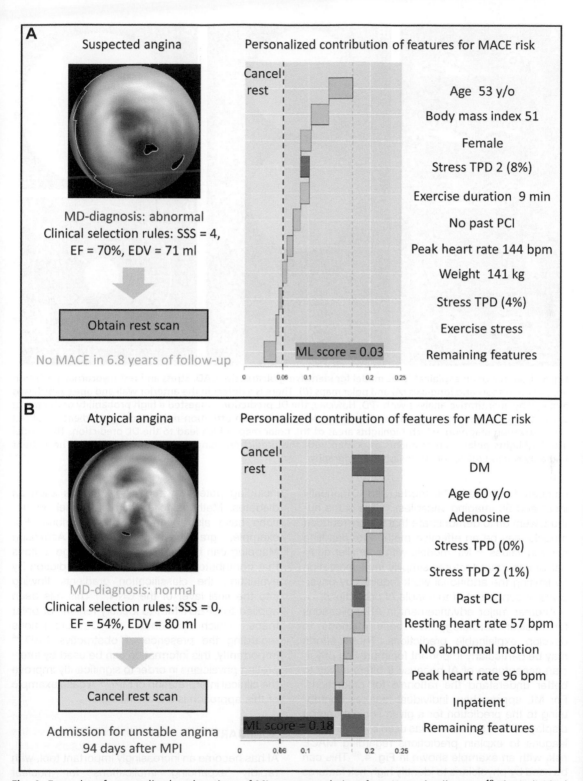

Fig. 4. Examples of personalized explanations of ML recommendations from Hu and colleagues.[49] The individual contributions of the top 10 features to the overall risk for each patient are shown (*blue bars* = decreasing risk, *red bars* = increasing risk). Gray dotted line indicates baseline cohort risk. Red dotted line indicates ML threshold, matching stress cancellation rate for the stringent clinical criteria. Panel *A* shows results for a patient with abnormal

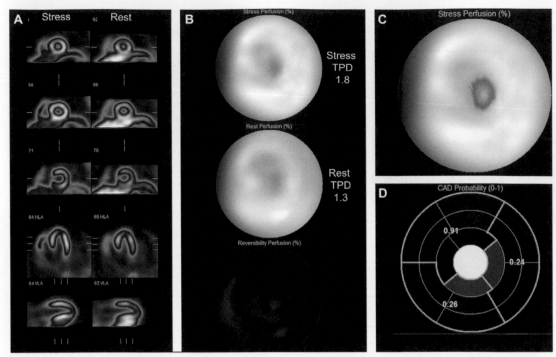

Fig. 5. Example of an explainable DL model for identifying obstructive CAD. Stress and rest myocardial perfusion are shown in short and long-axis (*A*) and polar maps (*B*). There is a defect in the anterior wall and apex, which was minimal by quantitative analysis with TPD. However, the DL prediction suggested a high probability of disease in the left anterior descending territory. The DL model generates an attention map (*C*) using gradient-weighted class activation mapping, which highlights areas of the polar map, which lead to the DL prediction. The model also highlights polar map segments associated with the prediction using a probability map (*D*). The patient had a 90% mid-LAD lesion on invasive angiography.

compared with the full ML model (with 40 manually input and 58 imaging variables).[55] The same authors went on to demonstrate that feature reduced models may be an effective method for handling missing values.[56] ML models with a smaller number of important features simplify implementation by limiting the additional work required by physicians or support staff to enable AI predictions.

Another major advancement in AI applications for nuclear cardiology has been methods to develop explainable predictions. These efforts may be particularly important for improving physician acceptance of AI because it offers a way to better understand the rationale for predictions. For ML approaches, individual features contributing to the prediction for a given subject can be displayed. This approach was used by Hu and colleagues to explain predictions regarding MACE risk, with an example shown in **Fig. 4**.[49] This can be used by physicians to identify high-risk features

including potentially modifiable factors such as diabetes. Methods to explain DL model predictions have also been recently described. For example, gradient-weighted Class Activation Mapping can be used to highlight image regions that contribute most to the final AI prediction by evaluating the classification gradients flowing into the final layer of the CNN.[57] This has been applied to SPECT MPI to identify regions of polar maps, which contribute to DL predictions regarding the presence of obstructive CAD.[44] Importantly, this information can be used by interpreting physicians in order to significantly improve the clinical interpretation of MPI.[58] A case example of this approach is shown in **Fig. 5**.

SUMMARY

AI has become an increasingly important tool, with rapidly expanding implications for nuclear

perfusion but at low-risk of MACE. Panel *B* shows a patient at higher risk of MACE despite having essentially normal myocardial perfusion by total perfusion deficit (TPD). (*From* Hu LH, Miller RJH, Sharir T, et al. Prognostically safe stress-only single-photon emission computed tomography myocardial perfusion imaging guided by machine learning: report from REFINE SPECT. Eur Heart J Cardiovasc Imaging. 2021;22(6):705-714. Figure 5.)

cardiology. When evaluating new AI techniques, it is critical to evaluate the training and testing regimens as well as considering the potential for clinical application. AI can significantly improve image reconstruction, potentially allowing reduction in radiation exposure or improvements in image quality. Clinically, AI could potentially be implemented to improve disease diagnosis or prediction of adverse events. Methods to improve the feasibility of implementing ML models and explain AI predictions are critical to improving clinical implementation.

CLINICS CARE POINTS

- When evaluating an AI model, it is critical to ensure that there was rigorous separation of training and testing data
- AI can improve image quality, facilitating lower radiation doses, or replace AC imaging
- AI models have higher accuracy for disease diagnosis and for risk estimation compared with standard image quantification
- Simplified ML models and explainable models may improve clinical translation of AI

DISCLOSURES

Dr R.J.H. Miller has received consulting fees and research support from Pfizer, United States.

REFERENCES

1. Dey D, Slomka PJ, Leeson P, et al. Artificial intelligence in cardiovascular imaging: JACC state-of-the-art review. J Am Coll Cardiol 2019;73:1317–35.
2. Obermeyer Z, Emanuel EJ. Predicting the future - big data, machine learning, and clinical medicine. N Engl J Med 2016;375:1216–9.
3. Segar MW, Patel KV, Ayers C, et al. Phenomapping of patients with heart failure with preserved ejection fraction using machine learning-based unsupervised cluster analysis. Eur J Heart Fail 2020;22:148–58.
4. Krittanawong C, Tunhasiriwet A, Zhang H, et al. Deep learning with unsupervised feature in echocardiographic imaging. J Am Coll Cardiol 2017;69:2100–1.
5. Betancur J, Commandeur F, Motlagh M, et al. Deep learning for prediction of obstructive disease from fast myocardial perfusion SPECT: a multicenter study. JACC Cardiovascular imaging 2018;11:1654–63.
6. Betancur J, Hu LH, Commandeur F, et al. Deep learning analysis of upright-supine high-efficiency SPECT myocardial perfusion imaging for prediction of obstructive coronary artery disease: a multicenter study. J Nucl Med 2019;60:664–70.
7. Lundervold AS, Lundervold A. An overview of deep learning in medical imaging focusing on MRI. Z Med Phys 2019;29:102–27.
8. Ramon AJ, Yang Y, Pretorius PH, et al. Improving diagnostic accuracy in low-dose SPECT myocardial perfusion imaging with convolutional denoising networks. IEEE Trans Med imaging 2020;39:2893–903.
9. Ronneberger O, Fischer P, Brox T. U-net: convolutional networks for biomedical image segmentation. In: Navab N, Hornegger J, Wells WM, Frangi AF, editors. MICCAI 2015;234–41.
10. Jung Y, Hu J. A K-fold averaging cross-validation procedure. J Nonparametr Stat 2015;27:167–79.
11. Cawley GC, Talbot NLC. On over-fitting in model selection and subsequent selection bias in performance evaluation. J Machine Learn Res 2010;11:2079–107.
12. Riley RD, Ensor J, Snell KI, et al. External validation of clinical prediction models using big datasets from e-health records or IPD meta-analysis: opportunities and challenges. BMJ 2016;353:i3140.
13. Miller RJH, Sabovčik F, Cauwenberghs N, et al. Temporal shift and predictive performance of machine learning for heart transplant outcomes. J Heart Lung Transplant 2022;41:928–36.
14. Miller R.J.H., Rozanski A., Slomka P.J., et al., Development and validation of ischemia risk scores, J Nucl Cardiol, 2022. doi: 10.1007/s12350-022-02976-9. Online ahead of print.
15. Van Calster B, Vickers AJ. Calibration of risk prediction models: impact on decision-analytic performance. Med Decis Making 2015;35:162–9.
16. Ramon AJ, Yang Y, Pretorius PH, et al. Initial investigation of low-dose SPECT-MPI via deep learning. IEEE Nucl Sci Symp 2018;1–3.
17. Song C, Yang Y, Wernick MN, et al. Low-dose cardiac-gated spect studies using a residual convolutional neural network. IEEE Int Symp Biomed Imaging 2019;1:653–6.
18. Wang B. and Liu H., FBP-Net for direct reconstruction of dynamic PET images, Phys Med Biol, 65 (23), 2020, 1-16.
19. Shiri I, AmirMozafari Sabet K, Arabi H, et al. Standard SPECT myocardial perfusion estimation from half-time acquisitions using deep convolutional residual neural networks. J Nucl Cardiol 2021;28:2761–79.
20. Dorbala S, Di Carli MF, Delbeke D, et al. SNMMI/ASNC/SCCT guideline for cardiac SPECT/CT and PET/CT 1.0. J Nucl Med 2013;54:1485–507.
21. Arsanjani R, Xu Y, Hayes SW, et al. Comparison of fully automated computer analysis and visual

scoring for detection of coronary artery disease from myocardial perfusion SPECT in a large population. J Nucl Med 2013;54:221–8.

22. Goetze S, Wahl RL. Prevalence of misregistration between SPECT and CT for attenuation-corrected myocardial perfusion SPECT. J Nucl Cardiol 2007; 14:200–6.

23. Ko C-L, Cheng M-F, Yen R-F, et al. Automatic alignment of CZT myocardial perfusion SPECT and external non-contrast CT by deep-learning model and dynamic data generation. J Nucl Med 2019; 60:570.

24. Shi L, Onofrey JA, Liu H, et al. Deep learning-based attenuation map generation for myocardial perfusion SPECT. Eur J Nucl Med Mol Imaging 2020;47: 2383–95.

25. Li T, Zhang M, Qi W, et al. Motion correction of respiratory-gated PET images using deep learning based image registration framework. Phys Med Biol 2020;65:155003.

26. Guo X, Zhou B, Pigg D, et al. Unsupervised inter-frame motion correction for whole-body dynamic PET using convolutional long short-term memory in a convolutional neural network. Med Image Anal 2022;80:102524.

27. Shi L, Lu Y, Dvornek N, et al. Automatic inter-frame patient motion correction for dynamic cardiac PET using deep learning. IEEE Trans Med Imaging 2021;40:3293–304.

28. Hagio T, Poitrasson-Rivière A, Moody JB, et al. Virtual" attenuation correction: improving stress myocardial perfusion SPECT imaging using deep learning. Eur J Nucl Med Mol Imaging 2022;49(9):3140–9.

29. Chen XC, Zhou B, Shi LY, et al. CT-free attenuation correction for dedicated cardiac SPECT using a 3D dual squeeze-and-excitation residual dense network. J Nucl Cardiol 2021;29(5):2235–50.

30. Shanbhag AD, Miller RJH, Pieszko K, et al. Deep learning-based attenuation correction improves diagnostic accuracy of cardiac SPECT. J Nucl Med 2022;jnumed(122):264429.

31. Trpkov C, Savtchenko A, Liang Z, et al. Visually estimated coronary artery calcium score improves SPECT-MPI risk stratification. Int J Cardiol Heart Vasc 2021;35:100827.

32. Wolterink JM, Leiner T, de Vos BD, et al. Automatic coronary artery calcium scoring in cardiac CT angiography using paired convolutional neural networks. Med Image Anal 2016;34:123–36.

33. Takx RA, de Jong PA, Leiner T, et al. Automated coronary artery calcification scoring in non-gated chest CT: agreement and reliability. PLoS One 2014;9: e91239.

34. Zeleznik R, Foldyna B, Eslami P, et al. Deep convolutional neural networks to predict cardiovascular risk from computed tomography. Nat Commun 2021;12: 715.

35. Isgum I, de Vos BD, Wolterink JM, et al. Automatic determination of cardiovascular risk by CT attenuation correction maps in Rb-82 PET/CT. J Nucl Cardiol 2018;25:2133–42.

36. Pieszko K, Shanbhag AD, Lemley M, et al. Reproducibility of quantitative coronary calcium scoring from PET/CT attenuation maps: comparison to ECG-gated CT scans. Eur J Nucl Med Mol Imaging 2022;49:4122–32.

37. Pieszko K, Shanbhag A, Killekar A, et al. Deep learning of coronary calcium scores from PET/CT attenuation maps accurately predicts adverse cardiovascular events. JACC Cardiovasc Imaging 2022. Epub ahead of print.

38. Miller RJH, Pieszko K, Shanbhag A, et al. Deep learning coronary artery calcium scores from SPECT/CT attenuation maps improves prediction of major adverse cardiac events. J Nucl Med 2022; jnumed(122):264423.

39. Eisenberg E, McElhinney PA, Commandeur F, et al. Deep learning-based quantification of epicardial adipose tissue volume and attenuation predicts major adverse cardiovascular events in asymptomatic subjects. Circ Cardiovasc Imaging 2020;13: e009829.

40. Arsanjani R, Xu Y, Dey D, et al. Improved accuracy of myocardial perfusion SPECT for the detection of coronary artery disease using a support vector machine algorithm. J Nucl Med 2013;54:549–55.

41. Eisenberg E, Miller RJH, Hu LH, et al. Diagnostic safety of a machine learning-based automatic patient selection algorithm for stress-only myocardial perfusion SPECT. J Nucl Cardiol 2021;29(5): 2295–307.

42. Miller RJH, Hauser MT, Sharir T, et al. Machine learning to predict abnormal myocardial perfusion from pre-test features. J Nucl Cardiol 2022;29(5): 2393–403.

43. Spier N, Nekolla S, Rupprecht C, et al. Classification of polar maps from cardiac perfusion imaging with graph-convolutional neural networks. Sci Rep 2019;9:7569.

44. Otaki Y, Singh A, Kavanagh P, et al. Clinical deployment of explainable artificial intelligence of SPECT for diagnosis of coronary artery disease. JACC Cardiovasc Imaging 2022;15:1091–102.

45. Miller RJH, Singh A, Otaki Y, et al. Mitigating bias in deep learning for diagnosis of coronary artery disease from myocardial perfusion SPECT images. Eur J Nucl Med Mol Imaging 2022. Epub ahead of print.

46. Togo R, Hirata K, Manabe O, et al. Cardiac sarcoidosis classification with deep convolutional neural network-based features using polar maps. Comput Biol Med 2019;104:81–6.

47. Halme HL, Ihalainen T, Suomalainen O, et al. Convolutional neural networks for detection of transthyretin

amyloidosis in 2D scintigraphy images. EJNMMI Res 2022;12:27.

48. Betancur J, Otaki Y, Motwani M, et al. Prognostic value of combined clinical and myocardial perfusion imaging data using machine learning. JACC Cardiovasc Imaging 2018;11:1000–9.

49. Hu LH, Betancur J, Sharir T, et al. Machine learning predicts per-vessel early coronary revascularization after fast myocardial perfusion SPECT: results from multicentre REFINE SPECT registry. Eur Heart J Cardiovasc Imaging 2020;21:549–59.

50. Hu LH, Miller RJH, Sharir T, et al. Prognostically safe stress-only single-photon emission computed tomography myocardial perfusion imaging guided by machine learning: report from REFINE SPECT. Eur Heart J Cardiovasc Imaging 2021 10;22(6):705–14.

51. Juarez-Orozco LE, Martinez-Manzanera O, van der Zant FM, et al. Deep learning in quantitative PET myocardial perfusion imaging: a study on cardiovascular event prediction. JACC Cardiovasc Imaging 2020;13:180–2.

52. Singh A, Kwiecinski J, Miller RJH, et al. Deep learning for explainable estimation of mortality risk from myocardial positron emission tomography images. Circ Cardiovasc Imaging 2022;15:e014526.

53. Singh A, Miller RJH, Otaki Y, et al. Direct risk assessment from myocardial perfusion imaging using explainable deep learning. JACC Cardiovasc Imaging 2022;S1936-878X(22):00484–93.

54. Haro Alonso D, Wernick MN, Yang Y, et al. Prediction of cardiac death after adenosine myocardial perfusion SPECT based on machine learning. J Nucl Cardiol 2019;26:1746–54.

55. Rios R, Miller RJH, Hu LH, et al. Determining a minimum set of variables for machine learning cardiovascular event prediction: results from REFINE SPECT registry. Cardiovasc Res 2022;118:2152–64.

56. Rios R, Miller RJH, Manral N, et al. Handling missing values in machine learning to predict patient-specific risk of adverse cardiac events: insights from REFINE SPECT registry. Comput Biol Med 2022;145:105449.

57. Selvaraju RR, Cogswell M, Das A, et al. Grad-cam: visual explanations from deep networks via gradient-based localization. IEEE Int Conf Comput Vis 2017;618–26.

58. Miller RJH, Kuronuma K, Singh A, et al. Explainable deep learning improves physician interpretation of myocardial perfusion imaging. J Nucl Med 2022;63(11):1768–74.

Stress-First Myocardial Perfusion Imaging

Sean R. McMahon, MD, Etee K. Patel, MD, W. Lane Duvall, MD*

KEYWORDS

• Myocardial perfusion imaging • Stress-first • Stress-only • Radiation reduction

KEY POINTS

- Normal stress-only myocardial perfusion imaging (MPI) studies have the same prognosis as full rest-stress MPI studies.
- Stress-only MPI studies decrease test time by 38% compared with conventional rest-stress protocols.
- Stress-only MPI studies decrease radiation exposure to the patient by 40% to 88% compared with conventional rest-stress protocols.
- Successful stress-first protocols require attenuation correction for maximal effectiveness.

INTRODUCTION

Myocardial perfusion imaging (MPI) most commonly consists of 2 sets of images: first, an image of radiotracer distribution obtained during resting hemodynamic conditions, and second, images obtained under stress conditions (exercise or pharmacologic). MPI studies are typically interpreted by first reviewing the stress images for any areas of decreased activity. The reader then compares these areas to the resting scan to determine whether the defect is reversible (ischemia) or fixed (infarction). When stress images are normal, however, the rest images become superfluous.

As far back as 1992,[1] nuclear cardiologists suggested reviewing stress MPI before deciding on the need to image the patient at rest. This stress-first strategy provides perfusion data prognostically equivalent to a full rest-stress study while saving time in the imaging laboratory and reducing radiation exposure in appropriately selected patients. Yet few nuclear cardiology laboratories employ a stress-first protocol, perhaps reflecting challenges inherent in this protocol compared with a rest-stress protocol. A 2011 American Society of Nuclear Cardiology survey of US laboratories was the most optimistic, suggesting that 23% of sites used stress-first protocols.[2] A multinational 2016 International Atomic Energy Agency Nuclear Cardiology Protocols Study (INCAPS) found that in North America only 7.7% of patients underwent a stress-first protocol, with 3.1% finishing as a stress-only protocol (**Table 1**).[3] This represented the lowest proportion of stress-first studies in the survey behind Oceania, Latin America, Asia, and Africa, with Europe attempting stress-first in 84.4% of patients and completing stress-only in 19.8%. A 2022 update to the INCAPS survey found that worldwide, stress-first single-photon emission computed tomography (SPECT) imaging comprised nearly 20% of cases from all regions except North America (range 19%-88%), where it continued to represent just 7% of cases (**Fig. 1**).[4]

In current clinical practice, most appropriately indicated diagnostic stress MPI studies are found to be normal, especially in patients with no prior history of coronary artery disease (CAD). In a study by Rozanski and colleagues[5] of 39,515 patients with no history of CAD who underwent diagnostic stress MPI from 1991 to 2009, the prevalence of normal MPI studies was noted to have increased among all subgroups from a prevalence rate of 59.1% in 1991, to 91.3% in 2009. The prevalence rate of normal studies reached as high as 97.1% among exercising patients without typical angina.

Division of Cardiology, Hartford Hospital, 80 Seymour Street, Hartford, CT 06102, USA
* Corresponding author.
E-mail address: Lane.Duvall@hhchealth.org

Cardiol Clin 41 (2023) 163–175
https://doi.org/10.1016/j.ccl.2023.01.005
0733-8651/23/© 2023 Elsevier Inc. All rights reserved.

Table 1
Data from International Atomic Energy Agency Nuclear Cardiology Protocols Study

	North America	Europe	Africa	Asia	Latin America	Oceania	Total
Stress-first imaging (%)	7.7%	84.4%	89.9%	68.2%	40.7%	21.0%	51.7%
Stress-only imaging (%)	3.1%	19.8%	32.4%	11.3%	5.1%	9.9%	11.9%
Effective dose							
Nonstress-only imaging (mSv)	12.0 ± 3.0	9.0 ± 2.5	12.8 ± 4.2	11.2 ± 2.6	12.4 ± 3.5	9.9 ± 3.0	11.0 ± 3.2
Stress-only imaging (mSv)	5.2 ± 3.0	3.9 ± 1.4	3.9 ± 2.4	3.7 ± 1.7	5.4 ± 1.9	2.3 ± 0.7	4.0 ± 1.9
Difference (mSv)	6.8	5.1	8.9	7.5	7.0	7.6	7.0
Percent decrease	56.7%	56.7%	69.5%	67.0%	56.5%	76.8%	63.6%

Abbreviation: ED, effective dose.
Modified from Mercuri M, Pascual TN, Mahmarian JJ, et al. Estimating the Reduction in the Radiation Burden From Nuclear Cardiology Through Use of Stress-Only Imaging in the United States and Worldwide. JAMA Intern Med. 2016;176(2):269-273.

In a multicenter study of 108,654 patients undergoing clinically indicated stress MPI studies, an overall increase in the prevalence of normal studies was seen from 1996 to 2012 in all patients (46.2% to 68.2%), patients without CAD (67.8% to 82%), and patients with CAD (25.3% to 39.2%).[6] A review of over 140,000 MPI studies between 2002 and 2014 showed a decrease in the frequency of ischemic MPI studies over the first 8 years, with a leveling off over the last 5 years.[7] The frequency of ischemic studies was somewhat higher than in the East Coast experience and substantially higher than in the West Coast experience.

With the increasing competition from other noninvasive tests for the diagnosis of CAD, it is imperative that more cost-effective and time-efficient strategies are developed for the initial evaluation of patients who are at low risk for abnormal findings during conventional rest-stress MPI studies, and stress-first protocols represent an attractive option. Stress-first protocols can be done in 1 day in nonobese patients using a low-dose stress dose followed by a high-dose rest dose if needed. In obese patients, stress-first protocols would use a high-dose stress dose on day 1 and a high-dose rest dose on day 2 if needed.

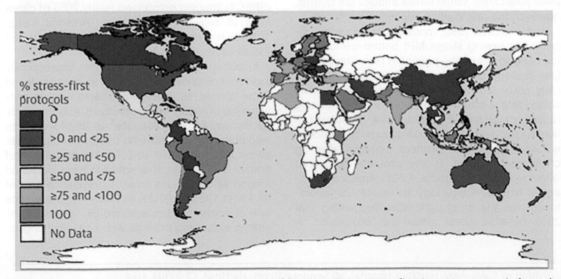

% stress-first protocols
- 0
- >0 and <25
- ≥25 and <50
- ≥50 and <75
- ≥75 and <100
- 100
- No Data

Fig. 1. The percentage of studies in each country world-wide utilizing stress-first imaging protocols from the 2022 INCAPS survey. (*From* Hirschfeld CB, Mercuri M, Pascual TNB, et al. Worldwide variation in the use of nuclear cardiology camera technology, reconstruction software, and imaging protocols. JACC Cardiovasc Imaging. 2021;14(9):1819-1828.)

Conventional SPECT cameras would use traditional doses and acquisition times, while newer high-efficiency cameras allow for faster acquisition and lower doses.

PROGNOSIS OF STRESS-ONLY STUDIES

The diagnostic accuracy of SPECT MPI for detecting flow-limiting CAD is well-established, such that patients are unlikely to undergo diagnostic angiography after a normal SPECT MPI result, and they have a benign 1-year prognosis.[8–10] This is a relevant issue for the clinician when interpreting stress-only SPECT MPI (ie, given a normal stress-only SPECT MPI, are the expected rates of cardiac events in the coming year similar to a full rest-stress MPI study?).

Since the initial publications comparing all-cause mortality and cardiac mortality between normal stress-only and rest-stress SPECT MPI studies,[11–13] several subsequent studies have continued to support a similar benign prognosis of normal stress-only studies. Gibson and colleagues initially reported on 729 patients with normal stress-only MPI with a mean follow-up of 22 months. There were 2 noncardiac deaths, no cardiac deaths, 1 nonfatal myocardial infarction (MI), and 3 episodes of unstable angina, resulting in an overall cardiac event rate of 0.6%.[11] Chang and colleagues[12] reported on 4.8 years of follow-up on 8034 patients who underwent stress-only SPECT imaging and 8820 patients who underwent both stress and rest imaging. Unadjusted and risk-adjusted all-cause mortality in the stress-only group was similar to that in the stress-rest and rest-stress groups (2.6% annualized mortality rate vs 2.9%). Duvall and colleagues[13] reported all-cause and cardiac mortality in a cohort of 4910 patients with a normal SPECT MPI study with a mean follow-up of 40 +/- 9 months. There

were 1673 patients with a normal stress-only study and 3237 with a normal rest-stress study. One-year cardiac mortality was 0.2% in the stress-only group and 0.1% in the rest-stress group, which was not significantly different after controlling for confounding variables.

A 2014 review cited 10 studies with a total of over 18,000 stress-only patients who all demonstrated annualized cardiac event rates less than 1% following a normal stress-only MPI.[14] The authors previously analyzed the pooled patient experience from the 4 studies including over 12,500 patients, directly comparing the prognosis of rest-stress and stress-only imaging.[12,13,15,16] This meta-analysis suggests the cardiac event rate is actually marginally lower following a normal stress-only MPI than following a normal rest-stress MPI, with a rate ratio of 1.2 (95% confidence interval [CI] 1.1–1.3, $P<.0001$) in favor of a normal stress-only study (Fig. 2). Low all-cause mortality and cardiac event rates following a normal stress-only MPI suggest that rest imaging may be omitted without any reduction in the prognostic value of the test.

ATTENUATION CORRECTION

Stress MPI studies have emerged as a mainstay for the diagnosis and prognosis of CAD; however, the presence of soft tissue attenuation often poses challenges for the correct interpretation of the images. With use of stress and rest electrocardiogram (ECG)-gated wall motion assessment,[17] position-dependent imaging,[18] and advancement in attenuation correction software and hardware technology,[19] the diagnostic accuracy of stress MPI studies has improved. Most importantly, attenuation correction (AC) software and hardware have been shown to decrease false positives and improve the prognostic ability of the results.[1] A

Meta Analysis of Studies Comparing Prognosis of Normal Stress-only to Normal Stress-Rest MPI

Rate ratio	Study name	Lower limit	Upper limit	Z-Value	p-Value	Rate ratio and 95% CI
1.139	Chang 2010	1.047	1.239	3.018	0.003	
1.337	Duvall 2010	0.951	1.879	1.673	0.094	
0.886	Ueyama 2012	0.512	1.534	-0.431	0.667	
2.431	Edenbrandt 2013	1.816	3.255	5.964	0.000	
1.206		1.116	1.304	4.708	0.000	

0.01   0.1   1   10   100

Rest-Stress Event Rate Lower   Stress-only Event Rate Lower

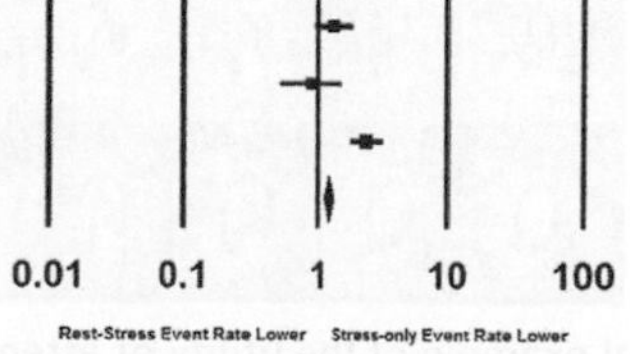

Fig. 2. Meta-analysis of studies investigating the prognosis of normal stress-only MPI studies. (*From* Hussain N, Parker MW, Henzlova MJ, Duvall WL. Stress-first Myocardial Perfusion Imaging. Cardiol Clin. 2016;34(1):59-67.)

meta-analysis of 17 studies on AC evaluating 1701 patients found that AC significantly increased the specificity for the detection of CAD compared with non-AC (80% vs 68%) and had a statistically higher diagnostic odds ratio (OR).[2] It is commonly held that the success of stress-first MPI protocols depends on AC to remove soft tissue artifacts as there are no rest images for comparison (**Fig. 3**). Current AC options include supine and prone imaging, scanning Gd-153 line sources, and CT.[20] However, AC technology comes at a significant cost and is not widely available as a result. The initial investment is substantial, and the annual maintenance costs continue to add to the expenditure. As a result, it has been reported that only 5% of installed SPECT systems have AC.[6] More recent data suggest that world-wide 26% of studies were acquired with AC and 7% with multiposition imaging, with identical percentages in North America.[4]

One of the major drawbacks of a stress-first MPI protocol is the need for some form of AC with its associated cost (Gd-153 line source or CT) or increased time of image acquisition (supine and prone images). ECG gating alone cannot substitute for actual AC, and has little added value for stress-first MPI studies as a given perfusion defect

with normal wall motion may still represent ischemia versus residual attenuation and thus a need for rest imaging. Heller and colleagues[21] assessed the impact of the use of ECG gating and AC on the perceived need for rest imaging and on the level of confidence of interpreting the results of stress-only MPI studies. Briefly, the application of ECG gating had little influence on the perceived need for rest imaging (77% without ECG gating vs 76% with) and on interpretation (37% vs 42%). However, the application of AC resulted in a statistically significant decrease in the perceived need for rest imaging (43% vs 77%, P-value <.005), and improved definitive interpretation (84% vs 37%, P-value <.005) without compromising the diagnostic accuracy of the test.

Another study demonstrated the clinical importance of AC, in which 58% of stress-only images were classified as abnormal without AC; however, after the application of AC, 83% of abnormal studies were reclassified as normal.[22] These US findings were mirrored in a first European study, where 49% of stress-first patients required rest images without AC, which decreased to 32% with AC,[23] and in another where the percentage of images interpreted as normal increased from

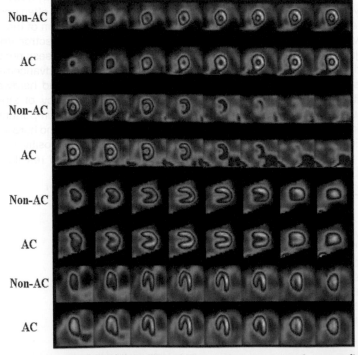
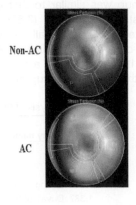

Fig. 3. Clinical example of the utility of attenuation correction for stress-first studies. A 57 year old male with an obvious inferior perfusion defect seen on the non-attenuation corrected stress images and polar plot. After the application of attenuation correction (Gd-153 scanning line source) the stress perfusion defect normalizes. AC, attenuation corrected.

45% without AC to 67% with the addition of AC.[24] Additional work has been done with newer high-sensitivity SPECT cameras and 2-position imaging for AC. In a small study of 152 patients, stress-only upright and supine high-efficiency SPECT were noninferior to attenuation corrected conventional SPECT with coronary angiography as the reference.[25] Another study found a similar benign prognosis with normal supine and prone stress-only and normal stress-rest imaging.[26]

PATIENT SELECTION

The determination of which patients are suitable candidates for stress-first MPI protocols is different laboratory to laboratory, with no universal standard. The first step in the appropriate selection of patients for any imaging protocol is of course to ensure that the study is appropriately indicated.[27,28] Once MPI is deemed appropriate, selecting patients for a stress-first protocol requires an initial evaluation of the patient's demographics, risk factors, and cardiac history. In general, patients with low-to-intermediate pretest probability for CAD (based on age, gender, risk factors, symptoms, and rest ECG) are suitable candidates for a stress-first or stress-only MPI protocol. Also suitable are patients with a high body mass index (BMI, >35 kg/m²) or weight over 250 lbs. Additionally, patients with recent negative (<3 years) noninvasive or invasive tests for the presence of obstructive CAD would seem to be suitable candidates.

An initial clinical scoring system was proposed to serve as a prediction model for determining which patients will undergo a successful stress-first Tc-99m MPI study and not require rest images in order to make selection of a stress-first protocol easier.[29] Clinical variables, most coronary risk factors, were individual assigned scores, and a higher tool score correlated with an unsuccessful stress-first MPI study. With use of this prediction model, patients were stratified into low-risk (−2 to <5), intermediate-risk (≥5 and <10), and high-risk (≥10) score groups. The low-risk cohort had a success rate of 92% for not requiring rest images, while the intermediate- and high-risk cohorts had 27% and 65% of patients requiring rest images, respectively.

In order to improve on this relatively unwieldy score and simplify the triage of patients to a stress-first protocol, this model was tested again in a new population and compared with using CAD status alone as the determination of imaging protocol.[30] A history of CAD was defined as a previous myocardial infarction, a history of percutaneous coronary intervention, or previous coronary artery bypass grafting. Simply assigning

all patients with no history of CAD to a stress-first protocol resulted in an 88% success rate for not needing subsequent rest images. Fifty-four percent of patients with known CAD did not require rest images.

Other investigators have attempted to design a simplified clinical tool to identify candidates for stress-first protocols.[31] Using a large derivation cohort of over 18,000 patients, Rouhani and colleagues assigned point values to age, clinical risk factors, and history of CAD to produce a variation on previous scores. As suggested by the accompanying editorial, the relatively cumbersome clinical tool could be simplified by removing measures of previous CAD such as known myocardial infarction or revascularization, and focus on the non-CAD clinical factors alone of age, gender, typical angina, smoking, hypertension, high cholesterol, and diabetes.[32] A simplified approach with a reasonable success rate based on lessons learned from all 3 clinical scores may then be to triage all patients without known CAD to a stress-first MPI protocol while patients with known CAD undergo a standard rest-stress protocol. This approach would be the most simplistic and practical to implement but would have the shortcoming that some patients with too many of the clinical variables used in the scoring tools would have a lower chance of a successful stress-first protocol (**Table 2**).

Table 2
Clinical and demographic variables with associated previously defined scores[29,31]

Variable	Weighting
Emergency department location	-
Age	++
Male gender	++
Diabetes mellitus	+
Hyperlipidemia	+
Hypertension	+
Current smoking	+
Congestive heart failure	++
Documented CAD	+++
History of myocardial infarction	+++
History of percutaneous coronary intervention	+++
History of coronary artery bypass graft	+++
Typical chest pain	+
Abnormal resting ECG	++

A thought-provoking quality improvement project undertaken at a Veterans Administration (VA) hospital in Gainesville Florida took the approach of starting a stress-first protocol at the institution by simply making all studies stress-first 31206046.[33] Four hundred twenty-four consecutive patients studied before the stress-first transition were compared with 716 consecutive patients receiving a stress-first protocol. Demographic characteristics on this population are lacking, but the VA patient population is not always comparable to community hospitals or practices. Of the stress-first patients, 59.1% became stress-only, and 40.9% were performed as stress-rest. This resulted in a substantial reduction in effective dose to the patient, with a median stress-only dose of 2.8 mSv compared with 14.1 mSv in the rest-stress group. Although no outcomes data were presented for these patients, the rate of normal studies was not different between cohorts (73.5% for the stress-first and 71.7% for the rest-stress cohort).

RADIATION REDUCTION

By using up-to-date software, modern camera technology, and stress-first imaging protocols, it has become possible to substantially reduce the effective dose delivered to patients in a high percentage of scenarios.[34] Stress-first imaging alone results in substantial reductions in radiation exposure to patients and laboratory staff when stress images are normal and no rest images are performed. In the INCAPS survey, the mean effective dose decreased 63.6% when a stress-only protocol was used.[3] The total effective dose for the patient will depend on if a conventional SPECT or a high-efficiency SPECT camera is used.

The 2016 American Society of Nuclear Cardiology (ASNC) guidelines[35] recommend for a 1-day rest-stress protocol on a conventional camera, a 8 to 12 mCi rest dose followed by a 24 to 36 mCi stress dose of Tc-99m, resulting in total effective dose of 8.4 to 12.6 mSv. For a larger patient, administering a high dose (18–30 mCi Tc-99m) at stress and canceling the rest scan decreases the total effective dose to 4.5 to 7.6 mSv, a 40% to 46% reduction in exposure. If the stress-first image is performed with the lower (8–12 mCi) dose, the effective dose is only 2.0 to 3.0 mSv, 76% less than the standard rest-stress protocol. Further dose reduction can be achieved with high-efficiency SPECT cameras (**Fig. 4**).[36,37] High-dose stress-only protocols of 9 to 15 mCi with a high-efficiency camera result in an effective dose of 2.3 to 3.8 mSv, a 70% to 73% reduction compared with a conventional 1-day rest-stress

study, and the low-dose (4–6 mCi) stress-first approach produces 1 to 1.5 mSv, a 88% reduction.

This reduced effective dose to patients is especially important in younger patients and women when it comes to the lifetime risk of developing cancer.[38] Although stress-first positron emission tomography (PET) imaging is feasible,[39] the short half-life and imaging time of Rb-82 make it a relatively impractical protocol. The longer half-life of N-13, and especially future F-18 labeled tracers such as flurpiridaz, would lend themselves better to a stress-first approach.[40]

In 2010, an ASNC Information Statement on recommendations for reducing radiation exposure suggested that by 2014 on average a total radiation exposure of no more than 9 mSv could be achieved in 50% of MPI studies.[41] Converting a laboratory to a stress-first approach, and the resultant stress-only studies can result in substantial progress toward meeting this ASNC goal. The INCAPS survey simulated various scenarios for reduction in effective dose in the United States based on adoption of different patterns of utilization of stress-only imaging.[3] If the United States utilized stress-only imaging at the same rate as Europe, there would be a projected 9.0% population reduction in radiation dose, while adopting practices similar to the top 10% of INCAPS laboratories estimates a 20.9% reduction in the mean effective dose from MPI. The best-case scenario would be performing stress-only in all normal cases, which would result in a 34.9% population reduction in radiation dose.

The radiation reduction seen with stress-first protocols has been demonstrated in practice, although often combined with other dose-reduction techniques such as high-efficiency SPECT. In a single health system study of almost 56,000 patients, the use of stress-only protocols resulted in reductions in effective dose of 6 to 11.5 mSv depending on the SPECT camera used (11.5 mSv reduction for stress-only on a high-efficiency camera, 10.1 mSv reduction for stress-only on a conventional camera with ½ time – ½ dose software, 6 mSv for stress-only on a conventional camera), and resulted in an impressively low mean effective dose of 1.9 +/- 1.8 mSv when stress-only protocols were performed with a high-efficiency SPECT camera.[42] The effects of the introduction of a stress-first protocol and high-efficiency SPECT technology were investigated in a single hospital in over 7000 patients and when the pre- and post-periods were compared, the mean Tc-99m administered activity per patient decreased from 36.5 to 23.8 mCi (34.7% reduction).[43] It was estimated that camera

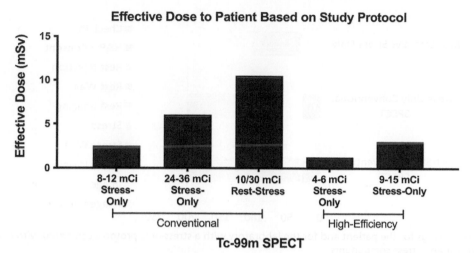

Fig. 4. Effective dose (mSv) to the patient based on imaging modality (conventional SPECT or high-efficiency SPECT) and study protocol (rest-stress or stress-only).[35]

technology was responsible for 39% of the reduction and stress-only protocols for 61%. Interestingly the benefit of radiation exposure reduction was also realized by laboratory staff. In this study, there was approximately a 40% reduction in radiation exposure to laboratory nurses and technologists based on badge dosimetry.[43] A year-long French experience with a stress-first protocol utilizing a high-efficiency camera in 2845 patients found that 37% of the overall population underwent a stress-only protocol, and 33% of patients had an abnormal perfusion study.[44] The mean effective dose was 3.5 +/- 2.1 mSv overall, and in a low-probability subgroup, 71% of patients finished with a stress-only study with a mean effective dose of 2.0 +/- 1.5 mSv.

TIME SAVINGS

A stress-first protocol that becomes a stress-only protocol also results in time savings for the patient and for the laboratory. The authors calculated the time it took to complete an SPECT MPI study from the time a patient checks into the laboratory at the reception desk to the time the study is interpreted based on guideline-specified waiting times, measured preparation and performance times in their laboratory, average exercise stress times, and standard imaging times with a conventional Na-I SPECT camera.[45] They found that a standard rest-stress SPECT MPI study took 203 minutes to perform, while a stress-only study took 126 minutes, resulting in a time savings of 77 minutes or a 38% time reduction compared with the standard protocol (**Fig. 5**). This time savings is immediately beneficial to the patient who has other shorter diagnostic modalities such as cardiac

CTA and stress echocardiography to choose from. It is also beneficial to the laboratory, potentially allowing the performance of additional MPI studies in the same workday, or allowing for a shorter workday, which may limit overtime expenditures.

Although a stress-first protocol has the potential to save time if rest images are not needed, concern has been raised regarding the risk of shine-through with low-dose stress images followed by high-dose rest images resulting in an underestimation of defect reversibility. This possible scenario involves stress-induced ischemia where the stress images are abnormal and the rest images are normal, but the rest/stress count density is not sufficiently great to minimize the contribution (shine-through) of the underlying stress defect.[46] Controversy remains as to whether the shine through phenomenon is clinically significant[46] or merely theoretic.[47] Current practice varies from as low as a 1:2 ratio between the low and high doses to as high as a 1:4 ratio. Also, the minimum recommended time to rest imaging after the stress dose varies considerably from a few minutes to several hours. A small study by Sharir and colleagues[37] looked at this issue of low-dose stress followed by high-dose rest using a high-efficiency SPECT camera. They found a 1-day low-dose 5 mCi/15 mCi stress-first protocol provided high diagnostic value compared with standard-dose 10 mCi/30 mCi stress-first protocol, and while not definitively answering the question, demonstrated that low-dose stress-first is a reasonable approach. More studies and modeling are needed to clarify and codify these issues with modern SPECT cameras and software.

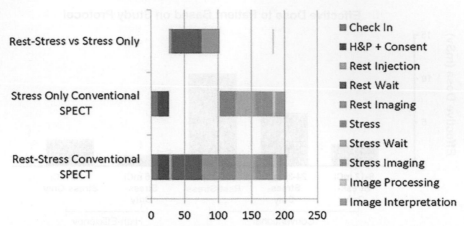

Fig. 5. Time savings for the patient and for the laboratory with a stress-only protocol compared with a full study including rest and stress components.

PROTOCOL MODIFICATIONS – BEYOND STRESS-FIRST

A protocol that uses a provisional dose of radiotracer and perfusion imaging in patients undergoing exercise stress-only when needed is an extension of the logic behind stress-first imaging that would further shorten test duration, decrease radiation exposure, and reduce health care costs. In this protocol, the patient would not have the isotope administered if at least 10 metabolic equivalent risk (MET) of exercise were achieved without symptoms or ECG changes. The cutoff of 10 MET was chosen based on work by Bourque and colleagues,[48] who demonstrated that low-to-intermediate risk patients achieving at least 10 MET with no ischemic ST segment depression have an annual mortality of only 0.1% and myocardial infarction rate of 0.4%. The most obvious application of a provisional protocol in routine clinical practice would be to downgrade negative high-level exercise MPI studies to an ETT, thereby avoiding unnecessary injections of isotope and saving time and resources. Another use would be to facilitate the efficient diagnosis of patients and encourage adherence to the current guidelines, encouraging the use of ETT.[27,28] In this case, by upgrading the study by adding imaging to an ETT when abnormal, a patient's evaluation can be efficiently completed in a single session as opposed to having the patient return for another stress and imaging session. This approach is similar to that employed in the What is the Optimal Method for Ischemia Evaluation in Women (WOMEN) trial, only more efficient.[49] A retrospective assessment of this protocol in over 5000 patients has found that few of these patients (5.9%) had abnormal perfusion images, and all had a benign prognosis at 5 years (1.1% all-cause

mortality).[50] A prospective evaluation of this protocol in almost 1000 patients referred for stress testing as part of their evaluation, showed that provisional injection of radioisotope saved time, reduced radiation exposure and health care costs as compared to standard imaging protocols, and conferred a low mortality, and fewer follow-up diagnostic tests.[51]

Other adjustments to the stress-first protocol have been proposed, including results of coronary artery calcium (CAC) scoring when interpreting stress images.[52] In a retrospective, hypothesis-generating study of 162 patients, Uretsky and colleagues had 2 readers interpret the stress images of a conventional rest-stress study without, and then with the results of the CAC score to determine the need for hypothetical rest images. They found that 72% of the patients felt to have probably normal stress perfusion did not need rest images, and 47% of the equivocal stress images did not need additional imaging when they had access to the CAC score. Because attenuation correction was not employed in this study, it is unclear how the use of attenuation correction would interact with the benefit of having a CAC score.

NEED TO REVIEW STRESS IMAGES

For the successful implementation of a stress-first MPI protocol, an experienced reader must be available to timely interpret the stress images and determine the need for rest images. In routine clinical practice, most cardiologists who interpret MPI studies have other concurrent clinical responsibilities, and the daily interpretation of studies is grouped together when all studies are completed for efficiency. These staffing and timing issues represent a major hurdle in the implementation of stress-first MPI protocols.

One solution would be remote or off-site reading options to review images on other computers or tablets. Current software by the major nuclear cardiology vendors all allow for fully functional image review away from the camera or stress laboratory. The use of laptop computers, tablets, or even smart phones to do this is now commonplace. The ability for the interpreting physician to quickly and conveniently review stress images while performing other clinical duties would allow for the use of stress-first protocols.

Another option to overcome the need for immediate stress image review is to take advantage of experienced nuclear technologists who are always available in the laboratory to review images. The ability of nuclear technologists and automated computer quantification to determine the need for rest images was compared with the physician gold standard in a multicenter study of 250 consecutive attenuation corrected stress-first studies.[53] Overall, 83.2% of patients (based on the gold standard) did not need any rest images, and nuclear technologists were able to correctly classify 91.6% of all patients. Using a cut off TPD score of at least 1.2%, cut off based on receiver operating characteristic (ROC) curve analysis, computer quantification classified 71.6% of patients correctly compared with gold standard. In a model whereby the computer or technologist could correct for the other's incorrect classification, 242 (96.8%) of the stress-first images were correctly classified. Several other studies at the same center have retrospectively assessed nuclear technologist's ability to determine the need for rest images and concluded that they are similar in ability to the physician gold standard.[54,55]

Finally, as artificial intelligence and machine learning progress in sophistication, initial interpretation using computer algorithms may soon be sufficient for most stress-first cases. In an initial study utilizing over 20,000 high-efficiency SPECT studies with patient clinical data and follow-up for major adverse cardiac events, researchers were able to demonstrate that machine learning algorithms could be used to cancel the rest images after reviewing the stress images and clinical data while preserving prognostic safety.[56] In another study of over 37,000 patients, a deep learning method outperformed a conventional quantitative software package with significantly higher area under the curve (AUC) interpreting stress-only SPECT (the majority performed on a conventional SPECT camera) using the final clinical diagnosis as the gold standard.[57] A recent study applied a machine learning algorithm to the stress-only images of 2079 patients undergoing high-efficiency SPECT, which had higher AUC and sensitivity than clinical reader interpretation or conventional automated total perfusion defect assessment for the prediction of obstructive CAD or high-risk CAD.[58]

FINANCIAL DISINCENTIVES

One significant deterrent to adopting a stress-first work flow has been the financial disincentive that can occur, specifically in an outpatient private practice setting. As separate CPT billing codes exist for SPECT MPI, single (78451) and SPECT MPI, multiple (78452) variable reimbursement is possible if the stress-first study becomes stress-only as opposed to a full stress-rest study. When using the Hospital Outpatient Prospective Payment (HOPPS) Medicare provides the same reimbursement for 1 or 2 sets of images. However, using global outpatient rates based on the 2022 Medicare Physician Fee Schedule (MPFS), there is a $131 or 28.2% reduction in reimbursement, when a single set of images is obtained versus 2 sets. With reimbursement already having been substantially reduced for MPI procedures over the past decade, many physicians are unable to contemplate a change in their practice that would result in further reimbursement reductions despite the advantages to the patients. Although stress-only imaging may free up staff and camera time to allow for performance of more tests in a given time period, this is difficult to realize on an outpatient basis given the complexities of scheduling these patients.

Further financial pressures comes into the picture when one considers the issue of unused rest doses (high dose for a same day study) that may have been prepared in advance. If these doses cannot be used on a subsequent patient, whether unit-doses from a radiopharmacy or doses made from an on-site generator, the cost of the dose will not be associated with a study for reimbursement. These pressures may be particularly felt by outpatient, lower-volume laboratories using unit doses that have less bargaining power with their radiopharmacy or less of an opportunity to use the doses on subsequent patients.

OTHER ISSUES

The definition of a normal stress MPI result that does not require rest imaging is somewhat up for debate. Most would agree that stress-only images require visually uniform radiotracer uptake, and often there is a less strict definition when attenuation correction is not available compared with attenuation correction.

Normal left ventricular size and function after stress have been an optional requirement of a normal stress-only study. Without rest imaging or other previous diagnostic imaging, one cannot definitively say that the ventricular dilatation is not secondary to transient ischemic dilatation. The same can be said for left ventricular dysfunction that may be ischemic in origin, although this would be less likely with normal perfusion. Lastly, the need for a negative ECG response to stress, or even lack of potential anginal symptoms during stress may also be considered necessary for a normal stress-only study. Although a post-hoc analysis by Chang and colleagues[12] suggested that prognosis was similar for patients with low and intermediate risk Duke treadmill scores in that cohort, and Edenbrandt and colleagues[16] did not find any differences in prognosis when left ventricular ejection fraction (LVEF) and ventricular volumes were abnormal in patients with normal perfusion findings; further work on a standard definition of a normal stress-only study is needed.

When stress images are not normal, rest imaging is generally recommended so that areas of abnormal stress perfusion can then be compared with the resting perfusion pattern to ascertain reversibility (ischemia) or persistence (attenuation artifact or infarction). If attenuation correction is utilized, the former becomes unlikely, and in patients with normal resting ECG and no personal history of infarction, the latter should also be rare. Therefore, patients with ischemic symptoms and electrocardiographic changes in combination with a significant perfusion defect at stress may benefit from proceeding directly to invasive coronary angiography and intervention without rest imaging.[14] Electrocardiographic evidence of ischemia and normal wall motion on the gated stress images may be important corroborating evidence of ischemia as opposed to artifact or infarction in such cases.

One final scenario is that of futile rest images. Abnormal stress images caused by left bundle branch block artifact represent a scenario where rest images are unlikely to clarify the diagnosis of CAD. A fixed defect may indicate a scar or left bundle branch block artifact, and a reversible defect may represent ischemia or left bundle branch block artifact. The rest images are unable to completely clarify the differential options, and are thus futile, still requiring other diagnostic testing. A similar difficulty in determining if the origin of a perfusion defect is from obstructive coronary disease or nonobstructive causes can be seen in patients with hypertrophic cardiomyopathy (supply-demand mismatch or fibrosis) and in pulmonary hypertension or significant right ventricular dysfunction (septal perfusion defects) and make rest images less helpful after abnormal stress images.

SUMMARY

Stress-first approaches to MPI provide diagnostically and prognostically accurate perfusion data equivalent to a full rest-stress study while saving time in the imaging laboratory and reducing the radiation exposure to patients and laboratory staff. Unfortunately, implementing a stress-first approach in a nuclear cardiology laboratory involves significant challenges such as the need for attenuation correction, triage of patients to an appropriate protocol, real-time review of stress images, and consideration of differential reimbursement. Despite it being best practice for both the patient and the laboratory, these impediments have kept the proportions of studies performed stress-first relatively unchanged in North America and world-wide in the last 10 years.

DISCLOSURE

The authors have nothing to disclose in relation to this article.

CLINICS CARE POINTS

- Normal stress-only and rest-stress SPECT MPI have the same benign prognosis as measured by low all-cause and cardiac mortality.

- Stress-first SPECT MPI protocols reduce the radiation exposure to patients and staff during testing.

- Stress-first SPECT MPI protocols save time in the imaging laboratory by providing a shorter test.

- Implementing a stress-first protocol involves significant challenges such as the need for attenuation correction, triage of patients to an appropriate protocol, real-time review of stress images, and consideration of differential reimbursement.

REFERENCES

1. Worsley DF, Fung AY, Coupland DB, et al. Comparison of stress-only vs. stress/rest with technetium-99m methoxyisobutylisonitrile myocardial perfusion imaging. Eur J Nucl Med 1992;19:441–4.

2. Einstein AJ, Tilkemeier P, Fazel R, et al, American Society of Nuclear C. Radiation safety in nuclear cardiology-current knowledge and practice: results from the 2011 American Society of Nuclear Cardiology member survey. JAMA Intern Med 2013;173: 1021–3.

3. Mercuri M, Pascual TN, Mahmarian JJ, et al. Estimating the reduction in the radiation burden from nuclear cardiology through use of stress-only imaging in the United States and worldwide. JAMA Intern Med 2016;176:269–73.

4. Hirschfeld CB, Mercuri M, Pascual TNB, et al. Worldwide variation in the use of nuclear cardiology camera technology, reconstruction software, and imaging protocols. JACC Cardiovasc Imaging 2021;14:1819–28.

5. Rozanski A, Gransar H, Hayes SW, et al. Temporal trends in the frequency of inducible myocardial ischemia during cardiac stress testing: 1991 to 2009. J Am Coll Cardiol 2013;61:1054–65.

6. Duvall WL, Rai M, Ahlberg AW, et al. A multi-center assessment of the temporal trends in myocardial perfusion imaging. J Nucl Cardiol 2015;22(3): 539–51.

7. Thompson RC, Allam AH. More risk factors, less ischemia, and the relevance of MPI testing. J Nucl Cardiol 2015;22:552–4.

8. Fleischmann KE, Hunink MG, Kuntz KM, et al. Exercise echocardiography or exercise SPECT imaging? A meta-analysis of diagnostic test performance. JAMA 1998;280:913–20.

9. Kim C, Kwok YS, Heagerty P, et al. Pharmacologic stress testing for coronary disease diagnosis: a meta-analysis. Am Heart J 2001;142:934–44.

10. Klocke FJ, Baird MG, Lorell BH, et al. ACC/AHA/ ASNC guidelines for the clinical use of cardiac radionuclide imaging–executive summary: a report of the American College of Cardiology/American Heart Association task force on practice guidelines (ACC/AHA/ASNC committee to revise the 1995 guidelines for the clinical use of cardiac radionuclide imaging). J Am Coll Cardiol 2003;42:1318–33.

11. Gibson PB, Demus D, Noto R, et al. Low event rate for stress-only perfusion imaging in patients evaluated for chest pain. J Am Coll Cardiol 2002;39: 999–1004.

12. Chang SM, Nabi F, Xu J, et al. Normal stress-only versus standard stress/rest myocardial perfusion imaging: similar patient mortality with reduced radiation exposure. J Am Coll Cardiol 2010;55:221–30.

13. Duvall WL, Wijetunga MN, Klein TM, et al. The prognosis of a normal stress-only Tc-99m myocardial perfusion imaging study. J Nucl Cardiol 2010;17: 370–7.

14. Gowd BM, Heller GV, Parker MW. Stress-only SPECT myocardial perfusion imaging: a review. J Nucl Cardiol 2014;21:1200–12.

15. Ueyama T, Takehana K, Maeba H, et al. Prognostic value of normal stress-only technetium-99m myocardial perfusion imaging protocol. Comparison with standard stress-rest protocol. Circ J 2012;76: 2386–91.

16. Edenbrandt L, Ohlsson M, Tragardh E. Prognosis of patients without perfusion defects with and without rest study in myocardial perfusion scintigraphy. EJNMMI Res 2013;3:58.

17. Taillefer R, DePuey EG, Udelson JE, et al. Comparative diagnostic accuracy of Tl-201 and Tc-99m sestamibi SPECT imaging (perfusion and ECG-gated SPECT) in detecting coronary artery disease in women. J Am Coll Cardiol 1997;29:69–77.

18. Berman DS, Kang X, Nishina H, et al. Diagnostic accuracy of gated Tc-99m sestamibi stress myocardial perfusion SPECT with combined supine and prone acquisitions to detect coronary artery disease in obese and nonobese patients. J Nucl Cardiol 2006;13:191–201.

19. Kluge R, Sattler B, Seese A, et al. Attenuation correction by simultaneous emission-transmission myocardial single-photon emission tomography using a technetium-99m-labelled radiotracer: impact on diagnostic accuracy. Eur J Nucl Med 1997;24: 1107–14.

20. Bateman TM, Cullom SJ. Attenuation correction single-photon emission computed tomography myocardial perfusion imaging. Semin Nucl Med 2005;35:37–51.

21. Heller GV, Bateman TM, Johnson LL, et al. Clinical value of attenuation correction in stress-only Tc-99m sestamibi SPECT imaging. J Nucl Cardiol 2004;11:273–81.

22. Mathur S, Heller GV, Bateman TM, et al. Clinical value of stress-only Tc-99m SPECT imaging: importance of attenuation correction. J Nucl Cardiol 2013;20:27–37.

23. Tragardh E, Valind S, Edenbrandt L. Adding attenuation corrected images in myocardial perfusion imaging reduces the need for a rest study. BMC Med Imaging 2013;13:14.

24. van Dijk JD, Mouden M, Ottervanger JP, et al. Value of attenuation correction in stress-only myocardial perfusion imaging using CZT-SPECT. J Nucl Cardiol 2017;24:395–401.

25. Jameria ZA, Abdallah M, Fernandez-Ulloa M, et al. Analysis of stress-only imaging, comparing upright and supine CZT camera acquisition to conventional gamma camera images with and without attenuation correction, with coronary angiography as a reference. J Nucl Cardiol 2018;25:540–9.

26. Gutstein A, Bental T, Solodky A, et al. Prognosis of stress-only SPECT myocardial perfusion imaging with prone imaging. J Nucl Cardiol 2018;25:809–16.

27. Hendel RC, Berman DS, Di Carli MF, et al. ACCF/ ASNC/ACR/AHA/ASE/SCCT/SCMR/SNM   2009

appropriate use criteria for cardiac radionuclide imaging: a report of the American College of Cardiology Foundation Appropriate Use Criteria Task Force, the American Society of Nuclear Cardiology, the American College of Radiology, the American Heart Association, the American Society of Echocardiography, the Society of Cardiovascular Computed Tomography, the Society for Cardiovascular Magnetic Resonance, and the Society of Nuclear Medicine. J Am Coll Cardiol 2009;53:2201–29.

28. Wolk MJ, Bailey SR, Doherty JU, et al. ACCF/AHA/ ASE/ASNC/HFSA/HRS/SCAI/SCCT/SCMR/STS 2013 multimodality appropriate use criteria for the detection and risk assessment of stable ischemic heart disease: a report of the American College of Cardiology Foundation Appropriate Use Criteria Task Force, American Heart Association, American Society of Echocardiography, American Society of Nuclear Cardiology, Heart Failure Society of America, Heart Rhythm Society, Society for Cardiovascular Angiography and Interventions, Society of Cardiovascular Computed Tomography, Society for Cardiovascular Magnetic Resonance, and Society of Thoracic Surgeons. J Am Coll Cardiol 2014;63: 380–406.

29. Duvall WL, Baber U, Levine EJ, et al. A model for the prediction of a successful stress-first Tc-99m SPECT MPI. J Nucl Cardiol 2012;19:1124–34.

30. Chaudhry W, Ahlberg AW, Mujtaba M, et al. Prediction of successful stress-first SPECT MPI using a clinical pre-rest scoring model. J Nucl Cardiol 2014;21:778.

31. Rouhani S, Al Shahrani A, Hossain A, et al. A clinical tool to identify candidates for stress-first myocardial perfusion imaging. JACC Cardiovasc Imaging 2020; 13:2193–202.

32. Hendel RC, Crawford MJ. Stress-only SPECT myocardial perfusion imaging for all? JACC Cardiovasc Imaging 2020;13:2203–5.

33. Winchester D, Jeffrey R, Wymer D, et al. Simplified approach to stress-first nuclear myocardial perfusion imaging: implementation of Choosing Wisely recommendations. BMJ Open Qual 2019;8(2): e000352.

34. Lecchi M, Malaspina S, Scabbio C, et al. Myocardial perfusion scintigraphy dosimetry: optimal use of SPECT and SPECT/CT technologies in stress-first imaging protocol. Clin Transl Imaging 2016;4:491–8.

35. Henzlova MJ, Duvall WL, Einstein AJ, et al. ASNC imaging guidelines for SPECT nuclear cardiology procedures: stress, protocols, and tracers. J Nucl Cardiol 2016;23:606–39.

36. Duvall WL, Croft LB, Ginsberg ES, et al. Reduced isotope dose and imaging time with a high-efficiency CZT SPECT camera. J Nucl Cardiol 2011;18:847–57.

37. Sharir T, Pinsky M, Pardes A, et al. Comparison of the diagnostic accuracies of very low stress-dose with standard-dose myocardial perfusion imaging: automated quantification of one-day, stress-first SPECT using a CZT camera. J Nucl Cardiol 2016; 23(1):11–20.

38. Berrington de Gonzalez A, Kim KP, Smith-Bindman R, et al. Myocardial perfusion scans: projected population cancer risks from current levels of use in the United States. Circulation 2010;122:2403–10.

39. McMahon SR, Kikut J, Pinckney RG, et al. Feasibility of stress only rubidium-82 PET myocardial perfusion imaging. J Nucl Cardiol 2013;20:1069–75.

40. Maddahi J, Lazewatsky J, Udelson JE, et al. Phase-III clinical trial of fluorine-18 flurpiridaz positron emission tomography for evaluation of coronary artery disease. J Am Coll Cardiol 2020;76:391–401.

41. Cerqueira MD, Allman KC, Ficaro EP, et al. Recommendations for reducing radiation exposure in myocardial perfusion imaging. J Nucl Cardiol 2010;17:709–18.

42. Al Badarin FJ, Spertus JA, Bateman TM, et al. Drivers of radiation dose reduction with myocardial perfusion imaging: a large health system experience. J Nucl Cardiol 2020;27:785–94.

43. Duvall WL, Guma KA, Kamen J, et al. Reduction in occupational and patient radiation exposure from myocardial perfusion imaging: impact of stress-only imaging and high-efficiency SPECT camera technology. J Nucl Med 2013;54:1251–7.

44. Perrin M, Djaballah W, Moulin F, et al. Stress-first protocol for myocardial perfusion SPECT imaging with semiconductor cameras: high diagnostic performances with significant reduction in patient radiation doses. Eur J Nucl Med Mol Imaging 2015;42: 1004–11.

45. Duvall WL, Naib T, Greco G, et al. Cost savings associated with the use of selective stress-only and CZT SPECT myocardial perfusion imaging. J Nucl Cardiol 2013;20:S57.

46. DePuey EG, Ata P, Wray R, et al. Very low-activity stress/high-activity rest, single-day myocardial perfusion SPECT with a conventional sodium iodide camera and wide beam reconstruction processing. J Nucl Cardiol 2012;19:931–44.

47. Herzog BA, Buechel RR, Katz R, et al. Nuclear myocardial perfusion imaging with a cadmium-zinc-telluride detector technique: optimized protocol for scan time reduction. J Nucl Med 2010;51:46–51.

48. Bourque JM, Charlton GT, Holland BH, et al. Prognosis in patients achieving >/=10 METS on exercise stress testing: was SPECT imaging useful? J Nucl Cardiol 2011;18:230–7.

49. Shaw LJ, Mieres JH, Hendel RH, et al. Comparative effectiveness of exercise electrocardiography with or without myocardial perfusion single photon emission computed tomography in women with

suspected coronary artery disease: results from the what is the Optimal Method for Ischemia Evaluation in Women (WOMEN) trial. Circulation 2011;124: 1239–49.

50. Duvall WL, Levine EJ, Moonthungal S, et al. A hypothetical protocol for the provisional use of perfusion imaging with exercise stress testing. J Nucl Cardiol 2013;20:739–47.

51. Duvall WL, Savino JA, Levine EJ, et al. Prospective evaluation of a new protocol for the provisional use of perfusion imaging with exercise stress testing. Eur J Nucl Med Mol Imaging 2015;42:305–16.

52. Uretsky S, Cohen R, Argulian E, et al. Combining stress-only myocardial perfusion imaging with coronary calcium scanning as a new paradigm for initial patient work-up: an exploratory analysis. J Nucl Cardiol 2015;22:89–97.

53. Chaudhry W, Ahlberg AW, Duvall WL. The ability of nuclear technologist to determine the need for rest imaging in a stress-first MPI protocol. J Nucl Cardiol 2014;21:772–3.

54. Johansson L, Lomsky M, Gjertsson P, et al. Can nuclear medicine technologists assess whether a myocardial perfusion rest study is required? J Nucl Med Technol 2008;36:181–5.

55. Tragardh E, Johansson L, Olofsson C, et al. Nuclear medicine technologists are able to accurately determine when a myocardial perfusion rest study is necessary. BMC Med Inform Decis Mak 2012;12:97.

56. Hu LH, Miller RJH, Sharir T, et al. Prognostically safe stress-only single-photon emission computed tomography myocardial perfusion imaging guided by machine learning: report from REFINE SPECT. Eur Heart J Cardiovasc Imaging 2021;22:705–14.

57. Liu H, Wu J, Miller EJ, et al. Diagnostic accuracy of stress-only myocardial perfusion SPECT improved by deep learning. Eur J Nucl Med Mol Imaging 2021;48:2793–800.

58. Eisenberg E, Miller RJH, Hu LH, et al. Diagnostic safety of a machine learning-based automatic patient selection algorithm for stress-only myocardial perfusion SPECT. J Nucl Cardiol 2022;29(5): 2295–307.

Obtaining a Coronary Artery Calcium Score with Myocardial Perfusion Imaging

Merrill Thomas, MD, MSc[a,b], Randall C. Thompson, MD[a,b],*

KEYWORDS

- Coronary artery calcium score • Myocardial perfusion imaging
- Single-photon emission computed tomography • PET

KEY POINTS

- A coronary artery calcium score can be diagnostic for coronary artery disease even in the presence of a normal myocardial perfusion imaging study.
- Irrespective of perfusion defects on myocardial perfusion imaging, coronary artery calcium scores have been shown to be prognostic for major adverse cardiovascular events.
- Clinicians alter medical management for coronary artery disease based on the coronary calcium scores.

INTRODUCTION

The most common indication for obtaining a myocardial perfusion imaging (MPI) study is chest pain concerning for coronary artery disease (CAD). MPI studies can detect flow-limiting CAD aiding in the diagnosis of myocardial ischemia or infarction; however, these tests are limited in their ability to diagnose nonobstructive CAD. The presence of CAD, whether obstructive or not, has important prognostic and management implications. The presence of coronary artery calcium (CAC) on gated chest computed tomography (CT) scans is diagnostic of coronary atherosclerosis and the extent of calcification roughly corresponds to the extent of coronary atherosclerosis and carries important prognostic value.[1,2] CT scanners are widely available and currently many nuclear cardiology laboratories have access to CAC scoring, or at least non-gated chest CT scans, through single-photon emission computed tomography (SPECT)-CT or PET-CT hybrid instrumentation or from nearby stand-alone CT scanners. Obtaining a concomitant CACscore at the time of MPI provides additional information on CAD not obtained by MPI alone.

DISCUSSION

Diagnosing Coronary Artery Disease

Although MPI has long been used as a valuable test in the detection and management of patients with CAD, one limitation is the inability to detect nonobstructive CAD. This has been shown in several studies in which patients with normal perfusion images have been found to have evidence of CAD. For example, following a normal SPECT MPI, Berman and colleagues[3] found 56% of patients had a CAC score ≥100 and only 22% of patients with a normal SPECT had no evidence of CAC. Similarly, Thompson and colleagues[4] identified 17.5% of patients with normal MPI as having CAD based on a CAC score ≥ 100, and in a study by Engbers and colleagues[5], of 3702 patients with normal SPECT, 69% had a CAC score greater than 0 with 15% having a CAC score ≥400, and 6% having a CAC score ≥1000.

Although MPI with PET is of higher spatial resolution and higher diagnostic accuracy than SPECT, even with PET MPI there can be extensive coronary calcifications that do not result in flow-limiting CAD.[6] For example, in a study by Bybee and colleagues[7], of 760 patients without known

[a] University of Missouri-Kansas City School of Medicine; [b] Saint Luke's Mid America Heart Institute, 4401 Wornall Road, Kansas City, MO 64111, USA

* Corresponding author. Saint Luke's Mid America Heart Institute, 4401 Wornall Road, Kansas City, MO 64111.
E-mail address: rthompson@saint-lukes.org

Cardiol Clin 41 (2023) 177–184
https://doi.org/10.1016/j.ccl.2023.01.006
0733-8651/23/© 2023 Elsevier Inc. All rights reserved.

CAD who were referred for PET MPI for suspected CAD and had normal myocardial perfusion, 64% were found to have coronary calcification with 30% having a CAC score ≥ 100. Thus, although a normal SPECT or PET MPI has traditionally been considered a marker of good short-term prognosis, clearly some patients with normal perfusion images have important preclinical CAD that warrants medical therapy and closer follow-up algorithms.

In addition, relative perfusion imaging with PET and SPECT normalizes the myocardial counts to the hottest pixel, and thus, there is a certain known rate of underdiagnosing multivessel CAD, and even false negative examinations.[8,9] The addition of a CAC score to MPI testing can identify the presence of significant coronary calcifications in multiple vessels, raising suspicion of important CAD in the correct clinical setting and potentially avoiding such misses.[8]

A summary of studies identifying CAD by elevated CAC score in patients with normal perfusion imaging is provided in **Table 1**. We also provide images from a 60-year-old patient who had normal digital PET myocardial perfusion images (**Fig. 1**A), normal left ventricular systolic function and normal quantitative myocardial perfusion reserve, but had a severely elevated CAC score at 3543 AU (**Fig. 1**B).

CAC scoring identifies and assesses the extent and location of calcified plaques in coronary arteries, whether flow-limiting or not, thereby supplementing information provided by the MPI. By combining the functional and anatomic assessment of MPI and CAC scoring, respectively, the sensitivity and specificity for diagnosing CAD may be improved compared with either test alone.[10] Similarly, a normal CAC score, given its strong negative predictive value, should be reassuring in ruling out CAD in a patient with a normal MPI.[4]

Prognostic Value of Coronary Artery Calcium

Many studies have shown the value of CAC scores in predicting outcomes.

Several studies have also shown that the prognostic value of the CAC score is complementary to the prognostic information on SPECT and PET MPI for both patients with ischemic and nonischemic studies. In a study by Chang and colleagues,[11] for patients with normal SPECT, a CAC score greater than 400 was associated with a 3.55-fold higher risk of events (revascularization, myocardial infarction, or death) compared with a CAC score less than 10. Engbers and colleagues[5] showed an increased risk of major adverse cardiovascular events (MACE) is present with increasing CAC score both in patients with normal and abnormal SPECT. For example, in patients with a normal SPECT, the annual event rate was 0.6% for patients with CAC score of 0 compared with 5.5%

Table 1
Frequency of abnormal coronary artery calcium score in patients with normal myocardial perfusion imaging studies

Study	Population	CAC Score Cutoffs Used	Frequency of Patients with Abnormal CAC
Berman et al,[3] 2004	1195 patients without known CAD who underwent SPECT MPI and CAC tomography within 6 mo of each other	0 1 to 9 10 to 99 100 to 399 400 to 999 ≥1000	22% 4% 18% 25% 20% 11%
Thompson et al,[4] 2005	200 patients referred for CAC tomography after normal SPECT or PET MPI	1 to 10 11 to 100 101 to 400 >400	69.0% 13.5% 11.0% 6.5%
Bybee et al,[7] 2010	760 patients without known CAD with normal PET/CT MPI and same setting CAC scoring	1 to 9 10 to 99 100 to 399 400 to 999 ≥1000	22.0% 31.0% 24.6% 14.0% 8.4%
Engbers et al.[5]	3702 patients without known CAD referred for SPECT and CAC and who had normal SPECT	>0 ≥400 ≥1000	69% 15% 6%

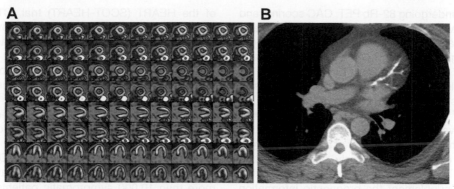

Fig. 1. A 60-year-old patient had normal digital PET myocardial perfusion images (*A*), normal left ventricular systolic function and normal quantitative myocardial perfusion reserve, but had a severely elevated coronary calcium score at 3543 AU (*B*). The patient was referred for aggressive coronary risk factor management.

in patients with a CAC ≥1000. In patients with an abnormal SPECT, the annual event rate was 0.4% for patients with a CAC score of 0 compared with 7.6% for patients with a CAC score ≥1000.[5]

Similar findings have been shown for CAC scoring in patients who undergo PET MPI. Schenker and colleagues[12] showed an increased risk of events with increasing CAC score in patients both with and without ischemia on PET MPI. Bybee and colleagues[7] found an annualized rate of death or myocardial infarction of 12.3% in patients with a normal PET MPI and a CAC score ≥1000. In the largest study of this type, Miller and colleagues[13] studied 2504 patients who

underwent PET MPI and CAC scoring. The risk stratifying value of CAC and total perfusion defect (TPD) were found to be complementary. During a median follow-up of 3.9 years, 594 patients had at least one MACE. Increasing CAC and ischemic TPD were associated with increased MACE, with the highest risk associated with CAC score greater than 1000. A summary of studies reporting annualized event rates in patients with normal MPI but elevated calcium scores is provided in **Table 2**.

Contemporary PET MPI includes measurement of absolute quantitation of myocardial perfusion, which is itself a very powerful prognostic marker. It should be noted that in one study of 5983

Table 2
Summary of studies reporting annualized event rates in patients with normal myocardial perfusion imaging

Study	Population	Prognostic Outcome	CAC Score Cutoff	Annualized Event Rate
Engbers et al,[5] 2016	3702 patients without known CAD referred for SPECT and CAC and who had normal SPECT	Late revascularization, nonfatal myocardial infarction, and all-cause mortality	0 ≥1000	0.6% 5.5%
Schenker et al,[12] 2008	516 patients who completed combined rest-stress PET and CAC scoring on a hybrid PET-CT scanner and who had normal PET	Death or myocardial infarction	0 ≥1000	2.6% 12.3%
Bybee et al,[7] 2010	760 patients without known CAD with normal PET/CT MPI and same setting CAC scoring	Death or myocardial infarction	≥1000	12.3%
Miller et al,[13] 2022	858 patients without known CAD who had CAC score and underwent PET with <1% ischemic total perfusion defect	Late revascularization, unstable angina, nonfatal myocardial infarction, and all-cause mortality	0 1 to 99 100 to 399 400 to 999 ≥1000	2.8% 3.2% 3.6% 6.4% 9.5%

patients undergoing 82-Rb PET, CAC scoring, and quantitative coronary blood flow, CAC score and myocardial blood flow reserve both had independent prognostic value in patients with normal and abnormal perfusion imaging.[14]

It should also be noted that the time frame of prognosis for MPI and CAC scores are not the same.[5,7,11] MPI studies provide prognostic information over the short term; however, after 1 to 3 years, the prognostic power of an MPI study reaches its expiration.[7] Routinely performing CAC scores, a measure of atherosclerotic burden, will therefore supplement the prognostic information available and better define longer-term risk of events.

Although the anatomic information of the CAC score adds complementary prognostic value to the physiology measure of MPI, it appears that combining two anatomic tests does not necessarily offer similar synergy. For example, the bulk of the prognostic value of a coronary CTA actually appears to be in the data provided by the CAC score. In a study by Mortensen and colleagues,[15] patients with nonobstructive CAD on CTA had similar risk of major cardiovascular events and death as patients with obstructive CAD when stratified by CAC scores.

Management Changes Based on Coronary Artery Calcium

Once CAD has been diagnosed by CAC score, studies have shown that clinicians alter medical therapy based on these results. Thompson and colleagues[4] found that patients with a normal MPI study who had a CAC ≥100 were significantly more likely to be given the advice to take lipid-lowering medication and aspirin compared with those with CAC scores of 0 at follow-up. In the study by Bybee and colleagues[7] of patients with a normal PET MPI and no known CAD, those with CAC were more likely to undergo optimization of medical therapy for CAD compared with those without CAC (53.3% vs 34.3%;). Taylor and colleagues[16] examined the association of CAC detected on a screening exam with subsequent statin and aspirin usage in a healthy male screening cohort. They found an independent 3-fold greater likelihood of statin and aspirin usage in the presence of CAC.

Early detection of CAD by CAC even in patients with a normal MPI allows for appropriate medical therapy and risk factor modification, maneuvers which have been shown to be effective in reducing death and myocardial infarction in patients with CAD.[17] For example, in the prospective randomized controlled Scottish Computed Tomography of the HEART (SCOT-HEART) trial, CT angiography was shown to improve the downstream use of preventive therapy, and this was associated with an approximately 45% relative risk reduction of fatal and nonfatal myocardial infarction.[18,19]

In addition, downstream testing may be reduced if CAC is not present. Le and colleagues[20] showed reduced rates of coronary angiography and revascularization in patients without CAC compared with those with CAC. Similarly, in the Coronary CT Angiography Evaluation for Clinical Outcomes: An International Multicenter registry that includes more than 10,000 symptomatic patients referred for coronary CT angiography, the 90-day revascularization rate was 1% in the CAC-absent group and 8.9% in the CAC-present group.[21]

Options for Obtaining a Calcium Score with Myocardial Perfusion Imaging

A formal CAC score can be obtained from a hybrid PET/CT or SPECT/CT camera or a dedicated CT scanner.

Visually Estimated Coronary Calcium on Low-Dose Attenuation Correction Computed Tomography

Although there is extensive literature and validation for coronary calcium scores from gated x-ray CT scans performed in a standard manner, obtaining a formal CAC score requires more expensive CT equipment, including hardware and software for ECG gating and a calcium scoring software package. Also, many patients undergoing MPI have already recently undergone chest CT scans, either with or without contrast, for other indications. As there is frequently not extra reimbursement for CAC scores and as moderate-to-severe CAC can usually be identified on non-gated chest CT scans and even low-dose x-ray transmission scans obtained for attenuation correction, there has been interest in visually estimating the presence of CAC from nonstandard studies. In one of the first studies in this space, Einstein and colleagues[22] evaluated the accuracy and reproducibility of visual estimation of CAC from CT attenuation correction (CTAC) scans performed for hybrid PET/CT and SPECT/CT MPI. Experienced readers estimated an Agatston score into six categories (0, 1 to 9, 10 to 99, 100 to 399, 400 to 999, and ≥1000). There was a high degree of association between the visually estimated CAC score and Agatston score with 63% of visually estimated scores in exactly the same category as the Agatston category and 93% varying by no more than 1 category. This held true for both women and men and for all vessels. Also, Mylonas and colleagues[23] showed visually estimated CAC scores from low-dose CTAC had good intraclass correlation with Agatston scores (0.84) and showed excellent interobserver agreement (kappa 0.941).

Trpkov and colleagues[24] took this a step further to show that visually estimated CAC scores were independently prognostic for MACE. In this study of 4720 patients who underwent SPECT/CT, calcium was visually estimated as absent, equivocal, present, or extensive. Increased risk of MACE was associated with visually-estimated categories of equivocal, present, and extensive. Patients with MACE were more likely to be in the visually-estimated extensive coronary calcium category (42.7% vs 18.8%), and patients without MACE were more likely to have absent visually-estimated calcium (32.7% vs 8.9%).

Le and colleagues[20] described their experience with combining visually estimated coronary calcium scores with PET MPI in clinical practice. They examined long term (up to 4 year) MACE, including all-cause death, myocardial infarction, and late revascularization (>90 days) in patients referred for PET MPI. Patients without visually apparent CAC on CT attenuation maps were less likely to undergo coronary angiography or revascularization. Even among patients with greater than 10% ischemia on PET MPI, those without visual CAC had substantially less high-grade CAD and revascularization compared with those with CAC. Visual CAC was predictive of risk of longer-term MACE even after adjusting for ischemic burden on PET MPI.

Although these studies show that there is good agreement between visually estimated scores and that visually estimated calcium can be prognostic of outcomes, there are limitations with visually estimating a CAC score on a low-dose CTAC. First, a visually estimated score is subjective. Second, the lack of ECG gating can introduce artifact into the images that can affect calcium scores. Third, there are patient populations such as obese patients in whom obtaining a visually estimated coronary calcium score on a low-dose CTAC can be difficult. For example, in their editorial, Thompson and Thomas provide an example of a 63-year-old woman with a body mass index of 40 who has no visible calcium on the low-dose CTAC but an Agatston score of 121 on formal CAC imaging.[25] In addition, in the study by Einstein and colleagues,[22] 22% of the 412 patients in whom coronary calcium was determined to be absent on the low-dose CTAC actually had an Agatston score greater than 0. Therefore, although the low-dose CTAC can provide a general idea on the extent of calcification and examining any available previously obtained chest CT scan can be useful, there is in all likelihood additional value in obtaining a formal CAC score in patients without known CAD undergoing MPI.

Recently, several investigators have used artificial intelligence to estimate CAC scores from nonstandard chest CT scans.[26–28] This emerging technology is already commercially available, uses deep learning, and promises to solve some of the limitations of visually estimating CAC scoring. For example, machine measurements would be expected to give much more reproducible scores than even expert human reviewers. To date, this technology is still considered in development, and in the United States, the service can be reported with a Current Procedural Terminology (CPT) Category III emerging technology code (CPT codes +0721T and + 0722T). However, at least one study suggests the human can outperform some AI derived automatic calcium scoring of low-dose CT attenuation maps.[27]

Diagnoses Other than Coronary Artery Disease

In addition to diagnosing CAD, relevant extracardiac findings are frequently identified on CT scans performed for coronary calcium scoring or CT transmission maps used for attenuation correction, and these images should be routinely reviewed.[29–33] These findings range from minor and incidental (such as small pulmonary nodules) to serious new diagnoses (such as lung or breast cancers). Sometimes findings may offer clues to the etiology of the patient's symptoms that prompted MPI stress testing to be performed, such as hiatal hernias, pleural effusions, elevated hemidiaphragm, pericardial thickening, interstitial lung disease or emphysema. **Table 3** lists some of the common findings that can be diagnosed on even low-resolution CT attenuation maps.

Table 3
Relevant diagnoses identifiable on computed tomography transmission maps

Cardiovascular	Other
Coronary calcifications	Pleural effusions
Thoracic aorta calcifications	Paralyzed diaphragm
Aortic aneurysm	Large lung masses
Pericardial effusions	Pneumonias
Pericardial calcifications	Pleural calcifications
Coronary anomaly	
Aortic arch anomaly	Interstitial lung disease
Dilated pulmonary artery	Lung abscess
	Breast mass

Downsides to Obtaining a Coronary Artery Calcium Score with Myocardial Perfusion Imaging

Although there are numerous benefits to obtaining a CAC score at the time of MPI stress testing, as described above, the downsides of obtaining the CAC score should be considered. There is a small amount of extra time for testing, generally about 30 s if the CAC score is obtained at the time of MPI on a hybrid PET or SPECT-CT camera. However, if a patient needs to have the CAC score performed in a separate department from the MPI study and must wait, the extra time can become an inconvenience. In general, the major limitation to this combined imaging approach is one of logistics. There is also a small amount of additional radiation exposure, normally about 1 mSv.

Cost of and Reimbursement for Coronary Artery Calcium Scoring

Although in the United States there is a billing code for reporting CAC scoring (CPT 75,571), most commercial insurance companies tend not to reimburse for the service, arguing that it is an uncovered screening test. When the CAC score is obtained at the time of MPI on an SPECT-CT or PET-CT camera, the incremental cost in time for the acquisition is quite small. Given the significant additional diagnostic and prognostic value of the combined approach to the patient, many laboratories simply accept that the CAC score part of the combined service might not be reimbursed, or they charge the patient only a modest additional fee. However, it is sometimes difficult to convince hospital leadership of the wisdom of this approach. In the United States, review of the CT attenuation maps for coronary calcium and other findings on cardiac PET-CT studies is considered part of the service and is included in the description of work of the billing codes. In this sense, reviewing these low-dose CT attenuation scans is obligatory. This is also the case with noncardiac PET and nuclear medicine SPECT. Currently in the United States, there are not separate codes to report *cardiac* SPECT-CT. All attenuation correction is included in the SPECT MPI CPT codes (78,451 and 78,452) when performed, and so SPECT MPI is billed the same way whether without attenuation correction, with line source attenuation correction, or using SPECT-CT instrumentation. As described above, there is considerable value in viewing the CT attenuation map images in these cases, and so it is strongly recommended to do so, even if not separately reimbursed.

SUMMARY

In patients undergoing MPI stress testing, obtaining a CAC score detects nonobstructive CAD, improves risk assessment, and leads to changes in management. Based on review of the available literature, consideration should be given to routinely obtaining a CAC score at the time of MPI stress testing in patients without known CAD.

CLINICS CARE POINTS

- A coronary artery calcium score can be diagnostic for coronary artery disease even in the presence of a normal myocardial perfusion imaging (MPI) study, leading to logical changes in patient management and follow-up algorithm.

- Coronary artery calcium scores have been shown to be prognostic for major adverse cardiovascular events, in a complementary fashion to perfusion defects on MPI.

- Clinicians alter medical management for coronary artery disease on the basis of coronary calcium scores.

- Visually estimating coronary calcium on the low-dose computed tomography (CT) performed for attenuation correction from hybrid PET/CT and single-photon emission computed tomography/CT imaging, and review of previously performed chest CT examinations, can provide a general idea to the extent of coronary calcification and is useful if formal coronary artery calcium scoring is not available.

- Adding a formal coronary artery calcium study to MPI stress testing does expose the patient to a small amount of additional radiation.

DISCLOSURES

M. Thomas and R.C. Thompson have nothing to disclose.

REFERENCES

1. Nasir K, Budoff MJ, Shaw LJ, et al. Value of multi-slice computed tomography coronary angiography in suspected coronary artery disease. J Am Coll Cardiol 2007;49:2070–1 [author reply 2071].
2. Budoff MJ, Shaw LJ, Liu ST, et al. Long-term prognosis associated with coronary calcification:

observations from a registry of 25,253 patients. J Am Coll Cardiol 2007;49:1860–70.

3. Berman DS, Wong ND, Gransar H, et al. Relationship between stress-induced myocardial ischemia and atherosclerosis measured by coronary calcium tomography. J Am Coll Cardiol 2004;44:923–30.

4. Thompson RC, McGhie AI, Moser KW, et al. Clinical utility of coronary calcium scoring after nonischemic myocardial perfusion imaging. J Nucl Cardiol 2005; 12:392–400.

5. Engbers EM, Timmer JR, Ottervanger JP, et al. Prognostic value of coronary artery calcium scoring in addition to single-photon emission computed tomographic myocardial perfusion imaging in symptomatic patients. Circ Cardiovasc Imaging 2016;9: e003966.

6. Parker MW, Iskandar A, Limone B, et al. Diagnostic accuracy of cardiac positron emission tomography versus single photon emission computed tomography for coronary artery disease: a bivariate meta-analysis. Circ Cardiovasc Imaging 2012;5:700–7.

7. Bybee KA, Lee J, Markiewicz R, et al. Diagnostic and clinical benefit of combined coronary calcium and perfusion assessment in patients undergoing PET/CT myocardial perfusion stress imaging. J Nucl Cardiol 2010;17:188–96.

8. Ghadri JR, Pazhenkottil AP, Nkoulou RN, et al. Very high coronary calcium score unmasks obstructive coronary artery disease in patients with normal SPECT MPI. Heart 2011;97:998–1003.

9. Berman DS, Kang X, Slomka PJ, et al. Underestimation of extent of ischemia by gated SPECT myocardial perfusion imaging in patients with left main coronary artery disease. J Nucl Cardiol 2007;14: 521–8.

10. Schepis T, Gaemperli O, Koepfli P, et al. Added value of coronary artery calcium score as an adjunct to gated SPECT for the evaluation of coronary artery disease in an intermediate-risk population. J Nucl Med 2007;48:1424–30.

11. Chang SM, Nabi F, Xu J, et al. The coronary artery calcium score and stress myocardial perfusion imaging provide independent and complementary prediction of cardiac risk. J Am Coll Cardiol 2009; 54:1872–82.

12. Schenker MP, Dorbala S, Hong EC, et al. Interrelation of coronary calcification, myocardial ischemia, and outcomes in patients with intermediate likelihood of coronary artery disease: a combined positron emission tomography/computed tomography study. Circulation 2008;117:1693–700.

13. Miller RJH, Han D, Singh A, et al. Relationship between ischaemia, coronary artery calcium scores, and major adverse cardiovascular events. Eur Heart J Cardiovasc Imaging 2022;23(11):1423–33.

14. Patel KK, Peri-Okonny PA, Qarajeh R, et al. Prognostic relationship between coronary artery calcium score, perfusion defects, and myocardial blood flow reserve in patients with suspected coronary artery disease. Circ Cardiovasc Imaging 2022;15: e012599.

15. Mortensen MB, Dzaye O, Steffensen FH, et al. Impact of plaque burden versus stenosis on ischemic events in patients with coronary atherosclerosis. J Am Coll Cardiol 2020;76:2803–13.

16. Taylor AJ, Bindeman J, Feuerstein I, et al. Community-based provision of statin and aspirin after the detection of coronary artery calcium within a community-based screening cohort. J Am Coll Cardiol 2008;51:1337–41.

17. Achenbach S, Ropers D, Pohle K, et al. Influence of lipid-lowering therapy on the progression of coronary artery calcification: a prospective evaluation. Circulation 2002;106:1077–82.

18. Investigators S-H, Newby DE, Adamson PD, et al. Coronary CT angiography and 5-year risk of myocardial infarction. N Engl J Med 2018;379:924–33.

19. Adamson PD, Williams MC, Dweck MR, et al. Guiding therapy by coronary CT angiography improves outcomes in patients with stable chest pain. J Am Coll Cardiol 2019;74:2058–70.

20. Le VT, Knight S, Min DB, et al. Absence of coronary artery calcium during positron emission tomography stress testing in patients without known coronary artery disease identifies individuals with very low risk of cardiac events. Circ Cardiovasc Imaging 2020; 13:e009907.

21. Villines TC, Hulten EA, Shaw LJ, et al. Prevalence and severity of coronary artery disease and adverse events among symptomatic patients with coronary artery calcification scores of zero undergoing coronary computed tomography angiography: results from the CONFIRM (Coronary CT Angiography Evaluation for Clinical Outcomes: an International Multicenter) registry. J Am Coll Cardiol 2011;58:2533–40.

22. Einstein AJ, Johnson LL, Bokhari S, et al. Agreement of visual estimation of coronary artery calcium from low-dose CT attenuation correction scans in hybrid PET/CT and SPECT/CT with standard Agatston score. J Am Coll Cardiol 2010;56:1914–21.

23. Mylonas I, Kazmi M, Fuller L, et al. Measuring coronary artery calcification using positron emission tomography-computed tomography attenuation correction images. Eur Heart J Cardiovasc Imaging 2012;13:786–92.

24. Trpkov C, Savtchenko A, Liang Z, et al. Visually estimated coronary artery calcium score improves SPECT-MPI risk stratification. Int J Cardiol Heart Vasc 2021;35:100827.

25. Thompson RC, Thomas GS. Power of adding coronary artery calcium scanning to myocardial perfusion imaging with positron emission tomography. Circ Cardiovasc Imaging 2020;13:e010286.

26. van Velzen SGM, Dobrolinska MM, Knaapen P. et al. Automated cardiovascular risk categorization through AI-driven coronary calcium quantification in cardiac PET acquired attenuation correction CT. J Nucl Cardiol. 2022. doi: 10.1007/s12350-022-03047-9.

27. Dobrolinska MM, Lazarenko SV, van der Zant FM, et al. Performance of visual, manual, and automatic coronary calcium scoring of cardiac 13N-ammonia PET/low dose CT. J Nucl Cardiol. 2022. doi: 10.1007/s12350-022-03018-0.

28. Atkins KM, Weiss J, Zeleznik R, et al. Elevated coronary artery calcium quantified by a validated deep learning model from lung cancer radiotherapy planning scans predicts mortality. JCO Clin Cancer Inform 2022;6:e2100095.

29. Horton KM, Post WS, Blumenthal RS, et al. Prevalence of significant noncardiac findings on electron-beam computed tomography coronary artery calcium screening examinations. Circulation 2002;106:532–4.

30. Osman MM, Cohade C, Fishman EK, et al. Clinically significant incidental findings on the unenhanced CT portion of PET/CT studies: frequency in 250 patients. J Nucl Med 2005;46:1352–5.

31. Schragin JG, Weissfeld JL, Edmundowicz D, et al. Non-cardiac findings on coronary electron beam computed tomography scanning. J Thorac Imaging 2004;19:82–6.

32. Coward J, Lawson R, Kane T, et al. Multicentre analysis of incidental findings on low-resolution CT attenuation correction images: an extended study. Br J Radiol 2015;88:20150555.

33. Coward J, Nightingale J, Hogg P. The clinical dilemma of incidental findings on the low-resolution CT images from SPECT/CT MPI studies. J Nucl Med Technol 2016;44:167–72.

Clinical Value of Positron Emission Tomography Myocardial Perfusion Imaging and Blood Flow Quantification

Marcelo F. Di Carli, MD[a,b,c,d],*

KEYWORDS

- Coronary artery disease • Myocardial perfusion imaging • Myocardial blood flow
- Myocardial flow reserve • Coronary microvascular dysfunction • Coronary allograft vasculopathy

KEY POINTS

- Accurate quantification of myocardial blood flow (MBF) and flow reserve is a unique strength of PET myocardial perfusion imaging and can be performed routinely by image postprocessing.
- A normal stress MBF and flow reserve (>2.0) have a very high negative predictive value and reliably exclude high-risk obstructive coronary artery disease (CAD).
- In the absence of obstructive CAD, reduced stress MBF and flow reserve (<2.0) are a marker coronary microvascular dysfunction.
- A global normal myocardial flow reserve (>2.0) identifies patients at consistently lower clinical risk. Conversely, a severely reduced flow reserve (<1.5) identifies patients at high clinical risk for adverse events.
- Recent evidence suggests that patients with angiographically obstructive CAD and a severe reduction in flow reserve (<1.6) may have a prognostic advantage from revascularization. This finding awaits confirmation by randomized clinical trials.
- Quantitative stress MBF and flow reserve provide accurate complementary value for the evaluation of coronary allograft vasculopathy (CAV) after heart transplantation and can be used for longitudinal monitoring of CAV.

Semiquantitative evaluation of regional myocardial perfusion has been standard practice in nuclear cardiology for almost a half century. This approach provides accurate and reproducible detection of flow-limiting stenosis. In addition, semiquantitative assessment of total perfusion deficit provides robust risk stratification that helps guide patient management. However, there is evidence that clinical presentations of patients with suspected or known coronary artery disease (CAD) are changing. Indeed, over the last 20 years, there has been a steady decline in the incidence of obstructive CAD on coronary angiography, a reduction in the incidence of acute presentations of myocardial infarction (MI), particularly with ST-segment elevation,[1] and an increase in hospitalizations with type 2 MI and heart failure with preserved ejection fraction.[2] Pathologically, this

a Cardiovascular Imaging Program, Department of Medicine, Brigham and Women's Hospital, Harvard Medical School, Boston, MA, USA; b Cardiovascular Imaging Program, Department of Radiology, Brigham and Women's Hospital, Harvard Medical School, Boston, MA, USA; c Division of Nuclear Medicine and Molecular Imaging, Department of Radiology, Brigham and Women's Hospital, Harvard Medical School, Boston, MA, USA; d Cardiovascular Division, Department of Medicine, Brigham and Women's Hospital, Harvard Medical School, Boston, MA, USA
* Brigham and Women's Hospital, Harvard Medical School, ASB-L1 037C, 75 Francis Street, Boston, MA 02115.
E-mail address: mdicarli@bwh.harvard.edu

Cardiol Clin 41 (2023) 185–195
https://doi.org/10.1016/j.ccl.2023.01.007
0733-8651/23/© 2023 Elsevier Inc. All rights reserved.

has been associated with an increased prevalence of diffuse atherosclerosis and coronary microvascular dysfunction (CMD). This may help explain, at least in part, the drop in diagnostic yields of radionuclide perfusion imaging[3] and invasive coronary angiography[4,5] over the last 2 decades. These observations parallel other epidemiologic shifts in the prevalence of cardiometabolic risk factors in the population, including the growth of obesity, glucose intolerance, and older age.[6] This epidemiologic change will demand advanced imaging tools to delineate the burden of atherosclerosis and its functional consequence to accurately phenotype clinical risk and guide management.

PET/computed tomography (CT) offers a set of quantitative tools that allow a comprehensive noninvasive evaluation of coronary atherosclerotic burden, myocardial perfusion, and left ventricular (LV) function. This review uses a series of case presentations to illustrate the current applications of myocardial perfusion PET/CT imaging in the evaluation and management of patients with suspected or known CAD.

COMPREHENSIVE DELINEATION OF CORONARY ARTERY DISEASE WITH HYBRID MYOCARDIAL PERFUSION POSITRON EMISSION TOMOGRAPHY/COMPUTED TOMOGRAPHY

The integration of quantitative PET and CT offers a powerful tool to noninvasively assess the diagnostic and prognostic interplay between the burden of atherosclerosis and its functional consequence across the spectrum of CAD. The extent and severity of coronary calcification, reflecting the burden of atherosclerosis in the coronary arteries, can be quantified by validated scoring techniques (eg, Agatston score). The nongated CT transmission scan used for attenuation correction of the PET data may also be used to assess the extent of coronary calcifications using semiquantitative visual analysis.[7]

The basic principle of radionuclide myocardial perfusion imaging (MPI) for detecting CAD is based on the ability of a perfusion tracer to identify a transient regional perfusion deficit in a myocardial region subtended by a coronary artery with a flow-limiting stenosis. The quantification of the total perfusion deficit and its degree of reversibility (reflecting ischemic myocardium) are key elements in the assessment of the extent and severity of focal flow-limiting CAD. However, this traditional measurement of ischemic burden is often insensitive to explain symptoms in patients with predominantly diffuse atherosclerosis and CMD.

Myocardial blood flow (MBF, measured in milliliters per minute per gram of myocardium) and myocardial blood flow reserve (MFR, defined as the ratio between stress and rest MBF) are important physiologic parameters that can be measured by routine postprocessing of myocardial perfusion PET images.[8] These absolute measurements of MBF provide a measure of the integrated effects of focal coronary stenoses, diffuse atherosclerosis, and microvascular dysfunction on myocardial perfusion, and, as such, the value obtained is a more sensitive and accurate measure of myocardial ischemia. As discussed later, these measurements of MFR have important diagnostic[9–13] and prognostic[14–23] implications in the evaluation and management[19,22,23] of the patients with known or suspected CAD.

INTEGRATING BLOOD FLOW QUANTIFICATION INTO ROUTINE EVALUATION OF SUSPECTED CORONARY ARTERY DISEASE

Prior meta-analyses[24–26] and prospective comparative effectiveness studies[27–29] support the notion that PET MPI is one of the most accurate noninvasive techniques for detecting flow-limiting CAD. The integration of quantitative MBF and MFR information into scan interpretation improves detection of the extent and severity of flow-limiting CAD by avoiding the pitfalls of spatially relative perfusion assessment associated with balanced reduction in myocardial perfusion (Fig. 1). In so doing, these quantitative measures of myocardial perfusion improve the sensitivity and negative predictive value of PET for ruling out high-risk angiographic CAD.[9–13] Indeed, an MFR > 2.0 is associated with a greater than 97% negative predictive value for ruling out high-risk angiographic CAD.[12]

Conversely, normal augmentation in stress MBF and MFR in symptomatic patients helps to confidently exclude obstructive CAD and CMD as the potential source of symptoms,[30] even in the presence of extensive atherosclerosis (Fig. 2). From a management perspective, the normal MBF and MFR avoid the need to pursue coronary angiography. On the other hand, the burden of coronary artery calcifications provides a guide for aggressive risk factor management, including lipid-lowering therapy.

Quantification of MBF and MFR also provides a powerful tool for incremental risk stratification and risk reclassification. Growing evidence from multiple single-center studies have demonstrated that a preserved MFR (>2.0) consistently associates with a low risk of adverse cardiac events, including

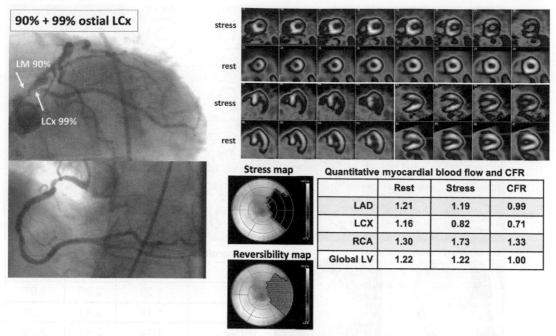

90% + 99% ostial LCx

LM 90%

LCx 99%

stress

rest

stress

rest

Stress map

Reversibility map

Quantitative myocardial blood flow and CFR

	Rest	Stress	CFR
LAD	1.21	1.19	0.99
LCX	1.16	0.82	0.71
RCA	1.30	1.73	1.33
Global LV	1.22	1.22	1.00

Fig. 1. Stress-rest myocardial perfusion PET images of a 68-year-old male patient presenting with chest pain and dyspnea (*upper right*). The images demonstrate a medium-sized perfusion defect of severe intensity throughout the lateral LV wall, showing complete reversibility consistent with severe ischemia in the left circumflex territory. This is also seen on the polar maps. However, the quantitative analysis showed severe reduction in stress MBF and coronary flow reserve (CFR, also called MFR), consistent with high-risk multivessel CAD (*lower right*). Subsequent coronary angiography showed severe left main and left circumflex obstructive lesions (*left panel*). CFR, coronary flow reserve; LAD, left anterior descending; LCx, left circumflex; LM, left main; RCA, right coronary artery.

cardiac death.[14–23,31] In contrast, a severe reduction in MFR consistently identifies patients at high risk of adverse cardiac events, even among those with normal MPI. For any amount of ischemic and/or scarred myocardium, a severely reduced global MFR is associated with a higher risk of death than in the setting of a relatively preserved flow reserve. PET measures of MFR improved risk stratification beyond comprehensive clinical assessment, LV ejection fraction, and semiquantitative measures of myocardial ischemia and scar, and in 1 study this led to clinically meaningful risk-reclassification of ~50% of intermediate-risk patients.[17] Importantly, stress MBF and MFR measurements provide robust complementary information that helps inform clinical risk and subsequent patient management. As shown in **Fig. 3**, concordant abnormal stress MBF and MFR identified the highest-risk patients (cardiac mortality: >3%/y), whereas concordant normal results identified the lowest-risk patients (cardiac mortality: <0.5%/y).[18] Discordantly low stress MBF (<1.8) with preserved MFR (>2.0) identifies patients with epicardial atherosclerosis that have a low risk of adverse events (<1%/y) in whom revascularization is unlikely to offer a prognostic advantage.[19,22,23] There is also evidence

that the quantitative blood flow information, a measure of coronary vascular health, helps with risk-reclassification of patients with cardiometabolic disease. For example, patients with diabetes without known CAD but abnormal MFR had a cardiac mortality risk comparable to that in nondiabetics with known CAD. Conversely, diabetics without overt CAD with relatively preserved MFR had an annual risk less than 1% that was comparable to subjects without diabetes or CAD (**Fig. 4**).

INTEGRATING NOVEL TOOLS TO DIFFERENTIATE OBSTRUCTIVE FROM NONOBSTRUCTIVE CORONARY ARTERY DISEASE

In patients with cardiometabolic disease, it can sometimes be challenging to ascertain if perfusion or MBF abnormalities are caused by obstructive versus diffuse nonobstructive atherosclerosis. From a clinical viewpoint, such distinction is very important to make decisions regarding referral to coronary angiography for possible revascularization.

Figs. 5 and **6** illustrate 2 patients with high-risk scan features, including severe regional and global abnormalities in MBF and MFR. In **Fig. 5**, the severe

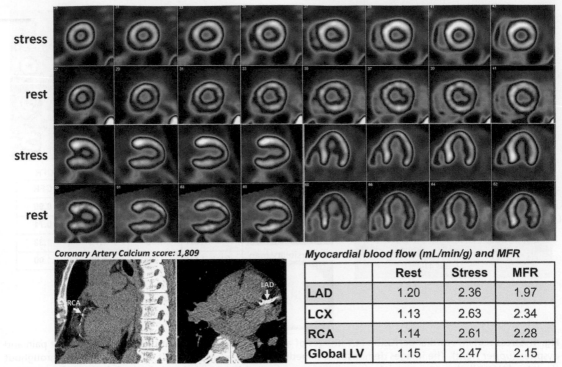

Coronary Artery Calcium score: 1,809

Myocardial blood flow (mL/min/g) and MFR

	Rest	Stress	MFR
LAD	1.20	2.36	1.97
LCX	1.13	2.63	2.34
RCA	1.14	2.61	2.28
Global LV	1.15	2.47	2.15

Fig. 2. Normal stress-rest myocardial perfusion PET study (*upper panel*) of a 57-year-old woman with a history of hypertension, dyslipidemia, and diabetes presenting with atypical chest pain. Her noncontrast gated CT scan showed extensive coronary artery calcifications and an Agatston score of 1809 (*lower left panel*). However, quantitative blood flow analysis showed normal stress MBF and MFR (*lower right panel*). These findings are consistent with diffuse atherosclerosis without flow-limiting disease or evidence of CMD.

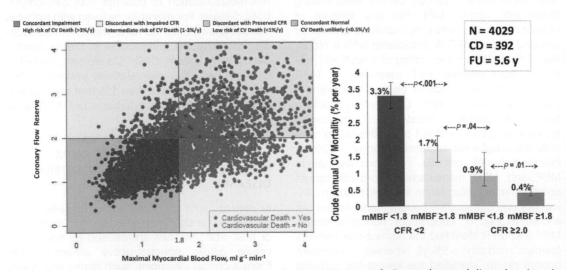

Fig. 3. Scatter plot of CFR and stress MBF by cardiovascular death (*left panel*). Concordant and discordant impairment of CFR and stress MBF identifies unique prognostic phenotypes of patients. A CFR < 2 and stress MBF < 1.8 mL g^{-1} min^{-1} were defined as impaired. Annualized CV mortality for the 4 groups based on concordant or discordant impairment of CFR and stress MBF (*right panel*). CV, cardiovascular; FU, follow-up; mMBF, median myocardial blood flow. (*From* Gupta A, Taqueti VR, van de Hoef TP, et al. Integrated Noninvasive Physiological Assessment of Coronary Circulatory Function and Impact on Cardiovascular Mortality in Patients With Stable Coronary Artery Disease. Circulation. Dec 12 2017;136(24):2325-2336.)

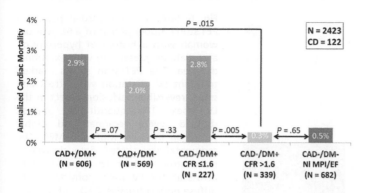

Fig. 4. Adjusted cardiac mortality among patients with CAD (history of coronary revascularization or MI) without diabetes (*orange*), diabetic patients without CAD who have impaired CFR (≤1.6; *blue*), diabetic patients without CAD who have preserved CFR (>1.6; *green*), and patients without diabetes or CAD with normal scans (no scar, ischemia, or LV dysfunction; *red*) presented as annualized cardiac mortalities. Data for patients with CAD and diabetes are also presented for comparison (*purple*). DM, diabetes mellitus; MPI/EF, myocardial perfusion imaging/ejection fraction; Nl, normal. (*From* Murthy VL, Naya M, Foster CR, et al. Association between coronary vascular dysfunction and cardiac mortality in patients with and without diabetes mellitus. Circulation. Oct 9 2012;126(15):1858-68.)

reduction in stress MBF and MFR is associated with large reversible perfusion defects. In addition, there is a significant drop in stress MBF from the base to the LV apex. Such gradient has been referred to as relative flow reserve, and it is calculated as the stress MBF in the distal segment divided by that in the proximal segment (a proxy for fractional flow reserve [FFR]).[32,33] In the example in **Fig. 5**, the so-called PET FFR was 0.64 in the LAD territory, indicating the presence of obstructive CAD (a PET FFR >0.8 suggests nonobstructive CAD). Thus, the association of a regional perfusion

abnormality and a concordant obstructive base to apical gradient is consistent with predominant obstructive CAD. In contrast, **Fig. 6** illustrates an example of a patient with marked transient cavity dilatation and a small apical perfusion defect and severely reduced stress MBF (without an obstructive gradient) and MFR. The diffusely reduced stress MBF without segmental gradient from base to apex suggests predominantly nonobstructive CAD. A gradient from base to apex can be seen in the presence of focal stenosis and severe diffuse atherosclerosis.

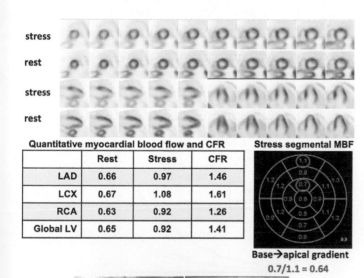

	Rest	Stress	CFR
LAD	0.66	0.97	1.46
LCX	0.67	1.08	1.61
RCA	0.63	0.92	1.26
Global LV	0.65	0.92	1.41

Base→apical gradient
0.7/1.1 = 0.64

Fig. 5. Stress-rest myocardial perfusion PET study (*upper panel*) of a 73-year-old man with a history of hypertension and chronic kidney disease presenting with heart failure and new regional wall motion abnormalities on echocardiography. The PET scan shows large, reversible perfusion defects throughout the anterior and anteroseptal walls, as well as the inferior wall, consistent with severe ischemia in the LAD and RCA territories. The quantitative analysis showed severe regional and global reduction in stress MBF and MFR. The segmental stress MBF data showed an obstructive base to apical gradient across the anterior and lateral walls, consistent with flow-limiting CAD (calculated from circles showing apical and basal flows). Subsequent coronary angiography showed a proximal total occlusion of the RCA (*arrow*) and >90% stenosis of the left main and LAD coronary arteries (*arrow*).

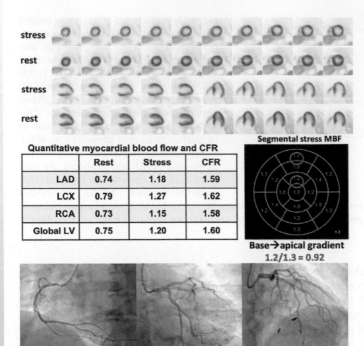

Quantitative myocardial blood flow and CFR

	Rest	Stress	CFR
LAD	0.74	1.18	1.59
LCX	0.79	1.27	1.62
RCA	0.73	1.15	1.58
Global LV	0.75	1.20	1.60

Segmental stress MBF

Base→apical gradient
1.2/1.3 = 0.92

Fig. 6. Stress-rest myocardial perfusion PET study (*upper panel*) of a 56-year-old woman with a history of hypertension and diabetes presenting with exertional dyspnea. The PET scan shows marked transient LV dilatation with stress and small, reversible perfusion defect in the LV apex. The quantitative analysis showed severe regional and global reduction in stress MBF and MFR. The segmental stress MBF data showed a nonobstructive base to apical gradient across all the LV walls, consistent with diffuse nonobstructive CAD. Subsequent coronary angiography showed nonobstructive CAD.

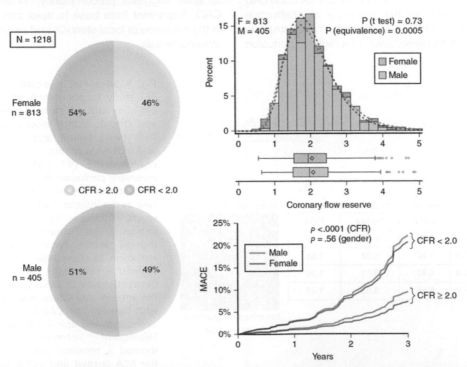

Fig. 7. Relative frequency of CMD in women and men (*left panel*). Distribution of CFR by sex (*top right panel*). Histogram (*top*) showing the distribution of CFR for men (*green*) and women (*pink*). Fitted log-normal distributions for men (*dashed green line*) and women (*dashed pink line*) are also displayed. Similar data are also shown in box plots (*bottom*). Adjusted cumulative rate of major adverse cardiac events by sex and CFR. The data are adjusted for the modified Duke clinical risk score and rest LV ejection fraction. (*From* Murthy VL, Naya M, Taqueti VR, et al. Effects of sex on coronary microvascular dysfunction and cardiac outcomes. Circulation. Jun 17 2014;129(24):2518-27.)

EVALUATION OF PATIENTS WITH ISCHEMIA WITHOUT OBSTRUCTIVE CORONARY ARTERY DISEASE

CMD is quite common in symptomatic patients with cardiometabolic risk factors,[30,34] especially women, and its presence identifies patients at higher risk of adverse cardiac events, including not only typical major adverse cardiac events (MACE) but also, importantly, heart failure events (**Fig. 7**).[30,35] Because the coronary microcirculation is beyond the resolution of coronary angiography, direct interrogation of coronary microvascular function by measuring MBF and/or microvascular resistance is necessary to establish the diagnosis of CMD[36] (**Fig. 8**). There are several noninvasive and invasive approaches for the evaluation of coronary vasomotor dysfunction,[37] each with advantages and limitations. Quantitative PET imaging is considered the most accurate and reproducible noninvasive technique to interrogate coronary microcirculatory function. An abnormal MFR by PET in a patient without obstructive CAD identifies

patients with CMD. Different thresholds for abnormality in MFR have been proposed depending on the technique used for evaluation of CMD. The consensus is that a flow reserve less than 2.0 in the absence of obstructive CAD is diagnostic of CMD. One important feature of CMD is it associates with diffuse nonobstructive atherosclerosis in the epicardial coronary arteries in greater than 80% of patients.[30,38,39] The association between extensive nonobstructive atherosclerosis and CMD increased clinical risk compared with either one alone.[40] This highlights the important complementary role of delineating atherosclerotic burden by either quantification of coronary artery calcifications or contrast CT angiography.

EVALUATION OF CORONARY ALLOGRAFT VASCULOPATHY

Cardiac allograft vasculopathy (CAV) is one of the leading causes of death in long-term orthotopic heart transplant (OHT) survivors and the principal cause of retransplantation after 1 year.[41] Annual

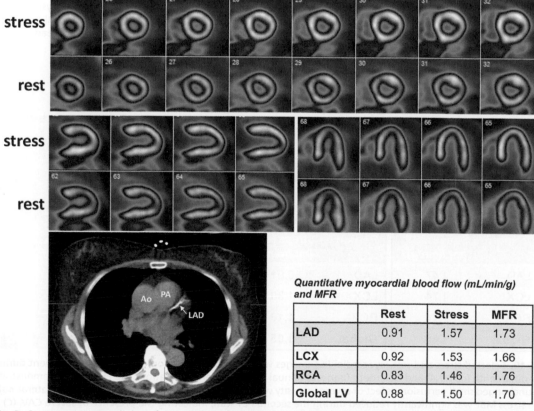

Quantitative myocardial blood flow (mL/min/g) and MFR

	Rest	Stress	MFR
LAD	0.91	1.57	1.73
LCX	0.92	1.53	1.66
RCA	0.83	1.46	1.76
Global LV	0.88	1.50	1.70

Fig. 8. Stress-rest myocardial perfusion PET study (*upper panel*) of a 76-year-old woman with a history of hypertension and dyslipidemia presenting with dyspnea and chest pain and nonobstructive CAD on recent coronary angiography. The PET scan is normal. The CT attenuation map shows moderate calcification in the LAD. The quantitative analysis showed moderate regional and global reduction in stress MBF and MFR, consistent with CMD. Ao, aorta; PA, pulmonary artery.

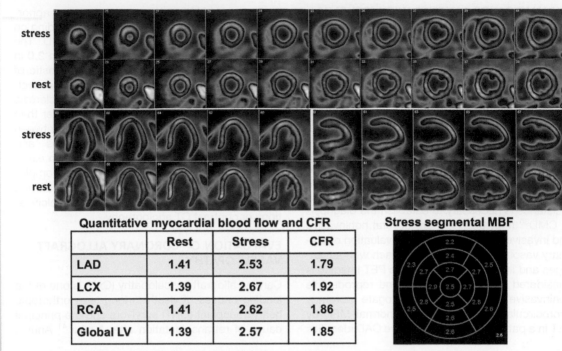

Quantitative myocardial blood flow and CFR			
	Rest	Stress	CFR
LAD	1.41	2.53	1.79
LCX	1.39	2.67	1.92
RCA	1.41	2.62	1.86
Global LV	1.39	2.57	1.85

Stress segmental MBF

Fig. 9. Stress-rest myocardial perfusion PET study (*upper panel*) of a 66-year-old man with a history of prior heart transplantation referred for routine surveillance of CAV. The PET scan is normal. The quantitative analysis showed normal regional and global stress MBF indicating no evidence of CAV. Rest MBF is elevated and consistent with the patient's elevated resting heart rate (common after heart transplantation) and hypertension, leading to a mildly reduced CFR.

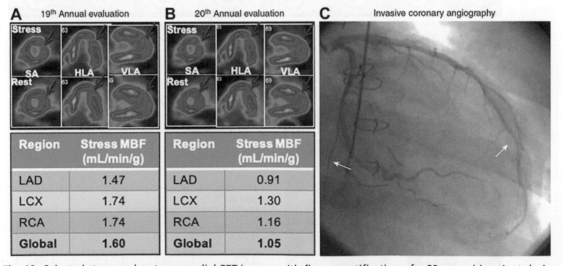

Fig. 10. Selected stress and rest myocardial PET images with flow quantification of a 22-year-old patient during her nineteenth (*panel A*) and twentieth (*panel B*) annual posttransplant evaluation. The PET images demonstrate an unchanged small perfusion defect of severe intensity with minimal reversibility in the apical anterolateral wall. The stress MBF was significantly reduced during the second PET scan, indicating the presence of severe CAV. (*C*) A selected view from invasive coronary angiography performed just 4 weeks after the twentieth annual evaluation demonstrated moderate obstructive CAV (*arrows*). HLA, horizontal long axis; SA, short axis; VLA, vertical long axis. (*From* Bravo P, Di Carli MF. Screening for transplant vasculopathy. In: Di Carli MF, editor. Nuclear Cardiology and Multimodal Cardiovascular Imaging. A companion to Braunwald's Heart Disease, 1st edition. Philadelphia: Elsevier; 2022. p. 307-17.)

surveillance with invasive coronary angiography to assess the presence and severity of CAV is the current standard of care. However, the high prevalence of renal dysfunction among OHT survivors makes this impractical in many patients. In addition, it is costly and not without risk for complications. Dobutamine stress echocardiography and single-photon emission computed tomography MPI are relatively insensitive for detection of CAV.[42,43]

Multiparametric PET provides the unique opportunity to quantify regional and global MBF (complementary to semiquantitative visual analysis) noninvasively, potentially serving as an indicator of the integrity and function of the large and small coronary vessels, which more closely reflect the pathobiology of CAV that is characterized by diffuse vessel narrowing, focal epicardial coronary stenoses, and obstructive microvasculopathy. There is growing, consistent evidence that flow quantification by PET is a very sensitive marker to rule out (**Fig. 9**) or rule in (**Fig. 10**) significant CAV and may offer advantages over other noninvasive imaging methods and invasive coronary angiography for longitudinal follow-up. Abnormalities in absolute stress MBF (in milliliters per minute per gram), MFR, and minimal coronary artery resistance, as measured by PET, have been proposed for diagnosis of CAV.[44–46] In addition, the quantitative PET approach also provides significant risk stratification beyond common standard clinical parameters.[44–46]

CLINICS CARE POINTS

- A stress myocardial blood flow and blood flow reserve > 2 exclude high risk angiographic CAD with a high negative predictive value.

- A myocardial blood flow reserve > 2 is associated with low clinical risk, whereas a blood flow reserve <1.5 is predictive of high clinical risk.

DISCLOSURE

The author has received an institutional grant from Gilead Sciences, United States and in-kind support from Amgen, United States.

REFERENCES

1. Yeh RW, Sidney S, Chandra M, et al. Population trends in the incidence and outcomes of acute myocardial infarction. N Engl J Med 2010;362(23): 2155–65.

2. Owan TE, Hodge DO, Herges RM, et al. Trends in prevalence and outcome of heart failure with preserved ejection fraction. N Engl J Med 2006; 355(3):251–9.

3. Rozanski A, Gransar H, Hayes SW, et al. Temporal trends in the frequency of inducible myocardial ischemia during cardiac stress testing: 1991 to 2009. J Am Coll Cardiol 2013;61(10):1054–65.

4. Jespersen L, Hvelplund A, Abildstrom SZ, et al. Stable angina pectoris with no obstructive coronary artery disease is associated with increased risks of major adverse cardiovascular events. Research Support, Non-U.S. Gov't. European Heart Journal 2012;33(6):734–44.

5. Maddox TM, Stanislawski MA, Grunwald GK, et al. Nonobstructive coronary artery disease and risk of myocardial infarction. JAMA 2014;312(17):1754–63.

6. Benjamin EJ, Virani SS, Callaway CW, et al. Heart disease and stroke statistics-2018 update: a report from the American Heart Association. Circulation 2018. https://doi.org/10.1161/cir.0000000000000558.

7. Einstein AJ, Johnson LL, Bokhari S, et al. Agreement of visual estimation of coronary artery calcium from low-dose CT attenuation correction scans in hybrid PET/CT and SPECT/CT with standard Agatston score. Comparative Study Multicenter Study Research Support, NIH, Extramural. J Am Coll Cardiol 2010;56(23):1914–21.

8. Murthy VL, Bateman TM, Beanlands RS, et al. Clinical quantification of myocardial blood flow using PET: joint position paper of the SNMMI Cardiovascular Council and the ASNC. J Nucl Med 2018;59(2): 273–93.

9. Danad I, Uusitalo V, Kero T, et al. Quantitative assessment of myocardial perfusion in the detection of significant coronary artery disease: cutoff values and diagnostic accuracy of quantitative [(15)O] H2O PET imaging. J Am Coll Cardiol 2014;64(14): 1464–75.

10. Johnson NP, Gould KL. Physiological basis for angina and ST-segment change PET-verified thresholds of quantitative stress myocardial perfusion and coronary flow reserve. JACC Cardiovasc Imaging 2011;4(9):990–8.

11. Kajander S, Joutsiniemi E, Saraste M, et al. Cardiac positron emission tomography/computed tomography imaging accurately detects anatomically and functionally significant coronary artery disease. Circulation 2010;122(6):603–13.

12. Naya M, Murthy VL, Taqueti VR, et al. Preserved coronary flow reserve effectively excludes high-risk coronary artery disease on angiography. J Nucl Med 2014;55(2):248–55.

13. Ziadi MC, Dekemp RA, Williams K, et al. Does quantification of myocardial flow reserve using rubidium-82

positron emission tomography facilitate detection of multivessel coronary artery disease? Research Support, Non-U.S. Gov't. J Nucl Cardiol 2012;19(4): 670–80.

14. Fukushima K, Javadi MS, Higuchi T, et al. Prediction of short-term cardiovascular events using quantification of global myocardial flow reserve in patients referred for clinical 82Rb PET perfusion imaging. J Nucl Med 2011;52(5):726–32.

15. Herzog BA, Husmann L, Valenta I, et al. Long-term prognostic value of 13N-ammonia myocardial perfusion positron emission tomography added value of coronary flow reserve. J Am Coll Cardiol 2009; 54(2):150–6.

16. Murthy VL, Naya M, Foster CR, et al. Association between coronary vascular dysfunction and cardiac mortality in patients with and without diabetes mellitus. Circulation 2012;126(15):1858–68.

17. Murthy VL, Naya M, Foster CR, et al. Improved cardiac risk assessment with noninvasive measures of coronary flow reserve. Comparative Study Research Support, NIH, Extramural Research Support, Non-U.S. Gov't. Circulation 2011;124(20):2215–24.

18. Gupta A, Taqueti VR, van de Hoef TP, et al. Integrated noninvasive physiological assessment of coronary circulatory function and impact on cardiovascular mortality in patients with stable coronary artery disease. Circulation 2017;136(24):2325–36.

19. Taqueti VR, Hachamovitch R, Murthy VL, et al. Global coronary flow reserve is associated with adverse cardiovascular events independently of luminal angiographic severity and modifies the effect of early revascularization. Circulation 2015; 131(1):19–27.

20. Tio RA, Dabeshlim A, Siebelink HM, et al. Comparison between the prognostic value of left ventricular function and myocardial perfusion reserve in patients with ischemic heart disease. Comparative Study. J Nucl Med 2009;50(2):214–9.

21. Ziadi MC, Dekemp RA, Williams KA, et al. Impaired myocardial flow reserve on rubidium-82 positron emission tomography imaging predicts adverse outcomes in patients assessed for myocardial ischemia. Research Support, Non-U.S. Gov't. J Am Coll Cardiol 2011;58(7):740–8.

22. Gould KL, Johnson NP, Roby AE, et al. Regional, artery-specific thresholds of quantitative myocardial perfusion by PET associated with reduced myocardial infarction and death after revascularization in stable coronary artery disease. J Nucl Med 2019; 60(3):410–7.

23. Patel KK, Spertus JA, Chan PS, et al. Myocardial blood flow reserve assessed by positron emission tomography myocardial perfusion imaging identifies patients with a survival benefit from early revascularization. Eur Heart J 2019. https://doi.org/10.1093/eurheartj/ehz389.

24. Mc Ardle BA, Dowsley TF, deKemp RA, et al. Does rubidium-82 PET have superior accuracy to SPECT perfusion imaging for the diagnosis of obstructive coronary disease?: a systematic review and meta-analysis. Meta-Analysis Research Support, Non-U.S. Gov't Review. J Am Coll Cardiol 2012;60(18): 1828–37.

25. Parker MW, Iskandar A, Limone B, et al. Diagnostic accuracy of cardiac positron emission tomography versus single photon emission computed tomography for coronary artery disease: a bivariate meta-analysis. Meta-Analysis Research Support, Non-U.S. Gov't Review. Circulation Cardiovascular Imaging 2012;5(6):700–7.

26. Takx RA, Blomberg BA, El Aidi H, et al. Diagnostic accuracy of stress myocardial perfusion imaging compared to invasive coronary angiography with fractional flow reserve meta-analysis. Circ Cardiovasc Imaging 2015;8(1). https://doi.org/10.1161/CIRCIMAGING.114.002666.

27. Neglia D, Rovai D, Caselli C, et al. Detection of significant coronary artery disease by noninvasive anatomical and functional imaging. Circ Cardiovasc Imaging 2015;8(3). https://doi.org/10.1161/CIRCIMAGING.114.002179.

28. Danad I, Raijmakers PG, Driessen RS, et al. Comparison of coronary CT angiography, SPECT, PET, and hybrid imaging for diagnosis of ischemic heart disease determined by fractional flow reserve. JAMA Cardiol 2017;2(10):1100–7.

29. Driessen RS, Danad I, Stuijfzand WJ, et al. Comparison of coronary computed tomography angiography, fractional flow reserve, and perfusion imaging for ischemia diagnosis. J Am Coll Cardiol 2019;73(2):161–73.

30. Murthy VL, Naya M, Taqueti VR, et al. Effects of sex on coronary microvascular dysfunction and cardiac outcomes. Circulation 2014;129(24):2518–27.

31. Taqueti VR, Solomon SD, Shah AM, et al. Coronary microvascular dysfunction and future risk of heart failure with preserved ejection fraction. Eur Heart J 2018;39(10):840–9.

32. Collet C, Sonck J, Vandeloo B, et al. Measurement of hyperemic pullback pressure gradients to characterize patterns of coronary atherosclerosis. J Am Coll Cardiol 2019;74(14):1772–84.

33. Gould KL, Nguyen T, Johnson NP. Integrating coronary physiology, longitudinal pressure, and perfusion gradients in CAD: measurements, meaning, and mortality. J Am Coll Cardiol 2019;74(14):1785–8.

34. Patel KK, Shaw L, Spertus JA, et al. Association of sex, reduced myocardial flow reserve, and long-term mortality across spectrum of atherosclerotic disease. JACC Cardiovasc Imaging 2022;15(9):1635–44. https://doi.org/10.1016/j.jcmg.2022.03.032.

35. Taqueti VR, Shaw LJ, Cook NR, et al. Excess cardiovascular risk in women relative to men referred for

coronary angiography is associated with severely impaired coronary flow reserve, not obstructive disease. Circulation 2017;135(6):566–77. https://doi.org/10.1161/circulationaha.116.023266.

36. Ong P, Camici PG, Beltrame JF, et al. International standardization of diagnostic criteria for microvascular angina. Int J Cardiol 2018;250:16–20.

37. Taqueti VR, Di Carli MF. Coronary microvascular disease pathogenic mechanisms and therapeutic options: JACC state-of-the-art review. J Am Coll Cardiol 2018;72(21):2625–41.

38. Khuddus MA, Pepine CJ, Handberg EM, et al. An intravascular ultrasound analysis in women experiencing chest pain in the absence of obstructive coronary artery disease: a substudy from the National Heart, Lung and Blood Institute-Sponsored Women's Ischemia Syndrome Evaluation (WISE). J Interv Cardiol 2010;23(6):511–9.

39. Lee BK, Lim HS, Fearon WF, et al. Invasive evaluation of patients with angina in the absence of obstructive coronary artery disease. Circulation 2015;131(12):1054–60.

40. Naya M, Murthy VL, Foster CR, et al. Prognostic interplay of coronary artery calcification and underlying vascular dysfunction in patients with suspected coronary artery disease. J Am Coll Cardiol 2013;61(20):2098–106.

41. Lund LH, Edwards LB, Kucheryavaya AY, et al. The registry of the International Society for Heart and Lung Transplantation: thirty-first official adult heart transplant report–2014; focus theme: retransplantation. J Heart Lung Transplant 2014;33(10):996–1008.

42. Wenning C, Stypmann J, Papavassilis P, et al. Left ventricular dilation and functional impairment assessed by gated SPECT are indicators of cardiac allograft vasculopathy in heart transplant recipients. J Heart Lung Transplant 2012;31(7):719–28.

43. Chirakarnjanakorn S, Starling RC, Popovic ZB, et al. Dobutamine stress echocardiography during follow-up surveillance in heart transplant patients: diagnostic accuracy and predictors of outcomes. J Heart Lung Transplant 2015;34(5):710–7.

44. Bravo PE, Bergmark BA, Vita T, et al. Diagnostic and prognostic value of myocardial blood flow quantification as non-invasive indicator of cardiac allograft vasculopathy. Eur Heart J 2018;39(4):316–23.

45. Chih S, Chong AY, Erthal F, et al. PET assessment of epicardial intimal disease and microvascular dysfunction in cardiac allograft vasculopathy. J Am Coll Cardiol 2018;71(13):1444–56.

46. Mc Ardle BA, Davies RA, Chen L, et al. Prognostic value of rubidium-82 positron emission tomography in patients after heart transplant. Cardiovasc Imaging 2014;7(6):930–7.

What Is New in Risk Assessment in Nuclear Cardiology?

Alessia Gimelli, MD[a],*, Suvasini Lakshmanan, MD[b],
Veronica Della Tommasina, MD[c], Riccardo Liga, MD, PhD[d,e]

KEYWORDS

- Myocardial perfusion scintigraphy • Risk assessment • Coronary artery disease
- Myocardial blood flow • Innervation • Calcification • Ischemia • Inflammation

KEY POINTS

- Risk stratification of patients has a key role in modern cardiology, guiding diagnostic choices and treatment algorithms.
- Myocardial perfusion imaging with single-photon emission computed tomography (SPECT) and positron emission tomography (PET) is still the workhorse of nuclear cardiology, with the global burden of inducible myocardial ischemia (>15% of the left ventricle indicating high risk according to recent appraisals) being among the most relevant markers of cardiac risk available in modern cardiology.
- The introduction of dedicated cardiac cameras equipped with calcium zinc telluride detectors has revolutionized the field of nuclear cardiac imaging, also allowing dynamic cardiac imaging and myocardial blood flow assessment in a PET-like fashion.
- SPECT innervation imaging (^{123}I-MIBG) has demonstrated superior risk stratification abilities in key categories of patients, such as those with heart failure, where denervation is identified as a major predictor of cardiac decompensation and arrhythmogenicity at follow-up.
- Among of the recent radiotracers introduced in nuclear cardiac imaging, 18F sodium fluoride PET has shown ability to unmask microcalcifications, both at the level of great vessels and cardiac structures, which predict major cardiovascular events, and aortic stenosis progression.

INTRODUCTION

Nuclear cardiology techniques allow in-depth evaluation of cardiac patients, offering superior diagnostic and prognostic capabilities in cardiac pathologies including ischemic heart disease (IHD) and heart failure (HF). A consistent body of literature has established the use of nuclear cardiology, not only for risk stratification of patients with known or suspected coronary artery disease (CAD), but also in the setting of cardiomyopathies, infiltrative myocardial disease, cardiac inflammation, and valvular heart disease. The already excellent results obtained with traditional cameras have been further reinforced by those obtained with the implementation of a series of innovations that have gradually revolutionized the field of nuclear cardiology, including the use of novel stress agents and modern single-photon emission tomography (SPECT) technologies, such as the diffusion of dedicated cardiac cameras equipped with cadmium-zinc-telluride (CZT) detectors.

This article highlights the role of nuclear cardiology in the risk assessment of patients with different

[a] Imaging Department, Fondazione Toscana Gabriele Monasterio, Via Moruzzi, 1, Pisa, Italy; [b] University of Iowa Hospitals and Clinics, 200 Hawkins Drive, Iowa city, IA 52242, USA; [c] Cardiology Unit, Ospedale Versilia – USL Toscana Nord-Ovest, SS1 Via Aurelia n. 335 - 55049 Lido di Camaiore LU, Italy; [d] Dipartimento di Patologia Chirurgica, Medica, Molecolare e dell'Area Critica, University of Pisa, Via Savi, 10 – 56126 Pisa, Italy; [e] University Hospital of Pisa, Via Savi, 10 – 56126 Pisa, Italy
* Corresponding author.
E-mail address: gimelli@ftgm.it

Cardiol Clin 41 (2023) 197–205
https://doi.org/10.1016/j.ccl.2023.01.008
0733-8651/23/© 2023 Elsevier Inc. All rights reserved.

kinds of cardiac disease and sheds light on recent advancements of nuclear imaging techniques in the cardiovascular field.

RISK STRATIFICATION IN PATIENTS WITH KNOWN OR SUSPECTED CORONARY ARTERY DISEASE

An appropriate management of CAD patients should start from the assessment of the individual risk of future major adverse cardiac events (MACE), which is still based on the evaluation of key demographic and laboratory parameters to derive a risk score for MACE in the coming 10- to 20-years.[1,2] This approach would allow designing a more individualized treatment strategy based on an evidence-based approach, where patients with a high risk profile for MACE at follow-up would be better selected for a more aggressive management, while lower risk subjects would be treated more conservatively with optimal medical therapy only.[1] For risk stratification of patients with suspected CAD, models based on the integration of cardiac symptoms (angina and/or dyspnea) with basic demographic data have been proposed and progressively perfected. An outcome-based risk assessment model strives for improved patient outcome and avoidance of complications from unnecessary procedures, with the aim of being cost-effective. However, further refinement of patients' risk stratification algorithms is needed to improve the overall diagnostic accuracy and prediction capabilities.

Nuclear cardiology, and in particular myocardial perfusion imaging (MPI) with SPECT has been generally regarded as a reference standard for the evaluation of myocardial perfusion. It allows the evaluation of presence and severity of myocardial perfusion abnormalities while maintaining an appropriate diagnostic accuracy for the detection of functionally significant CAD even in the most complex patient categories, such as morbid obesity, respiratory failure, and inability to exercise.[3]

These concepts have been questioned by the results of several comparative studies evaluating the diagnostic ability of the different noninvasive cardiac imaging techniques for the diagnosis of significant CAD, almost invariably reporting a limited accuracy of standard SPECT. In particular, the results of the PACIFIC study reported a low sensitivity (57%) for conventional SPECT imaging in detecting significant CAD, as determined by invasive coronary angiography (ICA) + fractional flow reserve (FFR), despite a moderate specificity (84%) and overall accuracy (77%).[4] Similar results were reported by the multicenter Evaluation of

Integrated Cardiac Imaging for the Detection and Characterization of Ischemic Heart Disease (EVINCI) study, showing only a 70% overall accuracy of standard SPECT, with a modest specificity (68%). As a consequence of those data, the assessment of coronary anatomy through computed tomography coronary angiography (CTCA) has been emphasized by recent guidelines, as highlighted in the NICE recommendations[5] and then in the ESC and American Heart Association (AHA) guidelines,[2,6] all stressing on the use of CTCA rather than MPI, particularly in patients at low-intermediate pretest likelihood of CAD. The main reasons for these apparently negative results concerning SPECT MPI diagnostic accuracy for the detection of significant CAD are twofold: first, standard SPECT imaging can only demonstrate the presence of an hemodynamically significant coronary stenosis.[7] Secondly, the resolution of standard SPECT is inadequate to characterize multivessel CAD causing balanced ischemia or CAD with superimposed endothelial/microvascular dysfunction due to cardiovascular risk factors, possibly further limiting the overall accuracy of the imaging technique.

The recent introduction of dedicated cardiac cameras equipped with CZT detectors has revolutionized the field of nuclear cardiac imaging. Several studies have demonstrated that the use of CZT cameras has increased significantly the diagnostic accuracy of MPI, particularly in some of the most complex categories of patients, such as those with diffuse CAD.[8] Moreover, the higher spatial and energy resolution of CZT cameras, plus the ability to acquire in list mode, and thus to obtain dynamic acquisition in a positron emission tomography (PET)- like fashion, have paved the way to myocardial blood flow (MBF) quantitation[9,10] (**Fig. 1**).

Myocardial blood flow estimates obtained by PET provide more diagnostic[11] and prognostic[12] information than relative perfusion analysis data alone, with a decreased flow reserve on PET imaging a powerful independent predictor of cardiac mortality.[13] Furthermore, quantitative estimates of MFR obtained with PET can be useful in identifying balanced ischemia, as in patients with proximal obstructive 3-vessel CAD.[14] Finally, the evaluation of MFR can be used to reclassify patients with normal MPI as having abnormal findings, allowing a better stratification of patients at risk of MACE.[15] Considering the limited clinical implementation of PET scanners caused by consistent operational costs and relatively complex technology, the possibility of obtaining comparable values of MBF and MFR with a CZT camera could have a great impact on clinical practice.

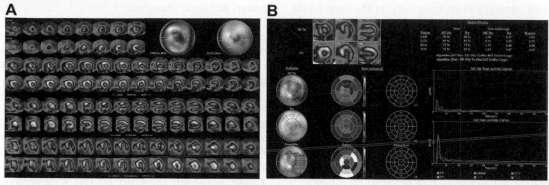

Fig. 1. A 68-year-old male patient with arterial hypertension and dyslipidemia complaining of atypical chest pain. A dynamic stress/rest single day CZT myocardial perfusion scintigraphy was performed (*A*). On quantitative myocardial perfusion analysis, a global mild MBF reduction was evident at rest (*B*). After dipyridamole infusion, MBF increased significantly in the left anterior descending (LAD) and right coronary (RCA) territories, while it remained severely impaired on the left circumflex (LCx) territory. Invasive coronary angiography showed a 90% stenosis of proximal LCx with nonobstructive CAD 50% on LAD and RCA.

The main technical limitation for quantitative perfusion imaging with CZT scanners is related to the use of 99mTc-labelled radiotracers that show a nonlinear myocardial extraction fraction, preventing the correct estimation of absolute myocardial perfusion parameters at higher flow rates. Despite this limitation, while a certain underestimation of hyperemic MBF data can be expected if compared with PET, the values of MBF and MFR obtained in all the published studies on dynamic CZT MPI seem comparable to PET and in line with invasive gold standards.

The first animal experimental study[16] showed that, compared with radioactive microspheres (being widely regarded as the gold standard for experimental measuring MBF), 201 TL or 99mTc labeled perfusion imaging agent CZT SPECT could be used to accurately measure MBF.

Accordingly, data obtained in patients with known or suspected CAD demonstrated an excellent reliability of CZT-derived myocardial perfusion parameters, increasing the accuracy of relative perfusion parameters in the detection of functionally significant CAD at ICA + FFR.[9,17]

Finally, recent data indicate that regional MBF obtained with a CZT camera could allow predicting vessels at risk of CAD progression even in the absence of obstructive CAD at baseline: an impaired regional MBF could identify those vessels that would more frequently require a late coronary revascularization.[18] Taken together, these data suggest the importance of the evaluation of MBF in a dedicated subgroup of patients, likely impacting patients' treatment strategies and possibly long-term outcome.

Those results might change the role of MPI in clinical practice. In fact, optimizing the accuracy of noninvasive imaging techniques while also

allowing the assessment of coronary functional abnormalities is gaining increasing relevance, not only in patients with CAD,[19] but in patients with microcirculatory abnormalities, where the quantitation of MBF and MFR is mandatory to stratify patient risk.[20]

The possibility of obtaining in a simple and inexpensive way an integrated assessment of semiquantitative evaluation and stress MBF and MFR might help improve the diagnostic and prognostic performances of MPI and also change the risk stratification abilities of SPECT imaging in patients with known or suspected CAD.

Last but not least, the use of machine learning techniques should be mentioned according to their impact on the prediction of MACE in patients undergoing SPECT MPI. These ML models combine clinical, stress, and imaging variables to improve prediction performance. ML models can potentially be used clinically to automatically select patients at low risk of MACE for rest scan cancellation, or improve prediction of MACE and revascularization.

Betancur and colleagues[21] developed an ML model using clinical, imaging, and stress test variables using 2689 patients from a single center, and improved MACE prediction compared with physician interpretation or quantitative analysis. This model was of great interest; however, it requires infrastructure that is not universally available, and the extracted data may still be incomplete or inaccurate.

More recently, Rios and Coll[22] showed interesting results on the use of ML models using only automatically extracted variables. According to the published results, this model had improved prognostic accuracy compared with standard interpretation methods and can be used clinically in an easy way. In the near future, the use of practical ML models combined with methods to explain risk predictions could help overcome key barriers to the broader clinical use of ML.

RISK ASSESSMENT IN PATIENTS WITH KNOWN OR SUSPECTED CORONARY ARTERY DISEASE: DOES THE EXTENT OF ISCHEMIA STILL MATTER?

The presence and increasing extent of inducible myocardial ischemia has not only represented a significant predictor of MACE,[23] but has also identified those patients who would have likely benefitted from targeted coronary revascularization.[24]

These concepts have been incorporated in current guidelines on the management of patients with chronic coronary syndromes that define as appropriate any coronary revascularization performed in the presence of greater than 10% inducible ischemia downstream.[2,6] However, the impact of revascularization on patient outcome remains controversial. In patients with multivessel disease, recent data obtained by randomized trials have potentially demonstrated a long-term better outcome with coronary artery bypass grafting (CABG) compared with percutaneous coronary intervention (PCI).[25] In line with this evidence, direct comparisons of PCI with medical therapy have failed to show a survival advantage for PCI.[26–29] In a recent observational analysis performed in patients with severe ischemia,[30] early revascularization with either PCI or CABG was associated with reduced all-cause mortality after adjusting for age and comorbidities. This was the first demonstration that the presence of severe ischemia could guide treatment choice in patients with chronic coronary syndromes, providing support for current guidelines that recommend decision making based on ischemia detection for revascularization.[2,6] Moreover, this study suggested that the presence of a myocardial ischemic burden involving more than 15% of the left ventricle would better stratify patient risk than the classic 10% threshold, also identifying those subjects who would more likely benefit from coronary revascularization. These results are concordant with the prior work of Hachamovitch and colleagues,[24] where the adjusted hazard ratios for medical therapy and revascularization lines crossed at 10% ischemia, while the 95% confidence intervals crossed at a higher ischemic threshold.

On the contrary, these findings may not seem in line with those of the ISCHEMIA trial, which used a lower ischemic threshold (>10%) to define the presence of significant inducible ischemia, possibly demonstrating why the study was unable to demonstrate any prognostic benefit of coronary revascularization in chronic coronary syndrome patients.[31,32]

There is emerging evidence that anatomy-based or combined anatomic and functional approaches to investigate patients with stable CAD may improve patient outcomes. The Scottish Computed Tomography of the Heart (SCOT-HEART) trial demonstrated that an anatomy-based approach obtained by CTCA, combined with a functional evaluation mainly by exercise testing (performed in 85% of enrolled patients) decreased rates of death or nonfatal MI compared with standard care.[33]

In the EVINCI study, the outcome of CAD patients with ischemia treated with early revascularization and of CAD patients without ischemia managed with medical treatment was comparable, further underscoring the prognostic importance of management appropriateness in chronic coronary syndromes patients at large.[19] Similarly, CAD patients without ischemia had higher event rates if they were managed with early revascularization. These data were confirmed by a recent study showing that an anatomic/functional phenotyping approach for clinical management was associated with a prognostic advantage at long-term follow-up.[34]

All these results emphasize the importance of the use of combined evaluation of coronary anatomy and ischemic burden to allow accurate disease phenotyping,[35,36] leading to targeted therapeutic intervention that might translate into a significant prognostic benefit[19,36] (**Fig. 2**).

THE ROLE OF INNERVATION IN THE EVALUATION OF RISK STRATIFICATION

Nuclear cardiac imaging techniques have traditionally represented the only way for the noninvasive evaluation of the activity of cardiac sympathetic terminals, by using specific radiotracers that are mainly analogs of catecholamines. Among those, norepinephrine analogs have traditionally represented the most widely used radiotracers for innervation imaging.

Both SPECT and PET imaging allow the evaluation of global and regional abnormalities of cardiac sympathetic activity. SPECT tracer MIBG (^{123}I-metaiodobenzilguanidine) and several PET radiotracers such as ^{11}C-metahydroxyephedrine, [^{11}C]-epinephrine, and [^{11}C]-phenylephrine are available to image cardiac sympathetic activity. A limitation of tracers labeled with ^{11}C is that because of short

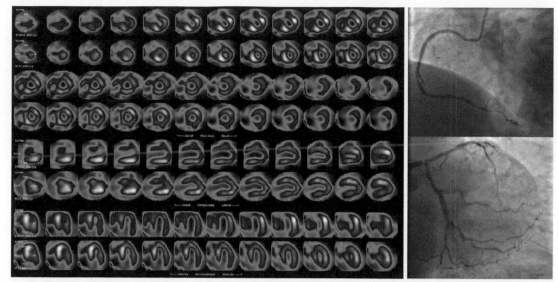

Fig. 2. A 72-year-old female patient with multiple cardiovascular risk factors, including diabetes mellitus and arterial hypertension. She complained of typical anginal chest pain. A stress/rest single day CZT myocardial perfusion scintigraphy (414 MBq, 11.2 mCi in total) was performed, showing inducible perfusion abnormalities at the level of multiple left ventricular walls, possibly indicative of hemodynamically significant multivessel CAD. Invasive coronary angiography revealed triple vessel coronary stenoses.

half-life, an onsite cyclotron is required for production, limiting their widespread use in clinical settings. Tracers labeled with the positron emitter ^{18}F have been introduced recently,[37] providing myocardial images of high quality and offering the possibility for reproducible quantification of intraneuronal retention by Patlak kinetic analysis.

Regarding SPECT imaging, MIBG ([123]I -metaiodobenzilguanidine) represents the radiotracer of reference for innervation imaging, being instrumental in demonstrating the presence of cardiac sympathetic dysfunction in different cardiac pathologies. In this context, the presence of an impaired MIBG uptake would identify patients at risk of adverse cardiac events on follow up.[38] Although planar acquisitions have been classically used to evaluate global cardiac MIBG uptake, the current imaging protocol should also include SPECT imaging to evaluate the regional distribution of the radiotracer. The application of CZT technology to innervation imaging has offered the advantage of improved image quality, repeated studies because of its low radiation exposure, and evaluation of regional myocardial MIBG kinetics in dynamic 3-dimensional datasets.[39]

Furthermore, improved spatial resolution of CZT SPECT scanners may facilitate simultaneous dual isotope evaluation of regional MIBG uptake in combination with myocardial perfusion, and this approach could be of help in patients' risk stratification, where the burden of viable myocardium with impaired innervation (innervation/perfusion mismatch) may identify patients at risk of adverse (arrhythmic) cardiac events (**Fig. 3**). However, more data are needed to be conclusive on this subject.

CARDIAC DEVICE IMPLANTATION

MIBG scintigraphy might be instrumental in the risk stratification of patients with heart failure.[40] Preliminary data seem to indicate a possible use of MIBG to identify who would benefit from ICD implantation despite the presence of borderline indications according to current guideline recommendations (ie, nonischemic dilated cardiomyopathy with left ventricular ejection fraction 30%–35%).[41] In these cases, the presence of a relatively preserved cardiac sympathetic tone might help to risk stratify high-risk patients and to eventually postpone the choice of ICD implantation.[41]

Specific interest has been given to the evaluation of cardiac sympathetic activity in patients eligible for cardiac resynchronization therapy. In these patients, the degree of sympathetic impairment predicted the magnitude of left ventricular reverse remodeling after cardiac resynchronization therapy and could, thus, identify positive responders to this therapy.[42] However, whether multiparametric nuclear cardiac imaging, comprising the evaluation of perfusion,

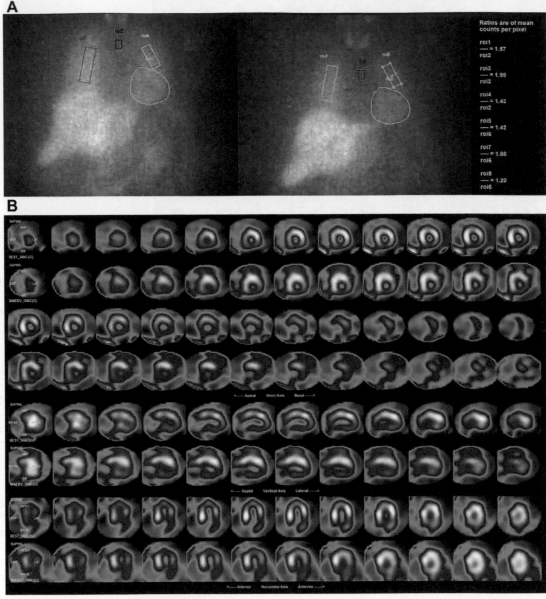

Fig. 3. A 58-year-old male patient with a history of myocarditis presenting to the emergency department because of a symptomatic sustained ventricular tachycardia. Coronary angiography was normal, and cardiac MRI excluded the recurrence of active myocardial inflammation. 123I-mIBG SPECT was performed for further characterization. Planar images demonstrated only a mildly reduced global 123I-mIBG uptake (A). Regional 123I-mIBG distribution was performed with a CZT camera and compared with myocardial perfusion. An area of inferior/inferolateral reduction in 123I-mIBG uptake was revealed, extending significantly over the region of the left ventricular scar, demonstrating the presence of a large area of innervation/perfusion mismatch (B).

dyssynchrony, and innervation, may help to identify responders to cardiac resynchronization therapy is still a matter of investigation.[43]

VENTRICULAR ARRHYTHMIAS

The evaluation of the integrity of cardiac sympathetic with MIBG scintigraphy has been classically applied for the stratification of patients at risk for ventricular arrhythmias (VA).[44]

Interestingly, patients with the highest arrhythmic risk are not necessarily those with a homogeneously depressed cardiac sympathetic activity, but rather patients showing a regionally jeopardized MIBG uptake that could possibly benefit from an ICD implantation.[45]

Moreover, the possibility to evaluate not only innervation, but also perfusion abnormalities, allows evaluation of the presence the so-called innervation/perfusion mismatch phenomenon, which, when located nearby scarred regions, has been identified as a likely source of VA. Consequently, these regions represent the ideal site for targeted therapeutic intervention, such as endocavitary ablations.

These data have been also confirmed by PET studies, which demonstrated that the presence of innervation/perfusion mismatch resulted as a major predictor of VA, colocalizing at the level of the electrically unstable border zone of a myocardial scar.[46]

CALCIFICATION IMAGING

Vascular calcification is a progressive pathologic process from which atherosclerosis originates. It is generally believed that calcified micronodules (<50 μm) are the first stage of vascular calcification that later merges into macroscopic deposits.[47] PET/CT imaging using ^{18}F-sodium fluoride (^{18}F-NaF) has been reported as the first noninvasive imaging modality to unmask vascular microcalcifications, with original studies demonstrating that ^{18}F-NaF uptake may identify culprit coronary plaques after myocardial infarction[48] and high-risk plaques on the carotid arteries.[49] Similarly, ^{18}F-NaF may unmask high-risk coronary plaques in stable CAD patients, paving the way for its possible clinical validation as a novel predictor of the future risk of a myocardial infarction. In this regard, it has been recently demonstrated that thoracic aortic ^{18}F-NaF is associated with the progression of atherosclerosis, and it was strongly associated with future coronary events (almost fivefold increased risk in patients with high uptake) but not ischemic stroke.

An innovative application of ^{18}F-NaF imaging has been the assessment of patients with aortic stenosis for the identification of subclinical valvular degeneration, either native or prosthetic, and the prediction of progressive deterioration of all the conventional echocardiographic measures.[50]

As in other aspects of nuclear cardiology, novel technical advancements (ie, PET/MR) will likely increase the diagnostic capabilities of ^{18}F-NaF imaging,[51] possibly extending its fields of application even further.[52] However, well-powered dedicated prospective studies will be needed to demonstrate the real clinical additive value of this innovative imaging technique.

SUMMARY

Accurate risk stratification of patients has a key role in modern precision medicine to guide downstream diagnostic and therapeutic interventions. In this regard, nuclear cardiac imaging techniques may quantitatively investigate major disease mechanisms of different cardiac pathologies, allowing the detection of early stages of cardiac and vascular diseases and, thus, identifying patients who would most likely benefit from early therapies, possibly directed at a subclinical stage of the underlying disease.

CLINICS CARE POINTS

- The management of patients with suspected CAD has varied greatly in the last decades, with most recent clinical guidelines favouring ICA only in patients with high-risk findings on non-invasive cardiac imaging.

- According to latest appraisals conventional SPECT imaging has a relatively lower accuracy than PET in unmasking the presence of hemodynamically significant CAD at ICA + FFR.

- The evidence of an area of ischemia >10% of the LV myocardium on MPI puts the patients at high risk of future adverse cardiac events (cardiac mortality >3% per year).

- Alterations of myocardial sympathetic innervation may be revealed already in the early stages of different cardiac pathologies - i.e., heart failure, cardiomyopathies - or as a result of some cardiovascular risk factors, such as arterial hypertension or diabetes mellitus.

- Vascular and even valvular (i.e., aortic valve) microcalcifications can be readily imaged with ^{18}F-NaF PET, possibly identifying high-risk coronary plaques.

DISCLOSURE

The authors have nothing to disclose.

REFERENCES

1. Visseren FLJ, MacH F, Smulders YM, et al. 2021 ESC guidelines on cardiovascular disease prevention in clinical practice. Eur Heart J 2021;42(34):3227–337.
2. Knuuti J, Saraste A, Capodanno D, et al. 2019 ESC guidelines for the diagnosis and management of chronic coronary syndromes. The Task Force for the Diagnosis and Management of Chronic Coronary Syndromes of the European Society of Cardiology (ESC). Eur Hear J 2020;41:407–77.
3. Verberne HJ, Acampa W, Anagnostopoulos C, et al. EANM procedural guidelines for radionuclide myocardial perfusion imaging with SPECT and

SPECT/CT: 2015 revision. Eur J Nucl Med Mol Imaging 2015;42:1929–40.

4. Danad I, Raijmakers PG, Driessen RS, et al. Comparison of coronary CT angiography, SPECT, PET, and hybrid imaging for diagnosis of ischemic heart disease determined by fractional flow reserve. JAMA Cardiol 2017;2:1100–10.

5. National Institute for Health and Clinical Excellence. Chest pain of recent onset: assessment and diagnosis of recent onset chest pain or discomfort of suspected cardiac origin. CG95. London: National Institute for Health and Clinical Excellence; 2010. Last Updated 2016. https://www.nice.org.uk/guidance/CG95. Accessed February 2023.

6. Gulati M, Levy PD, Mukherjee D, et al. 2021 AHA/ACC/ASE/CHEST/SAEM/SCCT/SCMR guideline for the evaluation and diagnosis of chest pain: a report of the American College of Cardiology/American Heart Association Joint Committee on Clinical Practice Guidelines. JACC (J Am Coll Cardiol) 2021; 78(22):221.

7. Herscovici R, Sedlak T, Wei J, et al. Ischemia and no obstructive coronary artery disease (INOCA): what is the risk? J Am Heart Assoc 2018;7:e008868.

8. Gimelli A, Liga R, Duce V, et al. Accuracy of myocardial perfusion imaging in detecting multivessel coronary artery disease: a cardiac CZT study. J Nucl Cardiol 2017;24:687–95.

9. Zavadovsky KV, Mochula AV, Boshchenko AA, et al. Absolute myocardial blood flows derived by dynamic CZT scan vs invasive fractional flow reserve: correlation and accuracy. J Nucl Cardiol 2021; 28(1):249–59.

10. Acampa W, Assante R, Mannarino T, et al. Low-dose dynamic myocardial perfusion imaging by CZT-SPECT in the identification of obstructive coronary artery disease. Eur J Nucl Med Mol Imaging 2020; 47(7):1705–12.

11. Valenta I, Dilsizian V, Quercioli A, et al. Quantitative PET/CT measures of myocardial flow reserve and atherosclerosis for cardiac risk assessment and predicting adverse patient outcomes. Curr Cardiol Rep 2013;15:344.

12. Herzog BA, Husmann L, Valenta I, et al. Long-term prognostic value of 13N-ammonia myocardial perfusion positron emission tomography. Added value of coronary flow reserve. J Am Coll Cardiol 2009;54:150–6.

13. Murthy VL, Naya M, Foster CR, et al. Improved cardiac risk assessment with noninvasive measures of coronary flow reserve. Circulation 2011;124:2215.

14. Ziadi MC, DeKemp RA, Williams K, et al. Does quantification of myocardial flow reserve using rubidium-82 positron emission tomography facilitate detection of multivessel coronary artery disease? J Nucl Cardiol 2012;19:670–768.

15. Fiechter M, Ghadri JR, Gebhard C, et al. Diagnostic value of 13N-ammonia myocardial perfusion PET:

added value of myocardial flow reserve. J Nucl Med 2012;53:1230–1.

16. Wells RG, Timmins R, Klein R, et al. Dynamic SPECT measurement of absolute myocardial blood flow in a porcine model. J Nucl Med 2014;55:1685–91.

17. Agostini D, Roule V, Nganoa C, et al. First validation of myocardial flow reserve assessed by dynamic 99mTc-sestamibi CZT-SPECT camera: head to head comparison with 15O-water PET and fractional flow reserve in patients with suspected coronary artery disease. The WATERDAY study. Eur J Nucl Med Mol Imaging 2018;45(7):1079–90. Available at: http://link.springer.com/10.1007/s00259-018-3958-7.

18. Liga R, Neglia D, Kusch A, et al. Prognostic role of dynamic CZT imaging in CAD patients: interaction between absolute flow and CAD burden. JACC (J Am Coll Cardiol): Cardiovascular Imaging 2022; 15(3):540–2.

19. Neglia D, Liga R, Caselli C, et al. Anatomical and functional coronary imaging to predict long-term outcome in patients with suspected coronary artery disease: the EVINCI-outcome study. Eur Heart J Cardiovasc Imaging 2020;21(11):1273–82.

20. Taqueti VR, Shaw LJ, Cook NR, et al. Excess cardiovascular risk in women relative to men referred for coronary angiography is associated with severely impaired coronary flow reserve, not obstructive disease. Circulation 2017;135:566–657.

21. Betancur J, Otaki Y, Motwani M, et al. Prognostic value of combined clinical and myocardial perfusion imaging data using machine learning. JACC Cardiovasc Imaging 2018;11(7):1000–9.

22. Rios R, Miller RJH, Hu LH, et al. Determining a minimum set of variables for machine learning cardiovascular event prediction: results from REFINE SPECT registry. Cardiovasc Res 2022;118(9):2152–64.

23. Gehi AK, Ali S, Na B, et al. Inducible ischemia and the risk of recurrent cardiovascular events in outpatients with stable coronary heart disease: the heart and soul study. Arch Intern Med 2008;168:1423–8.

24. Hachamovitch R, Rozanski A, Shaw LJ, et al. Impact of ischaemia and scar on the therapeutic benefit derived from myocardial revascularization vs. medical therapy among patients undergoing stress-rest myocardial perfusion scintigraphy. Eur Heart J 2011;32:1012–24.

25. Doenst T, Haverich A, Serruys P, et al. PCI and CABG for treating stable coronary artery disease. J Am Coll Cardiol 2019;73:964–76.

26. Boden WE, O'Rourke RA, Teo KK, et al. Optimal medical therapy with or without PCI for stable coronary disease. N Engl J Med 2007;356:1503–11.

27. Al-Lamee R, Thompson D, Dehbi HM, et al. Percutaneous coronary intervention in stable angina (ORBITA): a double-blind, randomised controlled trial. Lancet 2018;391:31–40.

28. Cleland JGF, Calvert M, Freemantle N, et al. The heart failure revascularisation trial (HEART). Eur J Heart Fail 2011;391:31–40.

29. Stergiopoulos K, Boden WE, Hartigan P, et al. Percutaneous coronary intervention outcomes in patients with stable obstructive coronary artery disease and myocardial ischemia. JAMA Intern Med 2014;174: 232–40.

30. Miller RJH, Bonow RO, Gransar H, et al. Percutaneous or surgical revascularization is associated with survival benefit in stable coronary artery disease. Eur Heart J Cardiovasc Imaging 2020;21: 961–97.

31. Hochman JS, Reynolds HR, Bangalore S, et al. Baseline characteristics and risk profiles of participants in the ISCHEMIA randomized clinical trial. JAMA Cardiol 2019;4:273–86.

32. Maron DJ, Hochman JS, Reynolds HR, et al. Initial invasive or conservative strategy for stable coronary disease. N Engl J Med 2020;382:1395–404.

33. Investigators S-H. Coronary CT angiography and 5-year risk of myocardial infarction. N Engl J Med 2018;379:924–33.

34. Liga R, Neglia D, Cavaleri S, et al. Prognostic impact of patients' management based on anatomic/functional phenotype: a study in patients with chronic coronary syndromes. J Nucl Cardiol 2022. https://doi.org/10.1007/s12350-022-03070-w.

35. De Bruyne B, Fearon WF, Pijls NHJ, et al. Fractional flow reserve–guided PCI for stable coronary artery disease. N Engl J Med 2014;371(13):12.

36. Liga R, Vontobel J, Rovai D, et al. Multicentre multidevice hybrid imaging study of coronary artery disease: results from the EValuation of INtegrated Cardiac Imaging for the Detection and Characterization of Ischaemic Heart Disease (EVINCI) hybrid imaging population. Eur Heart J Cardiovasc Imaging 2016;17(9):951.

37. Werner RA, Rischpler C, Onthank D, et al. Retention kinetics of the 18F-labeled sympathetic nerve PET tracer LMI1195: comparison with 11C-hydroxyephedrine and 123I-MIBG. J Nucl Med 2015;56(9): 1429–33.

38. Jacobson AF, Senior R, Cerqueira MD, et al. Myocardial iodine-123 meta-iodobenzylguanidine imaging and cardiac events in heart failure. Results of the prospective ADMIRE-HF (AdreView myocardial imaging for risk evaluation in heart failure) study. J Am Coll Cardiol 2010;55:2212–22.

39. Gimelli A, Liga R, Giorgetti A, et al. Assessment of myocardial adrenergic innervation with a solid-state dedicated cardiac cadmium-zinc-telluride camera: first clinical experience. Eur Heart J Cardiovasc Imaging 2014;15:575–85.

40. Nakajima K, Nakata T, Yamada T, et al. A prediction model for 5-year cardiac mortality in patients with chronic heart failure using 123I-metaiodobenzylguanidine imaging. Eur J Nucl Med Mol Imaging 2014; 41:1673–82.

41. Køber L, Thune JJ, Nielsen JC, et al. Defibrillator implantation in patients with nonischemic systolic heart failure. N Engl J Med 2016;375:1221–3.

42. Moreira RI, Abreu A, Portugal G, et al. Prognostic effect and modulation of cardiac sympathetic function in heart failure patients treated with cardiac resynchronization therapy. J Nucl Cardiol 2020;27:283–329.

43. Gimelli A, Liga R, Menichetti F, et al. Interactions between myocardial sympathetic denervation and left ventricular mechanical dyssynchrony: a CZT analysis. J Nucl Cardiol 2019;26(2):509–18.

44. Jacobson AF, Senior R, Cerqueira MD, et al. Myocardial iodine-123 meta-iodobenzylguanidine imaging and cardiac events in heart failure. Results of the prospective ADMIRE-HF (AdreView myocardial imaging for risk evaluation in heart failure) study. J Am Coll Cardiol 2010;55(20):2212–21.

45. Travin MI, Henzlova MJ, van Eck-Smit BLF, et al. Assessment of 123I-mIBG and 99mTc-tetrofosmin single-photon emission computed tomographic images for the prediction of arrhythmic events in patients with ischemic heart failure: intermediate severity innervation defects are associated with higher arrhythm. J Nucl Cardiol 2017;24:377–91.

46. Sasano T, Abraham MR, Chang KC, et al. Abnormal sympathetic innervation of viable myocardium and the substrate of ventricular tachycardia after myocardial infarction. J Am Coll Cardiol 2008;51: 2266–7.

47. Irkle A, Vesey AT, Lewis DY, et al. Identifying active vascular microcalcification by 18F-sodium fluoride positron emission tomography. Nat Commun 2015; 6:7495.

48. Joshi NV, Vesey AT, Williams MC, et al. 18F-fluoride positron emission tomography for identification of ruptured and high-risk coronary atherosclerotic plaques: a prospective clinical trial. Lancet 2014;383: P705.

49. Tzolos E, Dweck MR. 18F-Sodium fluoride (18F-NaF) for imaging microcalcification activity in the cardiovascular system. Arterioscler Thromb Vasc Biol 2020;40:1620–6.

50. Cartlidge TRG, Doris MK, Sellers SL, et al. Detection and prediction of bioprosthetic aortic valve degeneration. J Am Coll Cardiol 2019;73(10):110.

51. Andrews JPM, MacNaught G, Moss AJ, et al. Cardiovascular 18F-fluoride positron emission tomography-magnetic resonance imaging: a comparison study. J Nucl Cardiol 2021;28(5):1–12.

52. Andrews JPM, Trivieri MG, Everett R, et al. 18F-fluoride PET/MR in cardiac amyloid: a comparison study with aortic stenosis and age- and sex-matched controls. J Nucl Cardiol 2022;29(2):741–9.

Radionuclide Assessment of Sarcoidosis

Sanjay Divakaran, MD[a,b],*

KEYWORDS

- Cardiac sarcoidosis • Fluorodeoxyglucose (FDG) • Metabolic imaging • PET • Sarcoidosis
- Single-photon emission computed tomography (SPECT)

KEY POINTS

- The prevalence of cardiac involvement in patients with sarcoidosis is thought to be between 5% and 25%.
- Radionuclide imaging plays a critical role in establishing the diagnosis of cardiac sarcoidosis and in following the response to therapy.
- Prior studies have also shown the value of myocardial perfusion/metabolism imaging in risk stratification in cardiac sarcoidosis.

INTRODUCTION

Sarcoidosis is an inflammatory condition that can affect multiple organ systems.[1] It is characterized by non-caseating granulomatous inflammation and involves the pulmonary or reticuloendothelial system in 90% of cases.[2] The prevalence of cardiac involvement in patients with sarcoidosis is thought to be between 5% and 25%.[3–5] The hallmarks of cardiac sarcoidosis are heart failure or cardiomyopathy, atrioventricular nodal disease, and ventricular arrhythmia.[6] Radionuclide assessment is a vital component of management in suspected or known cases of cardiac sarcoidosis. Myocardial perfusion imaging (single-photon emission computed tomography/computed tomography, SPECT/CT, or PET/CT) and cardiac PET/ CT metabolic imaging play critical roles in establishing the diagnosis of cardiac sarcoidosis and following response to therapy.[7] Prior studies have also shown the value of radionuclide assessment of myocardial perfusion and metabolism in sarcoidosis in risk stratification. Finally, novel tracers bring the potential opportunity to improve the patient experience during metabolic imaging and improve the diagnostic accuracy of current

techniques. This review provides an overview of the techniques used in nuclear cardiology for the assessment of suspected or known cardiac sarcoidosis, how studies assist with regard to diagnosis, risk stratification, and monitoring response to therapy, and work that is on the horizon with novel tracers.

DISCUSSION
Technique and Interpretation

SPECT/CT or PET/CT myocardial perfusion imaging and cardiac perfusion and metabolism PET/CT imaging have contemporary roles in the diagnosis and management of cardiac sarcoidosis. [67]Gallium (^{67}Ga) imaging was used in the past to identify cardiac and extracardiac inflammation from active sarcoidosis. However, low sensitivity for cardiac sarcoidosis and the challenge of distinguishing myocardial versus pulmonary/mediastinal ^{67}Ga uptake (on SPECT without CT) have limited its use in present-day practice despite still having a presence in current guidelines.[8–10]

The exclusion of flow-limiting epicardial coronary artery disease is an important initial step in the assessment of suspected cardiac sarcoidosis

[a] Division of Cardiovascular Medicine and Cardiovascular Imaging Program, Brigham and Women's Hospital, 75 Francis Street, Boston, MA 02115, USA; [b] Harvard Medical School, Boston, MA, USA
* Corresponding author. Division of Cardiovascular Medicine and Cardiovascular Imaging Program, Brigham and Women's Hospital, 75 Francis Street, Boston, MA 02115.
E-mail address: sdivakaran@bwh.harvard.edu
Twitter: @sanjaydivakaran (S.D.)

Cardiol Clin 41 (2023) 207–215
https://doi.org/10.1016/j.ccl.2023.01.009
0733-8651/23/© 2023 Elsevier Inc. All rights reserved.

by radionuclide imaging. Both perfusion and metabolism abnormalities can be present in the setting of obstructive coronary disease. Rest perfusion abnormalities can be seen in cardiac sarcoidosis via [201]thallium and [99m]tecnetium SPECT/CT imaging. In addition, there is some literature that suggests resting perfusion defects can improve in cardiac sarcoidosis with vasodilator stress.[11,12] The utility of perfusion SPECT/CT imaging is highest when combined with metabolic PET/CT imaging. This is often done in centers where perfusion PET/CT is unavailable, or if insurance reimbursement for perfusion/metabolism PET/CT is a challenge. Areas of perfusion-metabolic mismatch (abnormal perfusion but increased fluorodeoxyglucose (FDG) uptake) are highly suggestive of inflammation.

Dietary preparation before imaging is critical for diagnostic metabolism PET/CT images for the evaluation of cardiac sarcoidosis. Normal myocardial cells have a variable affinity for glucose, depending on the dietary state, and therefore the presence of physiologic FDG uptake can render a study non-diagnostic. Unlike myocardial cells, inflammatory cells take up glucose in an insulin-independent fashion. Therefore, using dietary manipulation to create a low insulin state will promote myocardial free fatty acid metabolism. The goal is to have no background myocardial uptake of FDG so that if present, FDG uptake can be attributed to myocardial inflammation. Centers have different protocols for patient preparation, but the mainstays are at least two high-fat/low-carbohydrate meals the day before imaging, a prolonged fast, no exercise for 24 h before imaging, and a food log review the day of imaging by a technologist, nurse, or physician (**Table 1**).[13] Other methods used for patient preparation at some centers include intravenous unfractionated heparin infusion to induce lipolysis and increase free fatty acid levels and protein drinks just before imaging.

A typical perfusion/metabolism imaging protocol is shown in **Fig. 1**. After dietary preparation and food log review, rest perfusion imaging is performed with ^{13}N-ammonia or [82]Rubidium PET/CT or [99m]tecnetium or [201]thalium SPECT, ideally with CT attenuation correction (SPECT/CT). Rest-gated perfusion imaging should also be obtained at this time. After perfusion imaging, approximately 8 to 10 mCi of intravenous FDG is administered.[14] Dedicated, non-gated cardiac FDG PET/CT imaging, also ideally with attenuation correction, is acquired 90 min after injection (minimum 60 min) over 10 to 30 min depending on scanner properties and image acquisition mode. After cardiac metabolism imaging, whole-body FDG PET/CT image acquisition is performed using the same FDG injection and should include at least the chest and abdomen.

Detailed guidance regarding image interpretation can be found in the American Society of Nuclear Cardiology (ASNC)/Society of Nuclear Medicine and Molecular Imaging (SNMMI) guidelines.[7,14] After quality checks, visual interpretation includes assessing for the presence of perfusion abnormalities, focal FDG uptake, and the presence of regions of perfusion-metabolism mismatch in the left ventricle. Visual interpretation also includes assessing the dedicated cardiac imaging for right ventricular or atrial FDG uptake and interpretation of wall motion and left ventricular (LV) systolic function via rest-gated acquisition. Quantitative myocardial assessment of inflammation includes measuring the maximum standardized uptake value (SUV_{max}) in the myocardium and the volume of inflamed myocardium above an SUV threshold. Other metrics include the coefficient of variation, which is a marker of heterogeneous FDG uptake[15] and cardiometabolic activity, calculated as the volume of inflammation multiplied by the mean SUV_{max} of the involved myocardium (**Figs. 2 and 3**).[16]

Diagnosis

The utility of radionuclide imaging in the diagnosis of cardiac sarcoidosis is displayed in the 2017 Japanese Circulation Society (JCS) criteria[17] and the 2014 Heart Rhythm Society (HRS) expert consensus statement on cardiac sarcoidosis (**Table 2**).[18] In the JCS criteria, one of the major clinical criteria is abnormal myocardial uptake of ^{67}Ga or FDG. In the HRS criteria, if a patient has histologically confirmed extracardiac sarcoidosis, then cardiac involvement is probable (among other non-radionuclide imaging-based criteria) if myocardial FDG uptake is present on PET/CT in a pattern consistent with cardiac sarcoidosis or there is ^{67}Ga uptake in a pattern consistent with cardiac sarcoidosis.

As above, the HRS criteria delineate that the abnormalities on radionuclide imaging should be "in a pattern consistent with cardiac sarcoidosis." Radionuclide imaging findings suggestive of cardiac sarcoidosis include multiple noncontiguous perfusion abnormalities without associated FDG uptake, focal or focal on diffuse FDG uptake associated with a resting perfusion abnormality, multiple noncontiguous perfusion defects with associated FDG uptake (perfusion/metabolism mismatch), or multiple areas of focal FDG uptake and the presence of extracardiac FDG uptake.[19,20] Combining radionuclide imaging findings with cardiac MRI findings (such as the presence of late gadolinium enhancement (LGE) at the right ventricular insertion points with direct and contiguous extension across

Table 1
Patient preparation recommendations before fluorodeoxyglucose PET/computed tomography imaging in sarcoidosis

	Recommendation
Consume	• Meat fried in oil or butter without breading or broiled (chicken, turkey, bacon, meat-only sausage, hamburgers, steak, and fish) • Eggs (prepared without milk or cheese) • Oil (an option for patients who are vegan or are unable to eat and have enteral access) and butter • Clear liquids (water, tea, coffee, and diet sodas)
Acceptable	• Fasting for ≥18 h if the patient cannot eat and has no enteral access or if the patient has dietary restrictions preventing consumption of the advised diet
Avoid	• Vegetables, beans, nuts, fruits, and juices • Bread, grain, rice, pasta, and all baked goods • Sweetened, grilled, or cured meats or meat with carbohydrate-containing additives (some sausages, ham, and sweetened bacon) • Dairy products (milk and cheese) aside from butter • Candy, gum, lozenges, sugar, and sucralose • Alcoholic beverages, soda, and sports drinks • Mayonnaise, ketchup, tartar sauce, mustard, and other condiments • Dextrose-containing intravenous medications

From Chareonthaitawee P, Beanlands RS, Chen W, et al. Joint SNMMI-ASNC expert consensus document on the role of. J Nucl Cardiol. 10 2017;24(5):1741–1758.

the septum into the right ventricle) has been shown to have complementary value.[19]

Listed in **Box 1** are clinical scenarios in which referral for FDG PET/CT may be helpful in cases of suspected or known cardiac sarcoidosis.[7] In addition to offering complementary diagnostic utility, FDG PET/CT is particularly useful if cardiac MRI is suggestive of cardiac sarcoidosis to assess the presence of baseline myocardial inflammation and potentially identify FDG-avid extracardiac tissue that may be amenable to biopsy.

Risk stratification

In addition to a key role in the diagnosis of cardiac sarcoidosis, radionuclide imaging findings have prognostic value in patients with suspected and known cardiac sarcoidosis. In a retrospective study of 197 patients referred for FDG PET for suspected cardiac sarcoidosis not on immunosuppression at the University of Michigan, reduced left ventricular ejection fraction (LVEF), history of ventricular arrhythmia, and summed rest score (SRS) were associated with adverse events in a multivariable model.[21] In the subgroup of patients who met HRS criteria for the diagnosis of cardiac sarcoidosis (n = 52), only SRS was associated with adverse events. Of note, only 19 patients (10%) met the Japanese Ministry of Health and Welfare (JMHW) criteria for cardiac sarcoidosis

and only 64 (33%) had known histologically proven extracardiac sarcoidosis.[22]

In a retrospective study of 118 patients referred for FDG PET for suspected cardiac sarcoidosis at Brigham and Women's Hospital, the annualized rate of all-cause mortality or sustained ventricular tachycardia was 7.3%, 18.4%, and 31.9% for patients with normal myocardial perfusion and no myocardial FDG uptake, abnormal myocardial perfusion or focal myocardial FDG uptake, and abnormal myocardial perfusion and focal myocardial FDG uptake, respectively.[23] In one multivariable analysis from this study that included LVEF, JMHW criteria, and pattern of FDG PET abnormality, the presence of abnormal myocardial perfusion and focal FDG uptake had the strongest association with the composite outcome of all-cause mortality or sustained ventricular tachycardia. In another multivariable analysis from this study that included focal right ventricular FDG uptake, LVEF, and JMHW criteria, focal right ventricular FDG uptake remained associated with the composite outcome of all-cause mortality or sustained ventricular tachycardia. The cohort in this study consisted of 38 patients (34%) who met JMHW criteria and 30 (26%) who had histologically proven cardiac or extracardiac sarcoidosis.

In a study of 51 patients with suspected cardiac sarcoidosis who underwent hybrid FDG PET imaging and cardiac MRI at Barts Heart Centre, the

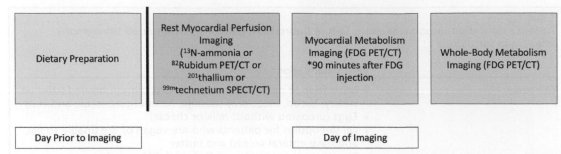

| Dietary Preparation | Rest Myocardial Perfusion Imaging (^{13}N-ammonia or ^{82}Rubidum PET/CT or ^{201}thallium or ^{99m}technetium SPECT/CT) | Myocardial Metabolism Imaging (FDG PET/CT) *90 minutes after FDG injection | Whole-Body Metabolism Imaging (FDG PET/CT) |

| Day Prior to Imaging | Day of Imaging |

Fig. 1. Recommended perfusion/metabolism imaging protocol. After at least two high-fat/low-carbohydrate meals the day before imaging, a prolonged fast, no exercise for 24 h before imaging, and a food log review the day of imaging by a technologist, nurse, or physician, patients undergo rest myocardial perfusion imaging. Then, 90 min after FDG administration, dedicated cardiac metabolic PET/CT is performed followed by whole-body imaging. SPECT, single-photon emission computed tomography.

presence of right ventricular FDG uptake and LGE on cardiac MRI were independent predictors of all-cause mortality, aborted sudden cardiac death, sustained ventricular arrhythmia, complete heart block, or heart failure hospitalization.[24] Thirty-three (65%) patients in this study met JMHW criteria and all patients had histologically proven cardiac sarcoidosis or extracardiac sarcoidosis. Finally, in a retrospective study of 203 patients referred for FDG PET imaging for suspected cardiac sarcoidosis at the Cleveland Clinic, the coefficient of variation and SRS in segments with abnormal myocardial FDG uptake were significantly associated with a composite endpoint of

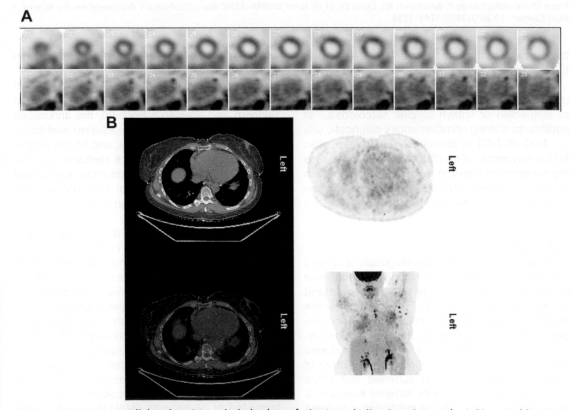

Fig. 2. Negative myocardial and positive whole-body perfusion/metabolism imaging study. A 61-year-old woman with biopsy-proven reticuloendothelial sarcoidosis and abnormal cardiac MRI was referred for a myocardial perfusion SPECT/CT and metabolism PET/CT study to evaluate for myocardial inflammation. (*A*). Dedicated cardiac imaging (top row = perfusion; bottom row = metabolism) shows normal myocardial perfusion and no evidence of focal myocardial inflammation. (*B*). Whole-body imaging shows extracardiac inflammation involving the lungs, spleen, and lymph nodes.

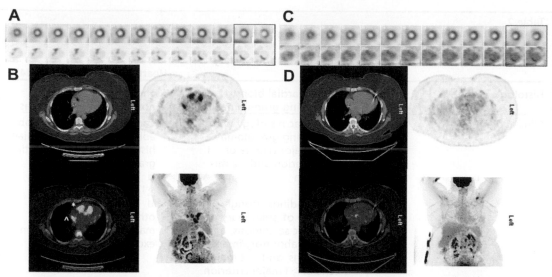

Fig. 3. Positive myocardial and negative whole-body perfusion/metabolism imaging study and response to therapy. A 53-year-old woman with biopsy-proven pulmonary sarcoidosis, uveitis, and cardiac sarcoidosis by cardiac MRI and a history of ventricular tachycardia was referred for a myocardial perfusion SPECT/CT and metabolism PET/CT to evaluate for myocardial inflammation. The patient was on methotrexate therapy at the time of imaging. In panels A and C, top row = perfusion; bottom row = metabolism. (A). Rest myocardial perfusion images showed a small-sized perfusion defect of moderate intensity involving the basal inferoseptal wall with corresponding FDG uptake (perfusion-metabolism mismatch; red box). There was also focal FDG uptake in the mid-inferoseptal wall and mid-anteroseptal wall of the left ventricle. Myocardial SUV_{max} was 20.5. Volume of inflamed myocardium using an SUV threshold of 2.7 was 114.4 cc. (B). There was also focal FDG uptake involving the right ventricular free wall (*) and the right atrium (). There was no evidence of extracardiac inflammation. (C). The patient returned for a repeat assessment 6 months after starting therapy with infliximab. There was a small perfusion defect of moderate intensity involving the basal inferoseptal wall with corresponding FDG uptake (perfusion-metabolic mismatch; red box). Both intensity and extent of myocardial inflammation were markedly reduced when compared with the prior study: myocardial SUV_{max} was 3.7 and the volume of inflamed myocardium using an SUV threshold of 2.7 was 0.6 cc. (D). There was no evidence of right ventricular, right atrial, or extracardiac inflammation.

all-cause death, cardiac transplantation, or ventricular arrhythmia requiring defibrillation after multivariable adjustment.[25] Thirty (15%) patients met JMHW criteria in this study and 146 (72%) had histologically proven extracardiac sarcoidosis.

Monitoring response to therapy

In addition to assisting in the diagnosis of cardiac sarcoidosis and identifying imaging biomarkers of risk, radionuclide imaging is used clinically to assess response to immunosuppressive therapy over time.[26] Changes in visual assessment of perfusion and metabolism, quantified intensity and volume of myocardial inflammation, LV systolic function, and extracardiac inflammation can be assessed serially by radionuclide imaging.[7] Importantly, this can be done in patients who have a cardiac implantable electronic device that may not be MRI conditional.

However, the data supporting the use of serial assessment by FDG PET/CT are limited/emerging.[27] In a study of 23 patients with cardiac sarcoidosis followed by a total of 90 serial FDG PET studies (median four per patient) over a median of 2.0 years at Brigham and Women's Hospital, the investigators found a significant inverse linear relationship between myocardial SUV_{max} and LVEF and volume of inflamed myocardium and LVEF using SUV thresholds of 2.7 and 4.1.[28] In a study of 20 patients with cardiac sarcoidosis who underwent catheter ablation for ventricular tachycardia with 92 serial FDG PET studies (3–10 per patient), lack of improvement in metabolic activity was the only variable associated with a composite endpoint of mortality, heart transplantation, hospitalization for heart failure, or implantable cardioverter defibrillator appropriate interventions.[29,30] In a study of 34 patients with cardiac sarcoidosis that included 128 FDG PET studies (median three per patient), 94 studies (73%) resulted in a change in therapy.[31] In a study that included 32 patients with cardiac sarcoidosis (17 meeting HRS criteria) who underwent FDG PET imaging before and after therapy with prednisone, 26 had a ≥ 25% reduction in myocardial SUV_{max} of

Table 2
Comparison of contemporary diagnostic criteria for cardiac sarcoidosis

	Japanese Circulation Society (2017)	Heart Rhythm Society (2014)
Histologic diagnosis	• Endomyocardial biopsy: noncaseating granulomas	• Endomyocardial biopsy: noncaseating granulomas
Clinical diagnosis	• Extracardiac histology with noncaseating granulomas and ≥2 major criteria or ≥1 major criterion and ≥2 minor criteria or • Clinical findings strongly suggestive of pulmonary or ophthalmic sarcoidosis, at least two laboratory/imaging findings, and ≥ 2 major criteria or ≥1 major criterion and ≥2 minor criteria	• Cardiac sarcoidosis is probable if there is extracardiac histology with noncaseating granulomas and • ≥1 clinical criterion and • other causes of cardiac manifestations have been excluded
Clinical criteria	1. Major a. High-grade atrioventricular block or fatal ventricular arrhythmia b. Basal thinning of the ventricular septum or abnormal ventricular wall anatomy c. Left ventricular ejection fraction < 50% d. Abnormal myocardial ^{67}Ga or FDG uptake e. Myocardial LGE by cardiac MRI 2. Minor f. ECG: NSVT, multifocal or frequent PVCs, bundle branch block, axis deviation, or abnormal Q-waves g. SPECT perfusion defects h. Endomyocardial biopsy: monocyte infiltration and moderate or severe myocardial interstitial fibrosis	1. Cardiomyopathy or heart block responsive to immunosuppression 2. Unexplained left ventricular ejection fraction <40% 3. Unexplained sustained ventricular tachycardia (spontaneous or induced) 4. Mobitz type II second-degree heart block or third-degree heart block 5. Patchy uptake on dedicated cardiac PET in a pattern consistent with cardiac sarcoidosis 6. LGE on cardiac MRI in a pattern consistent with cardiac sarcoidosis 7. Positive gallium uptake in a pattern consistent with cardiac sarcoidosis
Laboratory/imaging criteria	1. Bilateral hilar lymphadenopathy 2. High serum angiotensin-converting enzyme activity or elevated serum lysozyme levels 3. High serum soluble interleukin-2 receptor levels 4. Significant tracer accumulation in ^{67}Ga scintigraphy or FDG PET	

(continued on next page)

	Japanese Circulation Society (2017)	Heart Rhythm Society (2014)
	5. A high percentage of lymphocytes with a CD4/CD8 ratio of >3.5 in BAL fluid	
Isolated cardiac sarcoidosis	• Endomyocardial biopsy: noncaseating granulomas or • Clinical criterion (d) and ≥3 other major criteria	• Endomyocardial biopsy: noncaseating granulomas

Table 2
(continued)

Abbreviation: BAL, bronchoalveolar lavage; ECG, electrocardiogram; FDG, fluorodeoxyglucose; LGE, late gadolinium enhancement; MRI, magnetic resonance imaging; NSVT, nonsustained ventricular tachycardia; PVCs, premature ventricular contractions; SPECT, single-photon emission computed tomography.

Adapted from Terasaki F, Yoshinaga K. New Guidelines for Diagnosis of Cardiac Sarcoidosis in Japan. Annals of Nuclear Cardiology. 2017;3(1):42 to 45 and Birnie DH, Sauer WH, Bogun F, et al. HRS expert consensus statement on the diagnosis and management of arrhythmias associated with cardiac sarcoidosis. Heart Rhythm. Jul 2014;11(7):1305 to 23.

which 14 had complete resolution of myocardial inflammation.[32] Finally, in one study that included 91 patients with cardiac sarcoidosis in the final analysis, cox regression analysis identified the following independent baseline FDG PET/CT predictors of treatment response: LVEF > 40% (hazard ratio [HR]: 1.61; 95% confidence interval [CI]: 1.06–7.69; P = .031) and myocardial uptake index (defined as the product of LV SUV_{max} and the number of LV segments with abnormal uptake) > 30 (HR: 1.28, 95% CI 1.05–6.12; P = .010).[33] In addition, the baseline myocardial uptake index had a strong positive correlation (r = 0.887; P < .001) with change in LVEF following immunosuppressive therapy.

Novel Tracers

Somatostatin receptor type 2 imaging
In addition to being expressed in many neuroendocrine tumors, somatostatin receptor (SSTR) type 2 is expressed by macrophages, epithelioid cells, and giant cells in granulomatous inflammation in sarcoidosis.[34] In a study of 20 patients with sarcoidosis (12 with histologically-confirmed disease) who underwent both ^{67}Ga-scintigraphy and ^{68}Ga-DOTA-Tyr-octreotide (DOTATOC) PET/CT imaging, DOTATOC PET/CT was positive in 19, whereas ^{67}Ga-scintigraphy was positive in 17.[35] DOTATOC PET/CT also visualized more lesions in lymph nodes, uvea, and muscle when compared with ^{67}Ga-scintigraphy.

In a study of 13 patients with suspected active cardiac sarcoidosis (10 with histologically confirmed extracardiac disease) who underwent ^{68}Ga DOTATATE PET/CT a median of 37 days after FDG PET/CT, concordance of FDG and DOTATATE uptake was 54% in the heart and 100% for

thoracic nodal activity.[36] The authors concluded that SSRT type 2 imaging may be less sensitive for myocardial inflammation but comparable for extracardiac inflammation in sarcoidosis when compared with FDG imaging.

3′-deoxy-3′-^{18}F-fluorothymidine
3′-deoxy-3′-^{18}F-fluorothymidine (FLT) is a radiolabeled thymidine analog that was initially developed for imaging of cellular proliferation.[30] In a

---

Box 1
Clinical Scenarios in which referral for FDG PET/CT may be helpful in cases of suspected or known cardiac sarcoidosis.

-Assess response to therapy in patients with known cardiac sarcoidosis

-Patients with biopsy-proven extracardiac sarcoidosis and any of the following:

1. Abnormal cardiac MRI

2. Abnormal electrocardiogram

3. Abnormal echocardiogram

4. Nonsustained ventricular tachycardia on ambulatory monitoring

5. Syncope

-Patients with unexplained high-grade atrioventricular block

-Patients with ventricular tachycardia that is not fascicular or outflow tract in origin, or not secondary to structural heart disease

Adapted from Chareonthaitawee P, Beanlands RS, Chen W, et al. Joint SNMMI-ASNC expert consensus document on the role of. J Nucl Cardiol. 10 2017;24(5):1741 to 1758.

study that compared FDG and FLT PET imaging in 20 patients with newly diagnosed sarcoidosis, the sensitivity, specificity, and accuracy of FDG PET for detection of cardiac sarcoidosis was 85%, 100%, and 90% compared with 92%, 100%, and 95% for FLT PET.[37] In a prospective study that included 14 participants with sarcoidosis and 12 with cardiac sarcoidosis by HRS criteria, an agreement between FLT PET and FDG PET for the diagnosis of cardiac sarcoidosis was excellent ($\kappa = 0.86$).[38] Another prospective study of 14 participants that underwent both FDG PET and FLT PET within 2 weeks found that the SRS by ^{13}N-ammonia or [82]Rubidium PET strongly correlated with FLT SUV$_{total}$ but not with FDG SUV$_{total}$.[39] Given these findings, the investigators hypothesized that FLT may identify areas likely to develop a myocardial scar.

SUMMARY

In summary, radionuclide imaging has invaluable roles in the diagnosis of cardiac sarcoidosis and risk stratification. It is used in contemporary clinical practice to assess response to immunosuppressive therapy and guide management. Novel tracers continue to be developed and studied to improve the diagnostic accuracy of metabolic PET/CT imaging and improve the patient experience by obviating the need for dietary preparation.

CLINICS CARE POINTS

- Ketogenic dietary preparation before metabolism imaging is critical for diagnostic PET/computed tomography images for the evaluation of cardiac sarcoidosis.

- Several studies have shown the prognostic utility of myocardial perfusion/metabolism imaging in suspected and known cases of cardiac sarcoidosis.

- Current work to develop novel tracers in radionuclide myocardial inflammation imaging centers on eliminating the need for dietary preparation and improving specificity.

DISCLOSURE

Dr Divakaran was supported by a joint KL2/Catalyst Medical Research Investigator Training (CMeRIT) award from Harvard Catalyst and the Boston Claude D. Pepper Older Americans Independence Center (5P30AG031679–10) and the Khoury Innovation Award from the Brigham and Women's Hospital Heart and Vascular Center. He reports consulting fees from Kinevant Sciences.

REFERENCES

1. Iannuzzi MC, Fontana JR. Sarcoidosis: clinical presentation, immunopathogenesis, and therapeutics. JAMA 2011;305(4):391–9.
2. Birnie DH, Nery PB, Ha AC, et al. Cardiac sarcoidosis. J Am Coll Cardiol 2016;68(4):411–21.
3. Iwai K, Tachibana T, Takemura T, et al. Pathological studies on sarcoidosis autopsy. I. Epidemiological features of 320 cases in Japan. Acta Pathol Jpn 1993;43(7–8):372–6.
4. Perry A, Vuitch F. Causes of death in patients with sarcoidosis. A morphologic study of 38 autopsies with clinicopathologic correlations. Arch Pathol Lab Med 1995;119(2):167–72.
5. Hamzeh N, Steckman DA, Sauer WH, et al. Pathophysiology and clinical management of cardiac sarcoidosis. Nat Rev Cardiol 2015;12(5):278–88.
6. Gilotra NA, Griffin JM, Pavlovic N, et al. Sarcoidosis-related cardiomyopathy: current knowledge, challenges, and future perspectives state-of-the-art review. J Card Fail 2022;28(1):113–32.
7. Chareonthaitawee P, Beanlands RS, Chen W, et al. Joint SNMMI-ASNC expert consensus document on the role of. J Nucl Cardiol 2017;24(5):1741–58.
8. Futamatsu H, Suzuki J, Adachi S, et al. Utility of gallium-67 scintigraphy for evaluation of cardiac sarcoidosis with ventricular tachycardia. Int J Cardiovasc Imaging 2006;22(3–4):443–8.
9. Momose M, Kadoya M, Koshikawa M, et al. Usefulness of 67Ga SPECT and integrated low-dose CT scanning (SPECT/CT) in the diagnosis of cardiac sarcoidosis. Ann Nucl Med 2007;21(10):545–51.
10. Nakazawa A, Ikeda K, Ito Y, et al. Usefulness of dual 67Ga and 99mTc-sestamibi single-photon-emission CT scanning in the diagnosis of cardiac sarcoidosis. Chest 2004;126(4):1372–6.
11. Tellier P, Valeyre D, Nitenberg A, et al. Cardiac sarcoidosis: reversion of myocardial perfusion abnormalities by dipyridamole. Eur J Nucl Med 1985;11(6–7):201–4.
12. Tellier P, Paycha F, Antony I, et al. Reversibility by dipyridamole of thallium-201 myocardial scan defects in patients with sarcoidosis. Am J Med 1988;85(2):189–93.
13. Christopoulos G, Jouni H, Acharya GA, et al. Suppressing physiologic 18-fluorodeoxyglucose uptake in patients undergoing positron emission tomography for cardiac sarcoidosis: the effect of a structured patient preparation protocol. J Nucl Cardiol 2019;119(2):167–72.

14. Dilsizian V, Bacharach SL, Beanlands RS, et al. ASNC imaging guidelines/SNMMI procedure standard for positron emission tomography (PET) nuclear cardiology procedures. J Nucl Cardiol 2016; 23(5):1187–226.

15. Tahara N, Tahara A, Nitta Y, et al. Heterogeneous myocardial FDG uptake and the disease activity in cardiac sarcoidosis. JACC Cardiovasc Imaging 2010;3(12):1219–28.

16. Miller RJH, Cadet S, Pournazari P, et al. Quantitative assessment of cardiac hypermetabolism and perfusion for diagnosis of cardiac sarcoidosis. J Nucl Cardiol 2022;29(1):86–96.

17. Terasaki F, Yoshinaga K. New guidelines for diagnosis of cardiac sarcoidosis in Japan. Annals of Nuclear Cardiology 2017;3(1):42–5.

18. Birnie DH, Sauer WH, Bogun F, et al. HRS expert consensus statement on the diagnosis and management of arrhythmias associated with cardiac sarcoidosis. Heart Rhythm 2014;11(7):1305–23.

19. Vita T, Okada DR, Veillet-Chowdhury M, et al. Complementary value of cardiac magnetic resonance imaging and positron emission tomography/computed tomography in the assessment of cardiac sarcoidosis. Circ Cardiovasc Imaging 2018;11(1): e007030.

20. Divakaran S, Stewart GC, Lakdawala NK, et al. Diagnostic accuracy of advanced imaging in cardiac sarcoidosis. Circ Cardiovasc Imaging 2019;12(6): e008975.

21. Patel VN, Pieper JA, Poitrasson-Rivière A, et al. The prognostic value of positron emission tomography in the evaluation of suspected cardiac sarcoidosis. J Nucl Cardiol 2021. https://doi.org/10.1007/ s12350-021-02780-x.

22. Divakaran S, Blankstein R. FDG PET imaging in suspected cardiac sarcoidosis: diagnosis vs. prognosis. J Nucl Cardiol 2021. https://doi.org/10.1007/ s12350-021-02809-1.

23. Blankstein R, Osborne M, Naya M, et al. Cardiac positron emission tomography enhances prognostic assessments of patients with suspected cardiac sarcoidosis. J Am Coll Cardiol 2014;63(4):329–36.

24. Wicks EC, Menezes LJ, Barnes A, et al. Diagnostic accuracy and prognostic value of simultaneous hybrid 18F-fluorodeoxyglucose positron emission tomography/magnetic resonance imaging in cardiac sarcoidosis. Eur Heart J Cardiovasc Imaging 2018; 19(7):757–67.

25. Sperry BW, Tamarappoo BK, Oldan JD, et al. Prognostic impact of extent, severity, and heterogeneity of abnormalities on. JACC Cardiovasc Imaging 2018;11(2 Pt 2):336–45.

26. Giblin GT, Murphy L, Stewart GC, et al. Cardiac sarcoidosis: when and how to treat inflammation. Card Fail Rev 2021;7:e17.

27. Wand AL, Chrispin J, Saad E, et al. Current state and future directions of multimodality imaging in cardiac sarcoidosis. Front Cardiovasc Med 2021;8: 785279.

28. Osborne MT, Hulten EA, Singh A, et al. Reduction in 18F-fluorodeoxyglucose uptake on serial cardiac positron emission tomography is associated with improved left ventricular ejection fraction in patients with cardiac sarcoidosis. J Nucl Cardiol 2014;21(1): 166–74.

29. Muser D, Santangeli P, Castro SA, et al. Prognostic role of serial quantitative evaluation of. Eur J Nucl Med Mol Imaging 2018;45(8):1394–404.

30. Saric P, Young KA, Rodriguez-Porcel M, et al. PET imaging in cardiac sarcoidosis: a narrative review with Focus on novel PET tracers. Pharmaceuticals 2021;14(12). https://doi.org/10.3390/ph14121286.

31. Ning N, Guo HH, Iagaru A, et al. Serial cardiac FDG-PET for the diagnosis and therapeutic guidance of patients with cardiac sarcoidosis. J Card Fail 2019; 25(4):307–11.

32. Okada DR, Saad E, Wand AL, et al. Effect of corticosteroid dose and duration on 18-fluorodeoxyglucose positron emission tomography in cardiac sarcoidosis. JACC Cardiovasc Imaging 2020;13(5):1280–2.

33. Subramanian M, Swapna N, Ali AZ, et al. Pre-treatment myocardial. JACC Cardiovasc Imaging 2021; 14(10):2008–16.

34. ten Bokum AM, Hofland LJ, de Jong G, et al. Immunohistochemical localization of somatostatin receptor sst2A in sarcoid granulomas. Eur J Clin Invest 1999;29(7):630–6.

35. Nobashi T, Nakamoto Y, Kubo T, et al. The utility of PET/CT with (68)Ga-DOTATOC in sarcoidosis: comparison with (67)Ga-scintigraphy. Ann Nucl Med 2016;30(8):544–52.

36. Bravo PE, Bajaj N, Padera RF, et al. Feasibility of somatostatin receptor-targeted imaging for detection of myocardial inflammation: a pilot study. J Nucl Cardiol 2021;28(3):1089–99.

37. Norikane T, Yamamoto Y, Maeda Y, et al. Comparative evaluation of. EJNMMI Res 2017;7(1):69.

38. Martineau P, Pelletier-Galarneau M, Juneau D, et al. FLT-PET for the assessment of systemic sarcoidosis including cardiac and CNS involvement: a prospective study with comparison to FDG-PET. EJNMMI Res 2020;10(1):154.

39. Martineau P, Pelletier-Galarneau M, Juneau D, et al. Imaging cardiac sarcoidosis with FLT-PET compared with FDG/perfusion-PET: a prospective pilot study. JACC Cardiovasc Imaging 2019;12(11 Pt 1):2280–1.

Current Status of Radionuclide Imaging of Transthyretin Cardiac Amyloidosis

Anam Waheed, MD[a], Sharmila Dorbala, MD, MPH[a,b,c],*

KEYWORDS

- Cardiac amyloidosis • Transthyretin cardiac amyloidosis
- Single photon emission computed tomography • Bone avid tracer cardiac scintigraphy • 99mTc-PYP
- 99mTc-DPD • 99mTc-HDP

KEY POINTS

- Transthyretin (ATTR) cardiac amyloidosis is a significantly underdiagnosed cause of heart failure with preserved ejection fraction in older adults.
- ATTR cardiac amyloidosis can be diagnosed noninvasively using 99mTc-pyrophosphate/3,3-di-phosphono-1,2-propanodicarboxylic acid/hydroxy methylene diphosphonate (99mTc-PYP/DPD/HDP) cardiac SPECT, provided light chain amyloidosis is excluded.
- Quantitative 99mTc-PYP/DPD/HDP cardiac SPECT CT and amyloid binding cardiac PET are the next frontier of advancements in radionuclide imaging of cardiac amyloidosis.

INTRODUCTION

Amyloidosis is a disorder of protein misfolding with extracellular deposition of amyloid fibrils in a characteristic beta pleated sheet structure, leading to organ dysfunction and death.[1] Cardiac amyloidosis is usually a part of a multisystem disease but cases of isolated cardiac amyloidosis have also been described. The most common forms of cardiac amyloidosis are transthyretin (ATTR) amyloidosis and immunoglobulin-derived light chain (AL) amyloidosis. ATTR cardiac amyloidosis occurs when misfolded transthyretin (prealbumin), a protein synthesized by the liver, deposits as amyloid in the myocardial extracellular space.[2] There are 2 types of ATTR amyloidosis–wild type ATTR (ATTRwt) amyloidosis and hereditary amyloidosis (also known as variant amyloidosis or ATTRv; **Table 1**).

ATTRwt amyloidosis is the commonest form of amyloidosis. It is increasingly recognized as an underdiagnosed cause of heart failure with preserved ejection fraction (HFpEF) in the elderly affecting more than 1 in 10 older adults hospitalized with HFpEF and thickened ventricles.[3] It is a nonhereditary process with normal genetic sequence encoding the transthyretin protein. There is age-related destabilization of structurally normal homotetrameric transthyretin protein, leading to misfolding and tissue deposition of ATTR amyloid fibrils.[2] The exact reasons for destabilization of the transthyretin protein in ATTRwt amyloidosis are unknown.

a Division of Cardiovascular Imaging, Department of Radiology, Cardiovascular Division, Brigham and Women's Hospital, Boston, MA 02115, USA; b Division of Nuclear Medicine and Molecular Imaging, Department of Radiology, Brigham and Women's Hospital, Boston, MA 02115, USA; c Cardiac Amyloidosis Program, Division of Cardiology, Department of Medicine, Brigham and Women's Hospital, Boston, MA 02115, USA
* Corresponding author. Brigham and Women's Hospital, Harvard Medical School, 75 Francis Street, Boston, MA 02115.
E-mail address: sdorbala@bwh.harvard.edu
Twitter: @DorbalaSharmila (S.D.)

Cardiol Clin 41 (2023) 217–231
https://doi.org/10.1016/j.ccl.2023.01.010
0733-8651/23/© 2023 Elsevier Inc. All rights reserved.

Table 1
Types of cardiac amyloidosis

Type of Cardiac Amyloidosis	Associated Systemic Features	Prevalence
AL cardiac amyloidosis	Carpal tunnel syndrome Periorbital ecchymosis Macroglossia	Rare disease Annual age-adjusted incidence of 10.5 cases per million person-years (ref 14)
ATTR cardiac amyloidosis	Carpal tunnel syndrome Spontaneous tendon rupture Peripheral sensory and autonomic neuropathy	Overall prevalence unknown Val122Ile (pV142I)-associated ATTR found in 3.4% of self-identified African Americans (ref 7)

Hereditary ATTR (ATTRv) amyloidosis is a rare autosomal dominant condition, which occurs from a single mutation in transthyretin gene on chromosome 18.[4] Variant transthyretin protein produced by patients with transthyretin (TTR) gene mutations is unstable, increasing its propensity to misfold and form amyloid deposits.[2] Each of the TTR mutations is associated with different degrees of penetrance and varied clinical presentations.[2] The most common TTR mutations associated with cardiac amyloidosis include Val122ile (V122I or pV142I), Val30Met (V30M or pV50M), and Thr60Ala (T60 or pT80A).[5] The most common mutation seen in the United States is V122I,[6] which is a valine to isoleucine substitution at position 122. This mutation is seen in 3.4% of African Americans in the United States, and 1.5 million people carry the mutated allele.[7] Autopsy studies reveal this allele to be associated with increased deposition of amyloid after age 65.[7] Epidemiological studies reveal a greater prevalence of heart failure in patients with V122I mutation.[8]

Systemic light chain amyloidosis (AL amyloidosis) occurs when there is amyloid deposition composed of immunoglobulin AL fragments produced by a plasma cell dyscrasia. This is also associated with multiple myeloma, Waldenstrom macroglobulinemia, or monoclonal gammopathy of unknown significance (MGUS) causing overproduction of amyloidogenic ALs.[9]

Secondary amyloidosis (AA) has not been commonly reported to have cardiac involvement.[10]

CLINICAL PRESENTATION

Patients with amyloidosis have a variable clinical presentation depending on the type of amyloid and the organs involved. This makes the diagnosis of amyloidosis particularly challenging, especially if the clinician is not suspecting it and there is no single test to diagnose it.[9] Most patients experience vague symptoms such as fatigue, weight loss, and weakness.[9] Hepatic involvement and neuropathy occur

in up to 15% to 20% of patients.[5] Cardiac involvement can occur in more than 50% of patients.[11] Gastrointestinal tract infiltration with amyloid causes macroglossia, diarrhea, malabsorption, constipation, and dysmotility.

In ATTRwt amyloidosis, cardiac involvement with the development of congestive heart failure and arrhythmias is common.[12] Hereditary ATTR amyloidosis can present as a neuropathy predominant or a cardiac predominant process.[12] Extracardiac manifestations of ATTR amyloidosis include carpal tunnel syndrome, tendon rupture, and lumbar spinal stenosis.[13]

In AL amyloidosis, renal involvement manifesting as nephrotic syndrome is the most common presentation, followed by cardiac involvement.[10] Periorbital purpura—a purplish discoloration around the eyes—due to infiltration of small vessels and soft tissues can be seen.[10] Nerve involvement and autonomic dysfunction manifesting as orthostatic hypotension and neuropathy are also common.[14]

CARDIOVASCULAR MANIFESTATIONS OF AMYLOIDOSIS

Cardiovascular involvement is driven by interstitial amyloid deposition causing biventricular thickening, as well as cytotoxic and apoptotic changes to surrounding myocytes.[15] Myocardial infiltration with amyloid fibrils leads to diastolic dysfunction and a restrictive cardiomyopathy causing HFpEF.[15] Progressive reduction in left ventricular end diastolic volume can lead to a decrease in stroke volume and low but preserved ejection fraction.[12] Infiltration of the right ventricle leads to right ventricular thickening as well as right heart failure. Right ventricular involvement is a poor prognostic marker in patients with cardiac amyloidosis.[16] Valve thickening and regurgitation are common. Nearly 13% to 30% of patients with severe aortic stenosis have been shown to have concomitant cardiac ATTR amyloidosis on bone avid tracer cardiac scintigraphy studies.[17] Biatrial dilation in the setting of restrictive cardiomyopathy and atrial infiltration with amyloid fibrils often leads to the development of atrial fibrillation, which is the most common arrhythmia seen in cardiac amyloidosis.[15] Atrial dysfunction predisposes patients with amyloidosis to the risk of thromboembolism even in sinus rhythm.[15] Ventricular arrhythmias and sudden cardiac death are also seen. In addition, damage to the conduction system can lead to high-grade atrioventricular conduction blocks.[15] Notably, it is challenging, if not impossible, to definitively distinguish AL from ATTR amyloidosis based on clinical manifestations alone.

DIAGNOSIS OF CARDIAC AMYLOIDOSIS

The variability in clinical presentation, lack of physician awareness of the disease leading to low suspicion, and need for endomyocardial biopsy (until recently), had led to underdiagnosis, misdiagnosis, and delayed diagnosis of cardiac amyloidosis.[17] The prevalence of cardiac amyloidosis is severely underestimated, especially in older people.[18] The diagnosis is made more challenging because conditions such as hypertension, aortic stenosis, and hypertrophic cardiomyopathy cause left ventricular hypertrophy (LVH) and increased left ventricular wall thickness similar to cardiac amyloidosis.[15] However, early diagnosis is critical, given that untreated disease has a median survival of less than 6 months for AL cardiac amyloidosis[18] and 3 to 5 years for ATTR cardiac amyloidosis.[19] Emerging data suggest that there is more widespread use of noninvasive diagnosis with bone avid tracer cardiac scintigraphy,[20] and using that technique cardiac amyloidosis is being diagnosed at an earlier stage.[21]

Endomyocardial biopsy has, until recently, been considered the reference standard for diagnosing cardiac amyloidosis.[15] However, it is invasive and carries small procedural risks, and a lot of patients with advanced cardiac amyloidosis may not be candidates for this. In patients with early cardiac amyloidosis, sampling error can reduce the diagnostic accuracy of blind endomyocardial biopsy. In addition, procedural expertise is not available at all centers, defining a need to rely on the noninvasive diagnostic assessment of cardiac amyloidosis.[15]

Electrocardiogram is a widely available tool but has a low sensitivity for diagnosing cardiac amyloidosis. Typical findings include low-voltage QRS complexes or a pseudoinfarct pattern.[22] Low-voltage QRS despite the presence of LVH on imaging can be a differentiating factor from other causes of LVH. However, absence of low-voltage QRS complexes does not rule out amyloidosis, and some patients with coexisting hypertension may manifest LVH on ECG.[22]

N terminal pro brain natriuretic peptide (NT-proBNP) levels and troponin levels can be elevated in patients with cardiac amyloidosis.[17] Elevated NT-pro BNP and troponins in a patient with echocardiographic evidence of a restrictive cardiomyopathy, without other causes for elevated levels, should raise concern for cardiac amyloidosis.[13] No classic pathognomonic biomarker of ATTR cardiac amyloidosis has been discovered yet. A combination of monoclonal gammopathy on serum and urine immunofixation, elevated serum free ALs, abnormal kappa to lambda free AL ratio, has been found to have more than 95% sensitivity for the detection of AL amyloidosis.[23]

Transthoracic echocardiography is a widely available first-line tool for the initial evaluation of patients with suspected cardiac amyloidosis. Most of the clinical features of cardiac amyloidosis (described in the prior section on cardiovascular manifestations) are well imaged by echocardiography. Global longitudinal strain (GLS), a marker of myocardial deformation measuring the percentage of longitudinal shortening, has been observed to have a classic apical sparing pattern in cardiac amyloidosis with preserved strain in the apical segments and reduced strain at the mid-to-basal segments.[24] More recently, multiparametric echo scores have been proposed to improve the diagnostic accuracy of echocardiography for cardiac amyloidosis.[25] However, echocardiographic features, including apical sparing pattern of GLS, do not differentiate between amyloid and nonamyloid-related causes of left ventricular wall thickening and cannot distinguish AL and ATTR subtypes of amyloidosis. Echocardiographic features (GLS $\leq$ −14%, stroke volume index <33 mL/m^2) are powerful markers of mortality in patients with AL and ATTR cardiac amyloidosis.[26,27] A recent study demonstrated that patients with AL amyloidosis with sequential echocardiography demonstrating an improvement on GLS of more than 1% have better clinical outcomes (survival and heart failure hospitalizations), and the authors propose adding GLS to a risk score.[28]

Cardiac MRI (CMR), using gadolinium-based enhancing agents, is an extremely useful tool with a sensitivity of 100% and specificity of 80% to diagnose cardiac amyloidosis.[17] It provides tissue characterization as well as quantitative characterization of ventricular volumes and stroke volume. In addition, it provides an assessment of myocardial tissue characteristics by native and postcontrast T1 times and estimation of extracellular volume (ECV). These features are not specific for cardiac amyloidosis but if abnormal, they can be useful for risk stratification, assessment of disease progression, and monitoring response to therapy.[15] Abnormal gadolinium kinetics on the inversion scout sequence, with a characteristic pattern of myocardial nulling before nulling of the blood pool is seen in cardiac amyloidosis.[17,22] In addition, there is late gadolinium enhancement (LGE) from interstitial expansion of the extracellular space due to amyloid deposition. Diffuse, patchy, subendocardial, or transmural LGE may be present in cardiac amyloidosis.[5,10] However, none of the features on cardiac MRI can definitively distinguish between AL and ATTR amyloid subtypes. There are additional patient-specific limitations (atrial fibrillation, cardiac devices, reduced renal function, breath-holding difficulties) that may make the use of cardiac MRI for imaging assessment of cardiac amyloid difficult.[15]

RADIONUCLIDE IMAGING

Cardiac scintigraphy with ^{99m}Technetium-labeled (^{99m}Tc) bone avid tracers, ^{99m}Tc-pyrophosphate (PYP), and ^{99m}Tc-3,3-diphosphono-1,2-propanodicarboxylic acid (DPD) and ^{99m}Tc-hydroxy methylene diphosphonate (HDP), has come to play a key role in the diagnosis of ATTR cardiac amyloidosis.[17] The strength of ^{99m}Tc-PYP/DPD/HDP cardiac imaging lies in its ability to make a diagnosis without the need for an invasive endomyocardial biopsy. This test has transformed the field because patients with suspected ATTR cardiac amyloidosis can now be diagnosed noninvasively and treated with TTR stabilizing agents such as tafamidis[29] or diflunisal.[2] Noninvasive diagnosis of ATTR cardiac amyloidosis using ^{99m}Tc-PYP/DPD/HDP cardiac SPECT has also made possible screening studies that have uncovered the true epidemiology of cardiac amyloidosis.[30] Tracers currently available for imaging cardiac amyloidosis include ^{99m}Tc-PYP/DPD/HDP, amyloid-directed molecules, and amyloid-binding PET agents. Currently, ^{99m}Tc-bone avid tracer cardiac scintigraphy is the mainstay of cardiac amyloidosis imaging in clinical practice in the United States and forms the focus of this article.

^{99m}Technetium-LABELLED BONE AVID RADIOTRACERS

^{99m}Tc-labelled phosphate tracers, originally developed to image myocardial infarct and bone imaging, were discovered in the late 1970s to image cardiac amyloidosis. The mechanism of binding of bone avid radiotracers to amyloid fibrils is not known. It has been proposed to be mediated by the calcium-dependent P component of the amyloid fibrils, which binds to the technetium bone radiotracers in a calcium-mediated manner.[31] Comparison of these ^{99m}Tc-PYP/DPD/HDP in a metanalysis of 6 studies did not reveal any differences in the diagnostic accuracy of these radiotracers and showed a pooled sensitivity of 92% and a pooled specificity of 95%.[32] Currently, ^{99m}Tc-PYP and ^{99m}Tc-HDP are the 2 clinically used radiotracers in the United States, and ^{99m}Tc-DPD and ^{99m}Tc-HDP are used in Europe.

Investigations in the early 2000s revealed the ^{99m}Tc-labelled bone avid radiotracers have a significantly greater uptake in patients with ATTR than AL amyloidosis,[33] thereby improving the specificity to diagnose cardiac ATTR amyloidosis. This may be partly explained by the much higher degree of microcalcifications seen on endomyocardial biopsies in ATTR compared with AL amyloidosis.[34] Normal myocardium exhibits no uptake of bone avid radiotracers. Myocardial regions with prior acute infarction may exhibit an increased uptake of technetium-labelled radiotracers in the regional distribution of infarcts, whereas amyloidosis has more diffuse uptake.

WHO SHOULD BE REFERRED FOR TESTING FOR TRANSTHYRETIN CARDIAC AMYLOIDOSIS?

Patients aged older than 60 years with HFpEF and unexplained increase in wall thickness ($\geq$12 mm) should be referred for an assessment of cardiac amyloidosis.[13] This is particularly important in older persons of African American descent in whom HFpEF or unexplained increase in wall thickness should prompt the evaluation for cardiac amyloidosis.[13] Amyloidosis should also be suspected in elderly men with bilateral carpal tunnel syndrome, unexplained neuropathy, and heart failure, with echo or MRI features suggestive of infiltration.[13] In addition, patients with known or suspected familial amyloidosis, and those with echo or MRI features suggestive of infiltrative pathologic condition or cardiac amyloidosis should undergo radionuclide imaging to assess for cardiac amyloidosis.[15] A more recent European Society of Cardiology (ESC) working group recommendations suggest screening for cardiac amyloidosis in patients with left ventricular wall thickness of 12 mm or greater and 1 or more of the following features: heart failure in 65 years of age or older, aortic stenosis in 65 years of age or older, hypotension or normotension if previously hypertensive, sensory involvement, autonomic dysfunction, peripheral polyneuropathy, proteinuria, skin bruising, bilateral carpal tunnel syndrome, ruptured biceps tendon, subendocardial/transmural LGE or increased ECV, reduced longitudinal strain with apical sparing, decreased QRS voltage to mass ratio, pseudo Q waves on ECG, atrioventricular conduction disease, or possible family history.[35] In general, following suspicion based on echocardiography (or cardiac MRI), if AL amyloidosis is excluded (see "Importance of excluding AL amyloidosis" section), evaluation for ATTR cardiac amyloidosis by bone avid tracer scintigraphy is recommended. If AL amyloidosis evaluation is positive or equivocal, referral to a hematologist and biopsy of the involved organ is recommended.[13,35]

AMERICAN SOCIETY OF NUCLEAR CARDIOLOGY RECOMMENDED ^{99m}Tc-PYROPHOSPHATE/3,3-DIPHOSPHONO-1,2-PROPANODICARBOXYLIC ACID/ HYDROXY METHYLENE DIPHOSPHONATE IMAGING ASSESSMENT

American Society of Nuclear Cardiology (ASNC) has developed standardized protocols for ^{99m}Tc-PYP/DPD/HDP for cardiac amyloidosis.[17] No specific patient preparation is needed for the scan. After the radiotracer is injected intravenously, SPECT imaging (with or without planar imaging) is performed preferably after 2 to 3 hours, to assess radiotracer distribution in the myocardium at rest.[36] SPECT imaging (if available SPECT/CT) offers the advantage of being able to discern true myocardial uptake from counts in the blood pool, or counts added from overlying ribs, as well as focal uptake due to myocardial infarction and is recommended in all ^{99m}Tc-labelled bone radiotracer cardiac studies.[17] Images are inspected

visually and graded on a qualitative score comparing myocardial uptake to rib uptake. No myocardial uptake is Grade 0, myocardial uptake less than rib uptake is Grade 1, myocardial uptake equivalent to rib uptake is Grade 2 and myocardial uptake greater than rib uptake is Grade 3 (**Fig. 1**).

IMPORTANCE OF EXCLUDING LIGHT CHAIN AMYLOIDOSIS

A large international study of 1217 patients who were imaged with ^{99m}Tc-PYP, DPD, HDMP showed that a visual uptake of Grade 2 or 3 in patients, without evidence of a monoclonal gammopathy on serum and urine screening, had a 100% positive predictive value for ATTR amyloidosis.[36] If AL amyloid was not excluded, the specificity decreased to 91%.[36] Cases of AL amyloidosis with myocardial involvement with a positive ^{99}Tc-radionuclide scintigraphy scan have been reported in the literature and seen in clinical practice.[17,36] Therefore, it is key to exclude AL amyloid, even before referral to ^{99}Tc radiotracer amyloid scan. If the scan was performed, AL amyloidosis should be excluded irrespective of the scan results, as any grade PYP uptake (grade 0–grade 3) may represent AL cardiac amyloidosis.

A combination of serum protein immunofixation assay, urine protein immunofixation assay, and quantification of serum free ALs has a 99% sensitivity for diagnosing cardiac amyloidosis.[23] If a patient tests positive for AL amyloidosis on these tests or has a biopsy proven diagnosis of AL amyloidosis, radionuclide scintigraphy is not indicated and an involved organ biopsy with typing of amyloid fibrils will be necessary (**Fig. 2**).

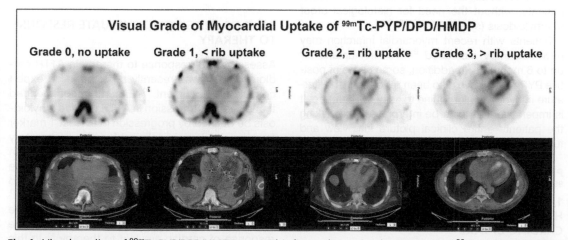

Visual Grade of Myocardial Uptake of ^{99m}Tc-PYP/DPD/HMDP

Grade 0, no uptake | Grade 1, < rib uptake | Grade 2, = rib uptake | Grade 3, > rib uptake

Fig. 1. Visual grading of ^{99m}Tc-PYP/DPD/HMDP scans. This figure shows visual assessment of ^{99m}Tc-PYP/DPD/HMDP scans. This research was originally published in JNM. Dorbala S, Park MA, Cuddy S et al. Absolute Quantitation of Cardiac (99m)Tc-Pyrophosphate Using Cadmium-Zinc-Telluride-Based SPECT/CT. Journal of nuclear medicine: official publication, Society of Nuclear Medicine 2021;62:716-722. © SNMMI.

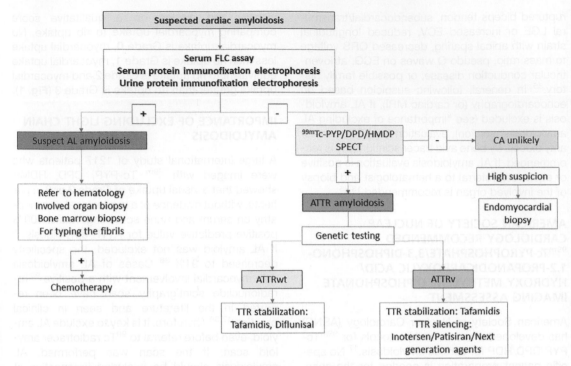

Fig. 2. An algorithmic approach to evaluation of cardiac amyloidosis. This figure shows an algorithmic approach to the evaluation for cardiac amyloidosis. ATTR, transthyretin amyloidosis; ATTRv, hereditary transthyretin cardiac amyloidosis; ATTRwt, wild type transthyretin cardiac amyloidosis; CA, cardiac amyloidosis; FLC, free light chain; TTR, transthyretin.

DIAGNOSTIC CRITERIA FOR CARDIAC AMYLOIDOSIS

Cardiac amyloidosis can be diagnosed by endo-myocardial biopsy or by extracardiac biopsy with typical cardiac imaging features. ATTR cardiac amyloidosis can be diagnosed noninvasively using 99mTc-PYP/DPD/HDP cardiac SPECT, in select patients, without the need for histological proof of amyloidosis (see **Table 1**).[13]

Patients with recent myocardial infarction may have regionally increased 99mTc-PYP uptake for up to 6 months.[37] In addition, some cases of positive PYP scans have also been reported in the literature in hydroxychloroquine toxicity.[38] Therefore, it is imperative that tests be interpreted while taking the patients entire clinical picture into view and further testing be sought if there is discordant data.

PROGNOSTIC SIGNIFICANCE OF 99mTc-PYROPHOSPHATE/3,3-DIPHOSPHONO-1,2-PROPANODICARBOXYLIC ACID/ HYDROXY METHYLENE DIPHOSPHONATE CARDIAC UPTAKE

Patients with no myocardial uptake of 99mTc-PYP/ DPD/HDP have significantly better survival compared with those with myocardial uptake.[39]

However, the degree of visually assessed myocardial uptake (Grade 1 vs Grade 2 vs Grade 3) of 99mTc-PYP/DPD/HDP has not been found to correlate with outcomes.[39] Whether semiquantitative imaging using standardized uptake value (SUV) type metrics provides prognostic value remains to be studied.

ROLE OF IMAGING TO EVALUATE RESPONSE TO THERAPY

Assessment of response to therapy in ATTR cardiomyopathy was recently reported in an expert consensus document.[40] Experts recommended that disease progression in ATTR cardiac amyloidosis be defined by progression in at least 1 marker from each domain: clinical/function, laboratory biomarker, and ECG/imaging.[40] Cardiac MRI with T1 mapping and ECV assessment can provide quantitative insight into amyloid burden and could potentially help evaluate changes over time.[41] However, currently there are limited data for the use of radionuclide scintigraphy to assess the response of cardiac amyloid to therapy.[41] In this document, the experts thought more data were needed before recommending serial MRI and radionuclide imaging for the assessment of

Table 2
Expert consensus recommendations for diagnosis of cardiac amyloidosis

Criteria for Diagnosis	Subtype
Histological Diagnosis of Cardiac Amyloidosis: Endomyocardial Biopsy[a]	
1. Endomyocardial biopsy positive for cardiac amyloidosis with Congo red staining with apple-green birefringence under polarized light; typing by immunohistochemistry and/or mass spectrometry at specialized centers	AL, ATTR, other subtypes
Histological Diagnosis of Cardiac Amyloidosis: Extracardiac Biopsy	

1. ATTR cardiac amyloidosis is diagnosed when below criteria are met:
  a. Extracardiac biopsy proven ATTR amyloidosis *and*
  b. Typical cardiac imaging features (as defined below)
	ATTR

2. AL cardiac amyloidosis is diagnosed when below criteria are met:
  a. Extracardiac biopsy proven AL amyloidosis *and*
  b. Typical cardiac imaging features (as defined below) *or*
  c. Abnormal cardiac biomarkers: abnormal age-adjusted NT-pro BNP or abnormal troponin T/I/Hs-troponin *with all other causes for these changes excluded*
	AL

Clinical Diagnosis of ATTR Cardiac Amyloidosis: ^{99m}Tc-PYP, DPD, HMDP	

3. ATTR cardiac amyloidosis is diagnosed when below criteria are met:
  a. ^{99m}Tc-PYP, DPD, HMDP Grade 2 or 3 myocardial uptake of radiotracer *and*
  b. Absence of a clonal plasma cell process as assessed by serum free light chains and serum and urine immunofixation *and*
  c. Typical cardiac imaging features (as defined below)
	ATTR

Typical Imaging Features of Cardiac Amyloidosis	
Typical cardiac echo or CMR or PET features: *Any* of the below imaging features *with all other causes for these cardiac manifestations, including hypertension, reasonably excluded.*	

1. Echo
  a. LV wall thickness >12 mm
  b. Relative apical sparing of global LS ratio (average of apical LS/ average of combined mid + basal LS > 1)
  c. ≥ Grade 2 diastolic dysfunction[b]
	ATTR/AL

2. CMR
  a. LV wall thickness > ULN for sex on SSFP cine CMR
  b. Global ECV >0.40
  c. Diffuse LGE[b]
  d. Abnormal gadolinium kinetics typical for amyloidosis, myocardial nulling before blood pool nulling
	ATTR/AL

3. PET: ^{18}F-florbetapir[b] or ^{18}F-florbetaben PET[b,c]
  a. Target to background (LV myocardium to blood pool) ratio >1.5
  b. Retention index >0.030 min^{-1}
	ATTR/AL

These consensus recommendations were based on moderate-quality evidence from one or more well-designed, well-executed nonrandomized studies, observational studies, registries, or meta-analyses of such studies. The PET recommendations were based on more limited data.

Abbreviations: AL, amyloidogenic light chain; ATTR, amyloidogenic transthyretin; CMR, Cardiac MRI; ECV, extracelullar volume; LGE, late gadolinium enhancement; LS, longitudinal strain; LV, left ventricular; SSFP, steady-state free precession; ULN, upper limit of normal, per reference at midcavity level ULN for women/men were 7 mm/9 mm (long axis) and 7 mm/8 mm (short axis), respectively.

[a] Endomyocardial biopsy should be considered in cases of equivocal ^{99m}Tc-PYP, DPD, HMDP scan. When ^{99m}Tc-PYP, DPD, HMDP is positive in the context of any abnormal evaluation for serum/urine immunofixation or serum-free AL assay, or MGUS, this should not be seen as diagnostic for ATTR cardiac amyloidosis. In these instances, referral to a specialist amyloid center for further evaluation and consideration of biopsy is recommended.

[b] Off-label use of FDA-approved commercial products.

[c] ^{18}F-flutemetamol not studied systematically in the heart. ^{11}C-Pittsurgh B compound is not FDA approved and not available to sites without a cyclotron in proximity.

From Dorbala S, Ando Y, Bokhari S et al. ASNC/AHA/ASE/EANM/HFSA/ISA/SCMR/SNMMI expert consensus recommendations for multimodality imaging in cardiac amyloidosis: Part 2 of 2-Diagnostic criteria and appropriate utilization. Journal of nuclear cardiology : official publication of the American Society of Nuclear Cardiology 2019;26:2065–2123.

response to therapy.[40] In a small study, Fontana and colleagues[41] found that percent injected dose of ^{99m}Tc-DPD reduced by a median of 19.6% in patients treated with patisiran for 12 months; however, given the smaller magnitude of changes in ECV (median decrease of 6%), the significance of this finding needs further study. Quantitative SPECT with the assessment of segmented maximal SUV and whole heart amyloid burden is being explored as a tool for the assessment of response to therapy in cardiac amyloidosis[42] but has not been validated for clinical use yet.

WHO SHOULD BE REFERRED FOR ENDOMYOCARDIAL BIOPSY FOR CARDIAC AMYLOIDOSIS?

Although the use of ^{99m}Tc-PYP/DPD/HDP cardiac SPECT has reduced the need for endomyocardial biopsy,[20] there are several instances where a biopsy may be considered. If a patient has echocardiographic and MRI features to suggest cardiac amyloidosis and a positive AL serological screening, further assessment with an endomyocardial biopsy is recommended, independent of the ^{99m}Tc-PYP/DPD/HMDP scan results. This is because patients with AL amyloidosis may have

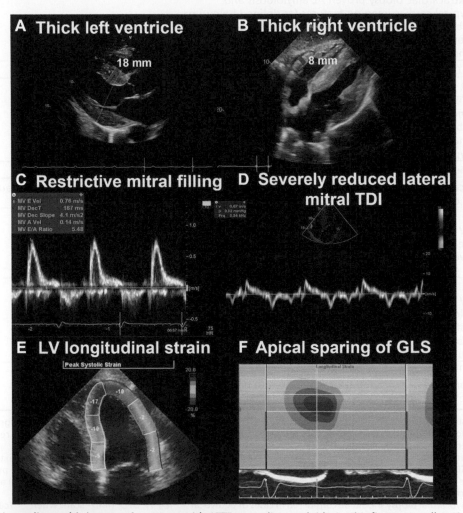

Fig. 3. Echocardiographic images of a patient with ATTRwt cardiac amyloidosis. This figure as well as **Figs. 4–6** are from a 68-year-old man with suspected cardiac amyloidosis eventually diagnosed with ATTRwt cardiac amyloidosis. Parasternal long axis and subcostal views demonstrate severely thickening of left (18 mm; *A*) and right ventricular walls (8 mm; *B*). Pulse wave Doppler velocity at the mitral valve leaflet tips, show rapid early diastolic filling with rapid equalization of pressures between the left atrium and left ventricle, leading to severely reduced late diastolic filling indicative of a restrictive filling pattern (*C*). Tissue Doppler velocity measured at the lateral mitral valve annulus revealed severely reduced velocities (7 cm/s) indicative of diastolic dysfunction (*D*). GLS was severely reduced −12% with a classical cherry on top pattern with preserved apical strain and severely reduced strain in the basal-to-mid segments (*E, F*).

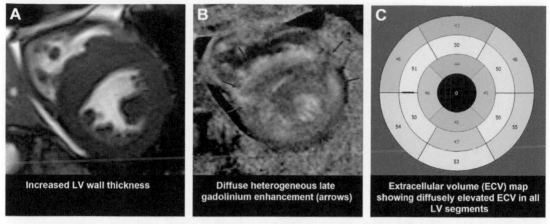

Fig. 4. Cardiac MRI images of a patient with ATTRwt cardiac amyloidosis. Midventricular short axis steady-state free precession MRI images shows severe concentric left ventricular wall thickening (20 mm, *A*). Corresponding midventricular short axis LGE images show diffuse patchy nearly transmural LGE of the myocardium (*B*). Extracellular volume (ECV) map derived from precontrast and postcontrast T1 times was severely abnormal (global ECV 49.5%) with segmentally increased ECV in all LV myocardial segments (*C*).

a negative bone avid tracer scan and either missed or delayed diagnosis of AL amyloidosis can prove fatal. Emerging evidence also suggests that patients with certain hereditary forms of amyloidosis[43] may manifest negative bone avid tracer SPECT. Thus, if there is a negative PYP scan in the context of abnormal TTR genotyping an endomyocardial biopsy is indicated. Finally, 99mTc-

MDP (methyl diphosphonate), a commonly used agent for bone scanning has low sensitivity to diagnose ATTR cardiac amyloidosis[44] and is not recommended for imaging cardiac amyloidosis. Select patients with a discordance between clinical presentation and laboratory or imaging findings can be referred for endomyocardial biopsy.

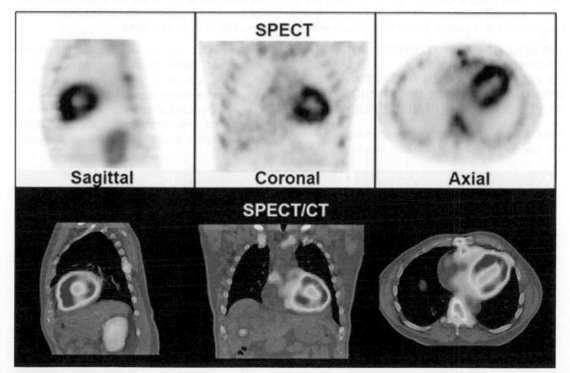

Fig. 5. 99m Tc-PYP SPECT Images of a patient with ATTRwt cardiac amyloidosis. 99mTc-pyrophosphate SPECT/CT scan in sagittal, coronal, and axial views shows grade 3 myocardial uptake (myocardial uptake greater than rib uptake, well seen on the top gray scale SPECT only images), which is diagnostic for cardiac amyloidosis.

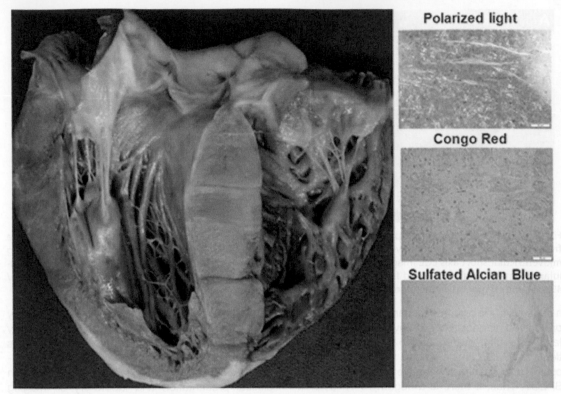

Fig. 6. Explanted heart with histopathological specimens of a patient with ATTRwt cardiac amyloidosis. Explanted heart images in a 4-chamber view showed severe biventricular thickening (left panel). The right panel shows tissue histopathological specimens from the explanted heart under polarized light, and stained with Congo Red and Sulfated Alcian Blue, showing findings characteristic of amyloid deposits. Mass spectrometry confirmed ATTRwt cardiac amyloidosis. (*Courtesy of* R Padera Jr., MD, PhD, Boston, MA.)

THE ROLE OF 99mTc-PYROPHOSPHATE/ 3,3-DIPHOSPHONO- 1,2-PROPANODICARBOXYLIC ACID/ HYDROXY METHYLENE DIPHOSPHONATE IN AMYLOIDOSIS/HEART FAILURE GUIDELINES

ASNC provided consensus recommendation for the use of imaging in cardiac amyloidosis.[13,17]

The diagnostic criteria for cardiac amyloidosis were defined (**Table 2**) and recommendation for appropriate utilization of imaging in cardiac amyloidosis were provided. Similarly, ESC Working Group on Myocardial and Pericardial Diseases[35] recommends radionuclide scintigraphy alongside serum and urine evaluation for AL amyloidosis in

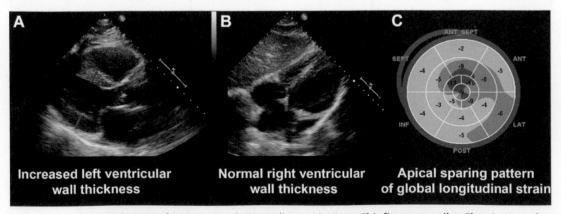

Fig. 7. Echocardiogram images of a patient with AL cardiac amyloidosis. This figure as well as **Figs. 8–10** are from a 59-year-old man with suspected cardiac amyloidosis eventually diagnosed with AL cardiac amyloidosis. Parasternal long axis (*A*) and subcostal (*B*) views of the echocardiogram demonstrate mild thickening of the left ventricular walls (14 mm) with normal thickness of the right ventricular walls. GLS imaging (*C*) shows the classical cherry on top pattern with preserved apical strain and reduced strain in the basal-to-mid segments.

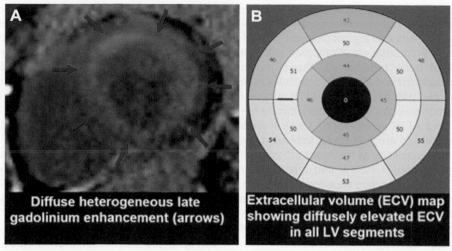

Fig. 8. Cardiac MRI images of a patient with AL cardiac amyloidosis. Cardiac MRI short axis view with LGE imaging shows diffuse nearly transmural LGE of the myocardium (*A*). Polar map showing segmental ECVs of LV myocardium shows a diffusely increased ECV (*B*).

patients with clinical scenarios suggestive of cardiac amyloidosis. An American Heart Association (AHA) Scientific Statement on the diagnosis of cardiac amyloidosis[5] suggests that in patients with clinical suspicion and echocardiographic features of amyloid, serum, and urine studies to screen for AL amyloid should be sent. If those studies are negative, then a ⁹⁹ᵐTc-PYP/DPD/HDP cardiac SPECT should be pursued.

POSITRON EMITTING AMYLOID TRACERS

PET tracers that bind to beta amyloid had been developed for brain imaging in Alzheimer

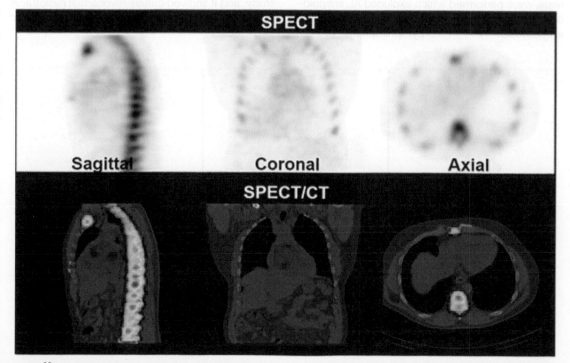

Fig. 9. ⁹⁹ᵐ Tc-PYP SPECT images of a patient with AL cardiac amyloidosis. The ⁹⁹ᵐ Tc-PYP SPECT/CT scan shows no myocardial uptake of radiotracer (Grade 0).

disease[45] but were also found in amyloid deposits in the heart. These radiotracers include ^{11}C-Pittsburgh B and ^{18}F-labelled agents (such as ^{18}F-florbetapir and ^{18}F-florbetaben). Compared with the ^{99m}Tc-labeled bone radiotracers, these tracers have been found to have higher myocardial uptake in AL compared with patients with ATTR amyloidosis but do not have the ability to discriminate between AL and ATTR amyloidosis. These tracers are also specific to amyloid fibrils, improving the accuracy and specificity of the results.[15] In addition, the advantage of PET is that it has higher spatial resolution and offers superior quantitation. Quantitation can potentially be useful to diagnose early amyloidosis and to assess response to therapy. A recent editorial summarized the results of PET amyloid tracers,[46] and a recent meta-analysis showed a sensitivity and specificity of more than 95% in diagnosing cardiac amyloidosis.[47] However, this imaging tool is still in investigational and is not used clinically.

ILLUSTRATIVE CASES
Case 1. ATTR Wild Type Cardiac Amyloidosis

A 68-year-old man presented with progressive heart failure. His echocardiogram (**Fig. 3**) and cardiac MRI (**Fig. 4**) showed characteristic features of cardiac amyloidosis. Serum free AL assay, as well as serum and urine immunofixation electrophoresis, were performed which excluded AL amyloidosis, increasing the suspicion for ATTR cardiac amyloidosis. A ^{99m}Tc-pyrophosphate SPECT

scan showed grade 3 myocardial uptake diagnostic for cardiac amyloidosis (**Fig. 5**). He was enrolled in the ATTR-ACT study evaluating tafamidis versus placebo. He eventually developed progressive heart failure requiring cardiac transplantation. ATTR wild type cardiac amyloidosis was confirmed on mass spectrometry analysis from the explanted heart (**Fig. 6**).

Case 2

A 59-year-old man with V122I mutation presented with heart failure. His echocardiogram (**Fig. 7**) and cardiac MRI (**Fig. 8**) showed characteristic features of cardiac amyloidosis. However, a ^{99m}Tc-pyrophosphate SPECT/CT scan was negative (Grade 0) (**Fig. 9**). His serum free AL levels were abnormally high with a lambda predominance, and serum and urine immunofixation electrophoresis confirmed a plasma cell dyscrasia. Given the V122I mutation (predisposing to ATTR cardiac amyloidosis), and evidence of a plasma cell dyscrasia, it was important to confirm the precise type of myocardial amyloidosis. An endomyocardial biopsy was performed and mass spectrometry confirmed cardiac amyloidosis of AL type. He responded well to chemotherapy with cyclophosphamide, bortezomib, dexamethasone and successfully attained hematological remission. An F18-florbetapir PET/CT scan (**Fig. 10**) was performed as part of a research study, and it showed diffuse myocardial radiotracer uptake in the left ventricle consistent with cardiac amyloidosis.

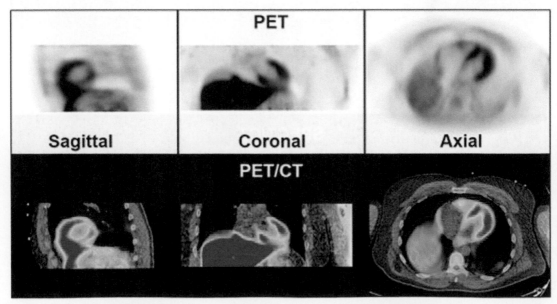

Fig. 10. ^{18}F-florbetapir PET/CT images of a patient with AL cardiac amyloidosis. This PET/CT scan shows diffuse myocardial uptake of ^{18}F-florbetapir in the left ventricle consistent with cardiac amyloidosis.

SUMMARY

Radionuclide imaging with bone avid tracers has been a major advancement in the diagnostic testing for cardiac amyloidosis. Bone avid tracer cardiac scintigraphy allows for a nonbiopsy diagnosis of ATTR cardiac amyloidosis and guides key therapeutic decisions. Patients with clinical symptoms, imaging findings, and laboratory data, suggesting ATTR cardiac amyloidosis, should be referred for ^{99m}Tc-PYP/DPD/HMDP cardiac scintigraphy. Bone avid tracer cardiac scintigraphy is gradually replacing endomyocardial biopsy and uncovering the true epidemiology of cardiac amyloidosis. Cardiac ATTR amyloidosis is now being diagnosed at an earlier stage, and by guiding appropriate novel therapies, bone avid tracer cardiac scintigraphy is likely to further improve clinical outcomes in cardiac amyloidosis.

CLINICS CARE POINTS

- The 2 most common forms of cardiac amyloidosis are transthyretin (ATTR) cardiac amyloidosis and light chain (AL) cardiac amyloidosis.

- ATTR cardiac amyloidosis is significantly underdiagnosed cause of HFpEF in older adults.

- Grade 2 or grade 3 myocardial uptake of ^{99m}Tc-PYP/DPD/HDP, can noninvasively diagnose ATTR cardiac amyloidosis with nearly 100% specificity, provided a plasma cell dyscrasia is excluded.

- Any grade myocardial uptake of ^{99m}Tc-PYP/DPD/HDP can be seen in AL amyloidosis and rapid exclusion of AL amyloidosis is thus critical before making a nonbiopsy diagnosis of ATTR cardiac amyloidosis.

- If clinical suspicion of cardiac amyloidosis remains high after a negative ^{99m}Tc-PYP/DPD/HDP SPECT, including patients with typical cardiac phenotype or genotype, further evaluation, including endomyocardial biopsy, should be considered.

- Quantitative cardiac ^{99m}Tc-PYP/DPD/HDP SPECT/CT and PET/CT with amyloid binding PET radiotracers are the next frontier for an early diagnosis and assessment of response to therapy.

DECLARATION OF INTEREST

Dr S. Dorbala has received research support from National Heart, Lung, and Blood Institute, National Institutes of Health, R01 HL130563, R01 HL150342, R01 159987, K24 157648, and American Heart Association grant AHA 16 CSA 28880004 and 19SRG34950011. Dr S. Dorbala has received consulting fees from Pfizer, GE Health Care, and investigator-initiated research grants from Pfizer, Attralus, and Phillips.

REFERENCES

1. Gilstrap LG, Dominici F, Wang Y, et al. Epidemiology of cardiac amyloidosis-associated heart failure hospitalizations among fee-for-service medicare beneficiaries in the United States. Circulation Heart failure 2019;12:e005407.
2. Ruberg FL, Grogan M, Hanna M, et al. Transthyretin amyloid cardiomyopathy: JACC STATE-OF-THE-ART REview. J Am Coll Cardiol 2019;73:2872–91.
3. Gonzalez-Lopez E, Gallego-Delgado M, Guzzo-Merello G, et al. Wild-type transthyretin amyloidosis as a cause of heart failure with preserved ejection fraction. Eur Heart J 2015;36:2585–94.
4. Wallace MR, Naylor SL, Kluve-Beckerman B, et al. Localization of the human prealbumin gene to chromosome 18. Biochem Biophys Res Commun 1985; 129:753–8.
5. Kittleson MM, Maurer MS, Ambardekar AV, et al. Cardiac Amyloidosis: evolving diagnosis and management: a scientific statement from the american heart association. Circulation 2020;142:e7–22.
6. Maurer MS, Hanna M, Grogan M, et al. Genotype and phenotype of transthyretin cardiac amyloidosis: THAOS (transthyretin amyloid outcome survey). J Am Coll Cardiol 2016;68:161–72.
7. Buxbaum JN, Ruberg FL. Transthyretin V122I (pV142I)* cardiac amyloidosis: an age-dependent autosomal dominant cardiomyopathy too common to be overlooked as a cause of significant heart disease in elderly African Americans. Genet Med 2017; 19:733–42.
8. Quarta CC, Buxbaum JN, Shah AM, et al. The amyloidogenic V122I transthyretin variant in elderly black Americans. N Engl J Med 2015;372:21–9.
9. Gertz MA. Immunoglobulin light chain amyloidosis: 2022 update on diagnosis, prognosis, and treatment. Am J Hematol 2022;97:818–29.
10. Lachmann HJ, Goodman HJ, Gilbertson JA, et al. Natural history and outcome in systemic AA amyloidosis. N Engl J Med 2007;356:2361–71.
11. Dubrey SW, Cha K, Anderson J, et al. The clinical features of immunoglobulin light-chain (AL) amyloidosis with heart involvement. QJM 1998;91:141–57.
12. Ruberg FL, Berk JL. Transthyretin (TTR) cardiac amyloidosis. Circulation 2012;126:1286–300.
13. Dorbala S, Ando Y, Bokhari S, et al. ASNC/AHA/ASE/EANM/HFSA/ISA/SCMR/SNMMI expert consensus recommendations for multimodality imaging in

cardiac amyloidosis: part 2 of 2-Diagnostic criteria and appropriate utilization. J Nucl Cardiol 2019;26: 2065–123.

14. Falk RH, Alexander KM, Liao R, et al. (Light-Chain) cardiac amyloidosis: a review of diagnosis and therapy. J Am Coll Cardiol 2016;68:1323–41.

15. Dorbala S, Cuddy S, Falk RH. How to image cardiac amyloidosis: a practical approach. JACC Cardiovascular imaging 2020;13:1368–83.

16. Patel AR, Dubrey SW, Mendes LA, et al. Right ventricular dilation in primary amyloidosis: an independent predictor of survival. Am J Cardiol 1997;80: 486–92.

17. Dorbala S, Ando Y, Bokhari S, et al. ASNC/AHA/ASE/ EANM/HFSA/ISA/SCMR/SNMMI expert consensus recommendations for multimodality imaging in cardiac amyloidosis: part 1 of 2—evidence base and standardized methods of imaging. Journal of Nuclear Cardiology 2019;26:2065–123.

18. Merlini G, Palladini G. Light chain amyloidosis: the heart of the problem. Haematologica 2013;98: 1492–5.

19. Grogan M, Scott CG, Kyle RA, et al. Natural history of wild-type transthyretin cardiac amyloidosis and risk stratification using a novel staging system. J Am Coll Cardiol 2016;68:1014–20.

20. Nativi-Nicolau J, Siu A, Dispenzieri A, et al. Temporal trends of wild-type transthyretin amyloid cardiomyopathy in the transthyretin amyloidosis outcomes survey. JACC CardioOncol 2021;3:537–46.

21. Poterucha TJ, Elias P, Bokhari S, et al. Diagnosing transthyretin cardiac amyloidosis by technetium Tc 99m pyrophosphate: a test in evolution. JACC Cardiovascular imaging 2021;14:1221–31.

22. Falk RH, Quarta CC, Dorbala S. How to image cardiac amyloidosis. Circulation Cardiovascular imaging 2014;7:552–62.

23. Palladini G, Russo P, Bosoni T, et al. Identification of amyloidogenic light chains requires the combination of serum-free light chain assay with immunofixation of serum and urine. Clin Chem 2009;55:499–504.

24. Phelan D, Collier P, Thavendiranathan P, et al. Relative apical sparing of longitudinal strain using two-dimensional speckle-tracking echocardiography is both sensitive and specific for the diagnosis of cardiac amyloidosis. Heart 2012;98:1442–8.

25. Boldrini M, Cappelli F, Chacko L, et al. Multiparametric echocardiography scores for the diagnosis of cardiac amyloidosis. JACC Cardiovascular Imaging 2020;13(4):909–20.

26. Milani P, Dispenzieri A, Scott CG, et al. Independent prognostic value of stroke volume index in patients with immunoglobulin light chain amyloidosis. Circulation Cardiovascular imaging 2018;11: e006588.

27. Barros-Gomes S, Williams B, Nhola LF, et al. Prognosis of light chain amyloidosis with preserved LVEF: added value of 2D speckle-tracking echocardiography to the current prognostic staging system. JACC Cardiovascular imaging 2017;10: 398–407.

28. Cohen OC, Ismael A, Pawarova B, et al. Longitudinal strain is an independent predictor of survival and response to therapy in patients with systemic AL amyloidosis. Eur Heart J 2022;43:333–41.

29. Maurer MS, Schwartz JH, Gundapaneni B, et al. Tafamidis treatment for patients with transthyretin amyloid cardiomyopathy. N Engl J Med 2018;379: 1007–16.

30. Aimo A, Merlo M, Porcari A, et al. 2022. P292 REDEFINING THE EPIDEMIOLOGY OF CARDIAC AMYLOIDOSIS. A SYSTEMATIC REVIEW OF SCREENING STUDIES. Eur Heart J, 24(Supplement_C), pp.suac012-281.

31. Pepys MB, Dyck RF, de Beer FC, et al. Binding of serum amyloid P-component (SAP) by amyloid fibrils. Clin Exp Immunol 1979;38:284–93.

32. Treglia G, Glaudemans A, Bertagna F, et al. Diagnostic accuracy of bone scintigraphy in the assessment of cardiac transthyretin-related amyloidosis: a bivariate meta-analysis. Eur J Nucl Med Mol Imaging 2018;45:1945–55.

33. Singh V, Falk R, Di Carli MF, et al. State-of-the-art radionuclide imaging in cardiac transthyretin amyloidosis. J Nucl Cardiol 2019;26:158–73.

34. Stats MA, Stone JR. Varying levels of small microcalcifications and macrophages in ATTR and AL cardiac amyloidosis: implications for utilizing nuclear medicine studies to subtype amyloidosis. Cardiovasc Pathol 2016;25:413–7.

35. Garcia-Pavia P, Rapezzi C, Adler Y, et al. Diagnosis and treatment of cardiac amyloidosis: a position statement of the ESC working group on myocardial and pericardial diseases. Eur Heart J 2021;42: 1554–68.

36. Gillmore JD, Maurer MS, Falk RH, et al. Nonbiopsy diagnosis of cardiac transthyretin amyloidosis. Circulation 2016;133:2404–12.

37. Olson HG, Lyons KP, Aronow WS, et al. Follow-up technetium-99m stannous pyrophosphate myocardial scintigrams after acute myocardial infarction. Circulation 1977;56:181–7.

38. Chang IC, Bois JP, Bois MC, et al. Hydroxychloroquine-Mediated Cardiotoxicity with a False Positive 99M-Technetium Labeled Pyrophosphate Scan for Amyloidosis. J Card Fail 2017;23(8):S46–7.

39. Hutt DF, Fontana M, Burniston M, et al. Prognostic utility of the Perugini grading of 99mTc-DPD scintigraphy in transthyretin (ATTR) amyloidosis and its relationship with skeletal muscle and soft tissue amyloid. European Heart Journal Cardiovascular Imaging 2017;18:1344–50.

40. Garcia-Pavia P, Bengel F, Brito D, et al. Expert consensus on the monitoring of transthyretin

amyloid cardiomyopathy. Eur J Heart Fail 2021;23:
895–905.

41. Fontana M, Martinez-Naharro A, Chacko L, et al.
Reduction in CMR derived extracellular volume
with patisiran indicates cardiac amyloid regression.
JACC Cardiovascular imaging 2021;14:189–99.

42. Dorbala S, Park MA, Cuddy S, et al. Absolute quantitation of cardiac (99m)Tc-pyrophosphate using
cadmium-zinc-telluride-based SPECT/CT. J Nucl
Med 2021;62:716–22.

43. Musumeci MB, Cappelli F, Russo D, et al. Low sensitivity of bone scintigraphy in detecting Phe64Leu
mutation-related transthyretin cardiac amyloidosis.
JACC Cardiovascular Imaging 2020;13:1314–21.

44. Perugini E, Guidalotti PL, Salvi F, et al. Noninvasive
etiologic diagnosis of cardiac amyloidosis using
99mTc-3,3-diphosphono-1,2-propanodicarboxylic
acid scintigraphy. J Am Coll Cardiol 2005;46:
1076–84.

45. Clark CM, Schneider JA, Bedell BJ, et al. Use of
florbetapir-PET for imaging beta-amyloid pathology.
JAMA 2011;305:275–83.

46. Singh V, Dorbala S. Positron emission tomography
for cardiac amyloidosis: timing matters. J Nucl Cardiol 2022;29:790–7.

47. Kim YJ, Ha S, Kim YI. Cardiac amyloidosis imaging
with amyloid positron emission tomography: a systematic review and meta-analysis. J Nucl Cardiol
2020;27:123–32.

Radionuclide Imaging of Infective Endocarditis

Paola Ferro, MD[a], Roberto Boni, MD[a], Francesco Bartoli, MD[b], Francesca Lazzeri, MD[b], Riemer H.J.A. Slart, MD, PhD[c], Paola A. Erba, MD, PhD[d],*

KEYWORDS

- Infectious endocarditis (IE)
- Infections associated with cardiovascular implantable electronic devices (CIED) • diagnosis
- Duke/ESC criteria • Echocardiography • PET/CT imaging • SPECT/CT imaging
- Labeled leukocyte (WBC) imaging

KEY POINTS

- Due to the increase use of intracardiac devices, prosthetic valves and the overall aging of the population nowadays a large spectrum of patient is at risk of developing IE.
- Early diagnosis is crucial to avoid severe complications and reduce mortality, but is still a challenging process and involves the evaluation of symptoms, laboratory tests, echocardiographic investigations and imaging such as 18F-PET/CT and WBC scintigraphy.
- each clinical scenario presents different diagnostic challenges and the various methods have different strength and weaknesses, therefore a multimodality multidisciplinary approach is needed.

The most recent epidemiological data show that the incidence of infective endocarditis (IE) varies from one country to another, within a range of 3 to 10 episodes/1,00,000 people per year.[1] IE still presents an unacceptably poor prognosis, with a mortality of about 17.1% despite the significant improvements in the diagnostic and therapeutic strategies, including an increasing proportion of older patients with more severe disease, changing epidemiological profiles.[1,2]

Prosthetic valve IE (PVE), cardiac device-related IE (CDRIE), nosocomial, staphylococcal, and enterococcal IE are currently the more frequent IE variants.[3] Indeed, infections on implantable devices and surgical biomaterials (PVE) have increased significantly during the last decades along with the increased number of devices implanted and are foreseen to represent the most common non-cardiac complication after cardiac surgery and device implants, affecting about 1.7 million patients each year, and are currently associated with nearly 1,00,000 deaths in the United States.[4,5] Infections associated with cardiovascular implants are critical as their infection risk[6,7] is nearly 5% in the first 2 months following cardiac surgery, with a 10-fold higher risk for mortality.[8]

IE diagnosis is challenging as a consequence of the broad spectrum of clinical presentation, ie, acute and rapidly progressive infection, subacute or chronic disease with low-grade fever, and nonspecific symptoms. In particular, clinical presentation is frequently atypical in elderly or immunocompromised patients.[9] Therefore, patients may refer initially to a variety of specialists who may consider a range of alternative diagnoses.

The authors have nothing to disclose.

[a] Nuclear Medicine Department ASST Ospedale Papa Giovanni XXIII Bergamo (Italy), Piazza OMS 1, Bergamo 24127, Italy; [b] Department of Translational Research and Advanced Technologies in Medicine and Surgery, Regional Center of Nuclear Medicine, University of Pisa, Via Roma 57, Pisa I-56126, Italy; [c] Medical Imaging Center, University Medical Center Groningen, Hanzeplein 1, 9713 GZ Groningen, the Netherlands; [d] Department of Medicine and Surgery, University of Milan Bicocca and Nuclear Medicine Unit ASST Ospedale Papa Giovanni XXIII Bergamo (Italy), Piazza OMS 1, Bergamo 24127, Italy

* Corresponding author. Regional Center of Nuclear Medicine, University Hospital of Pisa, Via Roma 57, Pisa I-56126, Italy.

E-mail address: paolaanna.erba@unimib.it

Cardiol Clin 41 (2023) 233–249
https://doi.org/10.1016/j.ccl.2023.01.011
0733-8651/23/© 2023 Elsevier Inc. All rights reserved.

The diagnostic criteria of the European Society of Cardiology (ESC)[10] and the American Heart Association (AHA)/American College of Cardiology[11] are based on the combination of major and minor diagnostic criteria. The major criteria consist of (i) the demonstration of the presence of a microorganism, generally by the detection of positive blood culture and (ii) identification of the infective process by imaging—echocardiography (ECHO), computed tomography (CT) , 18 Fluorine [18F]Fluorodeoxyglucose ([18F]FDG) [18F]FDG-PET/CT, and radiolabeled leukocyte single photon emission computed tomography (SPECT)/CT–of cardiac valves (native or prosthetic) or other prosthetic intracardiac material[3] and identification by imaging (whole-body CT, [18F]FDG-PET/CT, and cerebral MRI) of recent embolic events or infectious aneurysms (silent events)–this latter considered as a minor criterion.

ECHO is the main imaging technique used in IE as the first diagnostic test. Transthoracic echocardiography (TTE) and transesophageal echocardiography (TEE or TOE) are both used for documenting the presence of one of the major echocardiographic findings for the diagnosis of IE (ie, endocardial vegetations, abscess, or new dehiscence of a prosthetic valve).[12] ECHO is widely accessible. However, significant variations in the use and availability of TOE still exist.[13] Overall, the sensitivity of TTE and TOE are 70% and 96%, respectively, for the diagnosis of vegetation in native-valve endocarditis (NVE) and 50% and 92%, respectively, in PVE. For abscess detection, the sensitivity of TTE is about 50%, compared with 90% for TOE (with specificity >90% for both modalities).[14] TOE is especially useful for evaluating patients with suspected PVE,[15] and is also superior to TTE for detecting mechanical complications such as valve perforation and chordal rupture.[16] A negative TOE has a very high negative predictive value for IE, in particular, NV IE (86%–97%).[17] Echocardiographic imaging should be performed as soon as the diagnosis of IE is suspected. ECHO should be repeated 5 to 7 days after a first normal or inconclusive ECHO if the suspicion of IE remains high. It is worth remembering that ECHO findings provide prognostic implications, and help to guide the decision-making and patient follow-up while receiving antibiotic therapy and during the perioperative and postoperative period.[18] However, the detection of lesions in patients with PVE is more difficult than in patients with native valves, and normal or inconclusive findings results have been reported in up to 30% of cases.[18,19] False positive results can also occur.[19] Therefore, when ECHO fails to provide major diagnostic criteria or when it is necessary to better

assess the perivalvular extension of the disease, other non-invasive imaging modalities such as multislice computed tomography and nuclear imaging ([18F]FDG-PET/CT with or without CT-contrast agent and leukocyte scintigraphy)[20–24] are used to prove the local involvement at the cardiac valve/device level and to detect distant lesions related to the infectious process. To further enhance the value of an integrated multimodality approach, the clinical discussion of the imaging findings within the IE Team is necessary. With this approach, it is possible to overcome the potential limitations of each imaging procedure, thus optimizing the imaging results for the subsequent patient management.

CLINICAL SCENARIO
Fever and Bloodstream Infections in Patients with High Risk of IE

ECHO, the first-line and key imaging modality in IE should be performed in all patients with fever and positive blood culture and at higher risk of IE either on native-valve and prosthesis/CIED-based clinical presentation and risk factors. As the risk of IE in patients with bloodstream infections depends on the different bacterial species, strategies should be put in place to identify the subgroup of patients with high clinical risk. For example, given the high incidence of IE (6–32%)[25,26] among patients with *Staphylococcus aureus* bacteremia (SAB), risk scores were recently developed to identify patients at high risk for SA-IE, and those who should be evaluated with ECHO. Sensitivity was 77.6% (65.8–86.9), 85.1% (75.8–91.8), and 98.9% (95.7–100) for the POSITIVE, PREDICT, and VIRSTA scores, respectively. Negative predictive values (NPVs) were 92.5% (87.9–95.8), 94.5% (90.7–97.0), and 99.3% (94.9–100).[27] In patients with SAB and without any high-risk criteria defined as community-acquired SAB, high-risk cardiac conditions (prosthetic heart valve, prosthetic material, congenital heart disease, cardiac transplantation, prior IE, pacemaker, PM, or implantable cardioverter defibrillator, ICD) and intravenous drug, a normal TTE could rule out IE with high sensitivity (97%, 95% confidence interval [CI]87 – 100 %) and high negative predictive value (99%, 95% CI 96%–100%).[28]

On the contrary, in the presence of gram-negative bacteria (GNB), a very common cause of bloodstream infections,[29] only rarely IE is associated, a little more often CIED-related infection and, based on the little literature evidence, a substantially closer association to vascular graft infections is reported.[30] Therefore, in this circumstance, patients with no prosthetic material implanted or only a prosthetic heart valve should only undergo work-up for IE with TEE and [18F] FDG-PET/CT if signs suggestive of IE are present or when bloodstream infections relapse. In patients with CIEDs, special attention should be given to bloodstream infections with Pseudomonas and Serratia spp. because they can cause device infection in up to 50%. In other GNBs without IE suggestive signs, normal bloodstream infection treatment is a reasonable place to begin, and only in cases with relapse of bacteremia both ECHO and [18F]FDG-PET/CT are required to investigate for pocket and lead CIED infection.[30]

When ECHO fails to demonstrate valvular/perivalvular disease, other imaging techniques are used. cardiac (ECG)-gated cardiac CT(A) provides useful information on both valve and perivalvular IE lesions as well as complications such as perforation or valve aneurysm.[31] Excellent correlation with operative findings has been reported (96% sensitivity and 97% specificity) considering surgery as the reference standard in the "per valve" analysis.[32] ECHO continues to be superior to CT(A) for the detection of either small vegetations <10 mm (CT(A) sensitivity of 85% versus 96% of TOE) and leaflet perforations (CT(A) sensitivity of 48% versus 79% of TOE) or fistulae (CT(A) sensitivity of 86% versus 96% for TOE). The main strength of cardiac CT(A) is the detection of perivalvular lesions, such as abscesses and pseudoaneurysms with a reported sensitivity and specificity >95% when compared to surgical findings in left-sided valve IE, especially in the aortic localization[31,32] and a pooled sensitivity of 85% and 90% versus 64% and 77% of ECHO.[32–34] Nonetheless, it should be considered that data on the value of cardiac CT(A) in IE are relatively scarce, including few patients studied in highly experienced centers; therefore, this experience might not be valid for all centers managing patients with IE. Another additional major point of cardiac CT(A) is the assessment of noninfectious PV complications (ie, valve calcifications) and non-invasive coronary angiography is required preoperatively in patients with surgical indication. The role of whole-body CT in the identification of distant embolic events is discussed below.

Among the main relative limitations of CT(A), there are the high radiation exposure and the risk of nephrotoxicity associated with the use of iodinated contrast medium. However, the potential advantages of CT(A) should be always considered in a proper risk-benefit assessment.

In the presence of NVE, the value of [18F]FDG-PET/CT is limited[35–37] and the main added value of the technique is related to the detection of distant embolic events, a situation currently considered minor criteria in the 2015 ESC criteria (see further below).

In case of prosthetic material abnormal activity around the site of prosthetic valve implantation detected by [18F]FDG-PET/CT is a major criterion of the ESC 2015 diagnostic criteria. If PET/CT acquisition is combined with a cardiac CT (PET/CTA), the metabolic findings provided by the [18F]FDG uptake distribution and intensity might be added to the anatomic findings already described for cardiac CTA within a single imaging procedure. In a recent systematic review on the assessment of PVE, [18F]FDG-PET/CT sensitivity and specificity have been reported to range between 73% and 100% and 71% and 100%, respectively, with 67% to 100% positive (PPV) and 50% to 100% negative predictive values (NPV). Adding [18F]FDG-PET/CT to the modified Duke criteria increased sensitivity for a definite IE from 52% to 70% to 91% to 97%[38] by reducing the number of possible PVE cases. This finding has been confirmed in several series.[20,39–44] [18F] FDG-PET/CT has been reported to have similar sensitivities as ECHO for vegetations, perivalvular sequelae, and prosthetic valve dehiscence.[20] When [18F]FDG-PET/CTA, sensitivity and specificity for IE increased to 91%, with 93% PPV and 88% NPV.[42,45] In association with the Duke criteria, [18F]FDG-PET/CTA allowed reclassification of 90% of the cases initially classified as "possible" IE and provided a more conclusive diagnosis (definite/reject) in 95% of the patients. The presence of [18F]FDG-PET/CT uptake as a major criterion of the ESC 2015 had been shown in 40.9% of patients without major echo criteria.[46] Interestingly, in this study, when considering the subgroup of patients with high clinical suspicion of IE, the absolute increase in true positive using ESC criteria incorporation PET/CT findings instead of Duke criteria resulted higher than the absolute decrease in the false positive results. **Fig. 1** provides an example of PVE.

SPECT/CT with labeled leukocytes (WBC) presented a sensitivity ranging between 64% and 90%, associated with 36% to 100% specificity, 85% to 100% positive, and 47% to 81% NPVs.[22,39] In the case of an abscess, WBC SPECT/CT has been reported to have 83% to 100% sensitivity, 78% to 87% specificity, 43% to 71% positive, and 93% to 100% NPVs,[47] even in the early post-intervention phase.[22,47] Compared to [18F]FDG-PET/CT, WBC SPECT/CT has an excellent positive predictive value for the detection of perivalvular infection and abscesses in patients with suspected PVE sustained by pyogenic microorganisms. In addition, the intensity of WBC accumulation in the perivalvular area

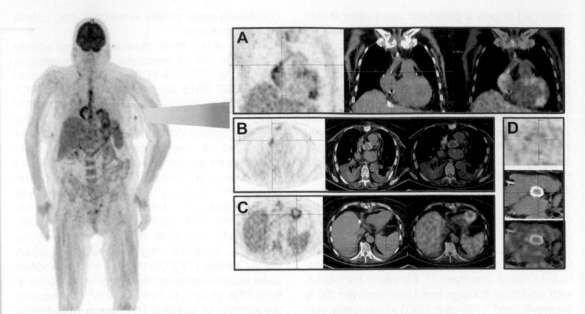

Fig. 1. A 71-year-old woman with aortic valve prosthesis and myectomy presented with fever and blood cultures positive for *E Coli* . Infectious endocarditis (IE) was suspected due to the presence of fever associated with relevant cardiac risk factors (prosthetic valve). Transesophageal echocardiography (TEE) showed a doubtful image on the prosthetic valve, suspected for IE but inconclusive. [18F]FDG-PET/CT images (MIP at left panel and emission, CT and superimposed PET/CT images in the coronal view (*A*) transaxial view at different levels (*B* and *C*) and details reconstructed aortic valve plain (*D*), Siemens Biograph mCT) showed normal tracer uptake at the aortic valve prosthesis and intense uptake at the pericardium at the level of the right atrium and the cardiac apical patch. Overall, these findings were suggestive for a normal prosthetic valve and pericarditis with cardiac patch infection.

represents an interesting marker of local infectious activity: patients with mild activity on the first scan disappearing on the second imaging evaluation seem to have a more favorable outcome.[47] This opens a very interesting perspective of the use of molecular multimodality imaging for the assessment of response to antimicrobial treatment. The most recent hybrid equipment allows performing CTA also during a WBC SPECT/CT scan. However, this potential further development has not been yet evaluated. **Fig. 2** provides an example of a WBC SPECT/CT scan.

Patients with Right-Sided IE

Involvement of the right heart is usually easy to detect using TTE because of the anterior location of the tricuspid valve and usually large vegetations,[48] although the right heart has many echocardiographically anomalous anatomic facets that may be difficult to distinguish from vegetations.[49] The eustachian and pulmonary valves should always be assessed. TEE is more sensitive in the detection of pulmonary vegetations,[50] associated left-sided involvement, central intravenous catheters and devices, prosthetic valve endocarditis, foreign bodies, unusual locations of right-side IE, and complications (eg, perivalvular

abscesses) after failing to respond to therapy.[51] TTE better defines the presence of prognostic features such as pericardial effusion, ventricular dysfunction, and increased pulmonary arterial pressure. TEE is superior to TTE in the detection and sizing of vegetations[52] and allows visualization of lead vegetations in the right atrium-superior vena cava area and other regions less well visualized by TTE.

CTA, [18F]FDG-PET/CT(A) (or [18F]FDG-PET/CT), and WBC SPECT/CT might be used in all the cases when right-sided IE (particularly PVE) is suspected. Contrast-enhanced CT may reveal pulmonary embolism, infarcts, and abscesses. Ventilation-perfusion scintigraphy may be an alternative to CT to screen patients for septic pulmonary embolism,[53] although [18F]FDG-PET/CT(A) and WBC SPECT/CT have largely replaced it, as they allow simultaneous assessment of right and left side valves, of sites of distant embolisms, and of potential portal of entry (POE) of the infection.[24]

IE in Patients with Congenital Heart Disease

The relative incidence of IE in patients with congenital heart disease is gradually increasing (currently representing about 10%–15% of the

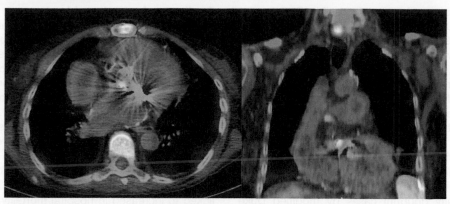

Fig. 2. Radiolabeled WBC scan in a patient with aortic and mitral mechanical prosthesis. The patient presents fever, increased C-reactive protein CRP and Erythrocyte Sedimentation Rate (ESR), negative Rheumatoid Factor (RF) and ECHO (both TEE and TOE). Positive urine culture with isolation of P. Mirabilis and positive blood culture with isolation of *Enterococcus faecalis* were found. SPECT/CT shows a focal area of increased uptake in the perivalvular aortic region, at the medial aspect (from left to right transaxial and coronal view, respectively).

cases) due to advances in surgical techniques that allow more patients to reach adulthood and to the relative reduction in post-rheumatic forms.[54]

Although the prevalence of IE in patients with congenital heart disease is higher than in the general population with valve disease but without congenital heart disease,[55] the risk is not evenly distributed within this cohort. In particular, it depends on the complexity of congenital heart disease—the greater the complexity, the greater the risk[56] and on specific factors for pediatric patients (peak at 10.3 years) and young adults (peak at 28.3 years),[57] respectively. Overall the risk of developing IE is strongly related to the past history of IE, the presence of multiple prosthetic materials, native abnormalities causing high-speed jets, and the Venturi effect, and it is more common in cyanotic heart disease and interventricular shunts.[58,59] This heterogeneity of clinical presentation is reflected in the mortality data, which are reported to range from 2% to 24%.[55,60,61] It should be noted, however, that the prognosis of patients with complex congenital heart disease is itself relatively severe and it is increased only slightly by concomitant IE (from 9 to 12.4 per 1000 patients). In contrast, the impact of IE in simple forms of congenital heart disease is substantial, doubling mortality (from 2.7 to 4.7 per 1000 patients).[56] In this context, early diagnosis is even more crucial despite being extremely clinically challenging, partly because of the patient's complex anatomical features, but also due to the often mild and nonspecific onset symptoms (such as persisting fever). Moreover, both in pediatric and adult patients, relatively low sensitivity of ECHO (TTE and TEE) and frequent negative blood cultures are reported in the literature.[45,62]

Indeed, in this setting, the limitations of ECHO in the assessment of right-sided IE, constituting 40% of congenital heart disease-IE generally extending to the lung valve prosthesis or the reconstructed conduit in the right ventricle are critical.[63] CTA is also technically challenging in this group of patients, in particular, due to the difficulty in selecting the best timing for the administration of the contrast medium during both the right and left phases.[64]

Therefore, [^{18}F]FDG-PET/CT has become more and more central for the evaluation of both intracardiac infections and distant disseminated disease.[65] Ishikita and colleagues[66] demonstrated in a 22-patient study that adding PET to the congenital heart disease-IE diagnostic process increases sensitivity from 39% to 88%, especially in evaluating right-sided IE, whereas negative PET results are associated with NVE and advanced age. Combining [^{18}F]FDG-PET/CT(A), Pizzi and colleagues[45] demonstrated to reclassify 86% of cases initially categorized as possible IE by ECHO in a population of 25 patients. More recently, Venet and colleagues[67] evaluated in a multicenter study conducted in eight tertiary care centers in France the performance of [^{18}F]FDG-PET for prosthetic pulmonic valve IE diagnosis in both children (n = 10; younger than 15 years of age) and adults (n = 49) with congenital heart disease. The underlying diagnoses included the tetralogy of Fallot sequence in 39%, double outlet right ventricle in 11%, aortic disease with pulmonic autograft (Ross) in 21% (with infection not of the pulmonic but of the neopulmonic valve), transposition in 9%, and truncus arteriosus in 5%. Active cardiac implanted electronic devices were present in 20% of patients. [^{18}F]FDG-PET/CT led to the reclassification of 57% of possible PVE by the modified Duke criteria to definitive IE, with a sensitivity of 79% and a positive predictive value of 92%. However, the specificity (73%) and negative predictive value (47%) were lower, potentially as a consequence of ongoing antibiotic treatment at the time of [¹⁸F]FDG-PET/CT in 55 of 59 (83%) patients. The study provides a valid and interesting data point in the scientific investigation of algorithms to diagnose a prosthetic pulmonic valve infection in a critically vulnerable group of patients with congenital heart defects. The high positive predictive value of [¹⁸F]FDG-PET/CT and its ability to reclassify doubtful cases by modified Duke criteria is particularly relevant. Early diagnosis of the disease without treatment delay is an important benefit, with favorable clinical and survival consequences. Of most importance in this patients' population is that the high spatial resolution of the technique allows excluding the involvement of other prosthetic material, resulting in better surgical planning and reducing the complexity or extensiveness of surgery or demonstrating multiple valve involvement from IE. **Fig. 3** provides an example of [¹⁸F]FDG-PET/CT in a patient with congenital heart disease–IE.

Finally, a consideration of radiation protection is mandatory, given the young age of patients and their frequent exposure to ionizing radiation: it is recommended to implement low-dose protocols. Even though it would reduce the radiation burden, PET/MR is currently not recommended due to the lower spatial resolution in comparison to CTA and the susceptibility to prosthetic artifacts, as well as the inability to perform the examination in patients with PM or ICD not MRI compatible.

Cardiovascular implantable electronic devices

The number of implanted cardiovascular implantable electronic devices (CIED), such as permanent pacemakers, implantable cardioverter/defibrillator, or cardiac resynchronization therapy devices with or without defibrillators, is estimated to exceed 1 million per year.[68] About 2% of patients over the age of 65 years have a CIED. Simultaneously, with the rise in device implants, the rate of infectious complications is also increasing by an estimated 5% per year,[69] reaching an incidence of 1.4 per 1000 device-years.[70] In addition to morbidity for patients, CIED infection has been linked to increased in-hospital mortality, by more than two-fold,[71,72] and higher rates of readmission up to 3 years following device implantation.[72–74] It is not surprising that CIED infections are estimated to cost over US \$500 million per year worldwide.[73,74]

Staphylococci are the main etiological agents (60%–80%), and *Staphylococcus aureus* is the most common cause of bacteremia and early-pocket infections. Superficial incisional infection from isolated pocket infection and pocket infections associated with lead infections and CIED systemic infections and/or IE represent different clinical entities that require different treatment management, and therefore, need to be differentiated. When dealing with systemic infection and IE complicating a CIED infection without local infection, the diagnosis may be more challenging as symptoms may be nonspecific and a long period may elapse between CIED implantation and symptom onset. In many cases, local and systemic symptoms coexist, but a systemic infection can also occur not associated with any local

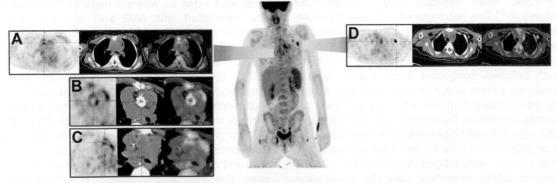

Fig. 3. An 11-year-old female patient, who previously underwent Konno surgery for aortic valve stenosis due to a congenital heart disease in Myhre syndrome, was admitted to further evaluate persistent fever and CRP elevation. TTE showed aortic valve restenosis. TEE was negative for valvular vegetations, but periprosthetic endoleak was reported. [18F]FDG-PET/CT images (MIP at the center and emission, CT and superimposed PET/CT images in transaxial view at different levels (*A* and *D*) and details reconstructed aortic valve plain (*B* and *C*), Siemens Biograph mCT) showed normal tracer uptake at the aortic valve prosthesis, moderate to intense uptake at the periprosthetic endoleak level, intense left axillary lymph node uptake. These findings were suggestive for infection in the endoleak site.

symptoms, as observed more frequently in late-onset infections. Patients with CIED infection may present with embolic involvement of the lungs and pleural space, frequently misdiagnosed as pulmonary infections.[75,76] CIED infections may also be revealed by other distant foci, such as vertebral osteomyelitis and discitis. In a recent international cohort, 10% of 2,781 episodes of IE were represented by device-related endocarditis.[77] When endocarditis is present, it is right-sided with the involvement of the tricuspid valve or the mural endocardium. Although the mitral and/or aortic valves are involved only in exceptional cases, in such instances, systemic embolism, stroke, congestive heart failure, and metastatic infections are more frequent and have a more severe prognosis.

The key issue for the successful treatment of definite CIED infections is the complete removal of all parts of the system and transvenous hardware, including the device and all leads.[78,79] This treatment concept applies to systemic as well as localized CIED pocket infections.[80] Patients with a cardiac implantable electronic device with superficial wound infections early after implantation, device exchange, or revision surgery should not undergo device and lead removal. Distinguishing between a superficial and a pocket infection can be a clinical challenge. Therefore, it is important to closely watch patients who are under suspicion of having a superficial infection. In such patients, oral antibiotic therapy (7–10 days) is reasonable.[71]

There is no standardized diagnostic tool for CIED endocarditis. The modified Duke criteria[81] and the ESC 2015 criteria[10] have generally been employed for the diagnosis. However, none represents a validated and standardized tool for diagnosis in this specific setting. Very recently, additional criteria merging the modified Duke criteria with the ESC 2015 criteria, known as the 2019 International CIED Infection Criteria, have been established (**Fig. 2** in Ref.[82]).

Identification of the microorganisms causing a CIED infection is pivotal for effective antibiotic therapy.

ECHO should be the first-line imaging tool to assess patients with CIED to identify lead vegetation and valvular involvement.[10] TTE and TEE are both recommended in case of suspected CIED infections. Although TTE better defines pericardial effusion, ventricular dysfunction, and pulmonary vascular pressure, TEE is superior for the detection and sizing of vegetations,[52] especially in the right atrium-superior vena cava area and in regions less well visualized by TTE. In the absence of typical vegetations of measurable size, both TTE and TEE may be false negative in CIED-related

IE. Lead masses in asymptomatic CIED carriers may be observed on TTE/TEE and do not predict CIED-related IE over long-term follow-up.[83,84] Therefore, once a lead mass is identified, careful clinical assessment to rule out either infection or non-bacterial lead-thrombotic endocarditis is needed, including serial TTE/TEE or additional imaging tests. In patients with CIED infections treated with percutaneous lead extraction, a TTE before hospital discharge is recommended to detect retained segments of the pacemaker lead, and to assess tricuspid valve function, right ventricular function, and pulmonary hypertension.[85]

Intracardiac ECHO is effective and has a high sensitivity for the detection of vegetation in cardiac devices.[86,87] Therefore, vegetation seen with intracardiac ECHO may be considered a major criterion for diagnosis. Recently, transvenous biopsy, guided by TEE, has been shown to be useful to distinguish vegetation from thrombus.[88]

It is important to consider that a normal ECHO does not rule out CIED-related IE.

Some radiographic and CT findings (ie, presence of fluid density between the heart and the device)[89] may suggest the presence of infection; however, these findings can be observed also in the postoperative or inflammatory changes, that are noninfectious. Furthermore, the absence of crumpling of patches in plain x-ray or fluid around the heart in the CT scan does not exclude the possibility of underlying infection at these sites.

WBC SPECT/CT and [^{18}F]FDG-PET/CT can be suggested in patients with CIED infections as a guide to clinicians for choosing the most suitable treatment, ie, conservative treatment (ESC class IIb recommendations).[10] PET/CT imaging may also contribute to assessing the mortality risk stratification after lead extraction. Patients with definite CIED infection without pocket involvement on [^{18}F]FDG-PET/CT had unfavorable outcomes, suggesting that the presence of an endovascular infection stemming from an unrecognized/distant site is associated with poor prognosis.[90]

WBC SPECT/CT allows the detection of additional unsuspected extracardiac sites of infection in up to 23% of patients with device-related sepsis,[91] although with some limitations in the case of small central nervous system (CNS) embolism. [^{18}F]FDG-PET/CT is used for identifying CIED infections,[92] particularly when the examination is performed to rule out device involvement during infection[93] and to define the embolic burden.[92,94–96] Recently, the performance of [^{18}F]FDG-PET/CT in CIED infections has been reported to improve when adopting ad-hoc- developed diagnostic criteria.[97] Similarly to what has been described for PVE, WBC SPECT/CT and

[^{18}F]FDG-PET/CT can be used to confirm or exclude infection, and to characterize the extension of the infectious process, including extracardiac workup. The value of [^{18}F]FDG-PET/CT in the diagnosis of CIED infection is confirmed by a large body of literature. The diagnosis of local infections is quite straightforward. A recent meta-analysis provides a pooled specificity and sensitivity in this subgroup of 93% (95% CI, 84%–98%) and 98% (95% CI, 88%–100%), respectively, and the area under the Receiver Operating Characteristic (ROC) curve was 0.98 for [^{18}F]FDG-PET/CT.[98,99] The largest study with labeled leukocyte scintigraphy (n = 63) reported a sensitivity of 94% and a specificity of 100%.[89] Using these imaging modalities, it is possible to distinguish between superficial and deep-pocket infection, the latter requiring removal of the generator rather than medical treatment. Non-attenuation-corrected images should be used for the final interpretation of the images. Semi-quantitative parameters such as semi-quantitative ratio of the maximum count rate of the pocket device over the mean count rate of lung parenchyma[97] or normalization of standardized uptake value $(SUV)_{max}$ around the CIEDs to the mean hepatic blood pool ratio activity[100] might help in differentiating mild postoperative residual inflammation up to 2 months after device implantation versus infection. The diagnostic accuracy for lead infections is lower, with an overall pooled sensitivity of 65% (95% CI, 53%–76%), specificity of 88% (95% CI, 77%–94%), and area under the curve of 0.861.[98] Such a finding is mainly related to the small size of the vegetations along the leads, which are often under the spatial resolution of the system.[92] The [^{18}F]FDG-PET/CT and WBC scintigraphy findings associated with Duke criteria also allowed reclassifying most of the cases initially classified as "possible" IE,[42] distinguishing infection limited to the pocket or leads from a more severe infection affecting the whole device,[101] and identifying patients requiring device extraction.[102] **Fig. 4** shows an example of CIED infection.

In addition, also in the case of CIED infections, accurate evaluation of the whole-body imaging might detect septic embolisms and identify the possible infection POE, impacting the subsequent therapeutic management and reducing the risk of relapse.[103] Indeed, in CIED infection, the detection of lung embolism, considered a major criterion of the Duke score, has been shown to increase the diagnostic sensitivity.[76]

CTA combined with PET may prove useful also for CIED infections in selected settings. [^{18}F] FDG-PET/CTA resulted in a high rate of reclassifications from "possible" to "definite" IE, improving the overall diagnostic accuracy with or without the Duke criteria in a series of patients with suspected pulmonary embolism or CIED infections.[42] Cardiac CTA may also add important information on remote vascular complications, including mycotic aneurysms, arterial emboli, and septic pulmonary infarcts, which add to the diagnostic criteria and affect the overall treatment strategy. In addition, pulmonary CTA may be useful in patients with recurrent pneumonia.[104] A wider use of contrast-enhanced CT is limited by the deleterious impact of contrast agents on kidney function, particularly as the patients are exposed to nephrotoxic antibiotic therapy.

Infections associated with left ventricular assist devices

Implantable left ventricular assist devices (LVAD) constitute a major medical advance for end-stage heart failure in selected patients.[105] This treatment is currently used as a bridge-to-transplantation, a bridge-to-recovery, or as destination therapy as the last resort in patients with neither prospect of recovery, nor of a heart transplant. Implantable LVAD intended for long-term use relies on a percutaneous driveline to carry electric signals and energy from the controller and batteries to the implanted pump. As with any other implantable foreign device, it is subject to LVAD-related infections.[106] The presence of a driveline piercing the skin places the patient at continual risk of infection that can affect the exit site, the subcutaneous tunnel, the abdominal pocket (if present), and the implanted pump, and that can disseminate through bloodstream infection. The transition from pulsatile to continuous-flow LVAD significantly improved the clinical outcome[107] and decreased the risk of infectious complications. Nonetheless, LVAD-related infections are still common with a prevalence that ranges from 23% to 58%, being associated with a high mortality rate (15%–44%).[91] The major sites of infection include the mediastinum drivelines and the device surface, identified as LVAD endocarditis.[108] The major pathogens involved in these emerging foreign device-related infectious diseases are–as it could be expected–the "big five": *Staphylococcus aureus*, Enterobacteriaceae, *Pseudomonas aeruginosa*, coagulase-negative Staphylococci, and *Corynebacterium sporigenous*.[109]

Due to the lack of large series in the literature, thus of specific guidelines, the management of LVAD infections is poorly standardized and mainly derived from the available recommendation of other CIEDs infections, prosthetic valves, or

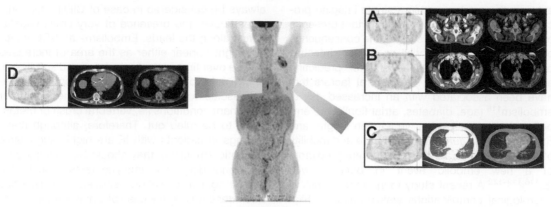

Fig. 4. [18F]FDG-PET/CT scan (Siemens Biograph mCT) in a 73-year-old male patient undergoing antibiotic therapy for Methicillin-sensitive Staphylococcus aureus (MSSA) endocarditis on mitral valve, to evaluate possible PM involvement and identify other septic foci. The images showed intense FDG activity at the PM pocket (*A*) and at the subcutaneous lead tract (*B*), compatible with infection. An additional infectious localization was noted in the anterior basal segment of the lower lobe of the left lung (*C*). Moderate uptake was seen at the mitral valve level (*D*), compatible with known endocarditis.

vascular prostheses, although their characteristics differ significantly.[110]

In this context, CT is the main diagnostic imaging test, based on the ability to detect edema as the primary sign of infection, a finding often nonspecific. The usefulness of WBC SPECT/CT and [18F]FDG-PET/CT for the diagnosis of LVAD-related infection has been shown in small series under routine clinical conditions and proved the ability to precisely localize and accurately assess the extent of a suspected infection,[91] with 100% sensitivity and 94% specificity of 94% for [18F]FDG-PET/CT.[111,112] A recent systematic review identified a total of four studies involving 119 scans assessing diagnostic performance.[112] Axial (n = 36) and centrifugal (n = 83) flow LVADs were represented. Pooled sensitivity was 92% (95% CI: 82%–97%) and specificity was 83% (95% CI: 24%–99%) for FDG-PET/CT in diagnosing LVAD infections. The summary receiver-operating characteristic curve analysis demonstrated an area under the curve of 0.94 (95% CI: 0.91–0.95).

A SUVmax cut-off of five has been recommended to help diagnose LVAD infection.[113] The use of the metabolic volume has recently been reported to be associated with increased diagnostic accuracy as compared to the SUV_{max} in a series of 48 patients. In particular, the NPV and sensitivity increased up to >95% by using the metabolic volume compared with 87.5% when using SUV_{max}.[114]

Patient with Embolic Events Without Definite IE

Extracardiac manifestations of IE (both NVE and PVE) are reported in 30% to 80% of patients.

The most frequent events are embolic stroke or septic embolization to bone, spleen, or kidneys, although only some of these are symptomatic.[2,115] The majority of embolisms take place within the first 14 days after treatment initiation,[116] thus, appearing as the initial symptom leading to the diagnosis, and are frequently recurrent.[116] Localization of the emboli and their cerebral/extracerebral proportion vary according to the studies, in particular, in consideration of the frequency and modalities of imaging, and the proportion of right-sided and left-sided IE.

The search for asymptomatic embolic events through systematic extracardiac imaging has become very important, because the detection of asymptomatic embolic events is now considered a minor Duke criterion in the 2015 ESC criteria.[10] This represents another main difference between the ESC and the AHA recommendations, in which only symptomatic extracardiac localizations of IE are considered as Duke classification minor criteria.[117]

The panel of imaging modalities used routinely to evaluate patients with extracardiac infective processes includes dental radiography, abdominal ultrasound, CT scan of the brain, whole-body CT, or MRI scan. The CT scan (including the brain) has long been considered the main imaging technique for the diagnosis of embolic events in IE patients; MRI is a valuable alternative in case of cerebral embolism, with the advantage of higher sensitivity in detecting recent ischemic lesions, and small ischemic or hemorrhagic lesions, without the use of iodine contrast. A noticeable advantage of [18F]FDG-PET/CT and WBC SPECT/CT is the possibility to perform the extracardiac workup within a single imaging procedure, thus, revealing the concomitant presence of extracardiac infection sites as the consequence of septic embolism, as well as primary infective processes. ECHO is also useful for predicting embolic events. Among the several factors that have been associated with an increased risk of embolism[118] (age, diabetes, atrial fibrillation, embolism before antibiotics, vegetation length, and *Staphylococcus aureus* infection size and mobility of the vegetations) are the most potent predictors of a new embolic event in patients with IE.[116,119–122] A recent study found that the risk of neurological complications was particularly high in patients with very large vegetation (>30 mm length).[123] The 2015 ESC guidelines recommend urgent surgical therapy in case of large (>10 mm) vegetation following one or more embolic episodes, and when the large vegetation is associated with other predictors of a complicated course.[10]

BRIEF TECHNICAL CONSIDERATIONS ON PATIENT PREPARATION, RADIOPHARMACEUTICALS PREPARATION, ACQUISITION PROTOCOLS, POST-ACQUISITION IMAGE PROCESSING, AND IMAGE READING/INTERPRETATION
Labeled Leukocyte SPECT/CT

In the case of IE, the procedure for labeled leukocyte scintigraphy is very similar to the one used for any other infection. No specific patient preparation is required, besides the standard preparation for WBC imaging.

The general rules for the radiolabeling of WBC preparation are also applied.

An important aspect of WBC imaging in cardiovascular infections is the image acquisition protocol, which should include planar acquisitions at 30 minutes (early images), at 4 to 6 hours (delayed images), and at 20 to 24 hours (late images) after reinjection of the radiolabeled leukocytes (most frequently ^{99m}Tc-HMPAO-WBC in the current clinical practice) with a mandatory SPECT/CT acquisition as part of the standard imaging protocol.[22,23] SPECT/CT images are used not only to confirm and localize findings at planar images consistent with infection (area or increased accumulation intensity or size over time), but also to increase diagnostic accuracy.

Rarely, false positive findings have been described for WBC imaging in IE and CIED infections, even in the case of very early infections. On the other hand, false negative scans have been observed in the presence of IE caused by non-pyogenic strains.[22] The same limitation must

always be considered in case of CIED infections, in particular, the presence of very small vegetation(s) along the leads. Embolisms at WBC imaging might appear either as the area of increased uptake over time in the brain, lung, and soft tissue, or as a cold spot when spleen embolism and spondylodiscitis occur, which requires other benign or malignant conditions (ie, vertebral crush or metastasis) to be ruled out. Therefore, although these findings in patients with IE are highly suggestive of septic embolism, they should be confirmed by additional diagnostic imaging tests. Due to the limited spatial resolution, reduced sensitivity has been described in the case of small embolisms.[124]

[^{18}F]FDG-PET/CT

For [^{18}F]FDG-PET/CT patient preparation, some specific aspects of the imaging protocol and imaging reading should be adapted. An extensive review of the main critical technical issues is provided in the "Recommendation on nuclear and multimodality imaging in IE and CIED infections" released by the European Association of Nuclear Medicine (EANM).[23] Briefly, we will discuss here some crucial points for a correct imaging procedure.

Patient preparation is very important to reduce the physiological uptake of [^{18}F]FDG in the myocardium. This can be achieved by the application of a proper fat-enriched, low-carbohydrate diet followed by fasting. Additionally, the use of intravenous heparin approximately 15 minutes before [^{18}F]FDG injection can be helpful.[125] There is a general agreement that a high-fat, low-carbohydrate diet for at least two meals with a fast of at least 4 hours is the minimum to obtain a suppression of physiologic myocardial utilization of glucose.

Efforts should be made to decrease blood glucose to the lowest possible level, although hyperglycemia does not represent an absolute contraindication for performing the study.[126,127]

The [^{18}F]FDG activity recommended in the joint EANM/SNMMI guidelines on PET imaging in inflammation/infection is 2.5 to 5.0 MBq/kg (175–350 MBq in a 70 kg standard adult).[126] Although antimicrobial treatment is expected to decrease the intensity of [^{18}F]FDG uptake,[128] there is no evidence at this stage to routinely recommend treatment discontinuation before performing PET/CT. On the contrary, corticosteroid treatment should be discontinued or at least reduced to the lowest possible dosage in the 24 hours preceding the exam.[129]

Image acquisition generally starts after an uptake time of 45 to 60 minutes. The emission time/

bed position depends on the sensitivity of the scanner. Whole-body images including the lower limbs are suggested to detect complications of IE, such as mycotic aneurysms that may require specific treatment by embolization to prevent rupture.[130] An additional separate bed position on the cardiac region is useful to record ECG-gated images. Diagnostic angio-CT (CTA) scan might be also performed to maximize the diagnostic information provided by the exam. The technical requisites for performing PET/CTA with a hybrid PET/CT scanner are arterial phase ECG-gated CTA with at least a 64-detector row CT scanner for the evaluation of left-sided prosthetic IE and a prospective, ECG-gated, venous phase CTA sequence for CIED infections/right side IE.[42] Image reconstruction with and without attenuation correction is recommended to identify potential reconstruction artifacts. Metal artifact reduction techniques are useful to minimize overcorrection, even if they do not always recover complete PET image quality.

Metabolic activity is evaluated both qualitatively and quantitatively. A focal or heterogeneous [^{18}F] FDG uptake distribution on visual assessment generally indicates active infection. Quantitative assessment supports visual information, but as many factors may affect measurements, the values obtained should be considered only a guide and not conclusive data.[23,131] SUV_{max} and the ratio of the prosthetic material SUV_{max} to the mean SUV of the blood pool or the liver (SUV_{ratio} or target-to-background ratio) can be used[100] with a cut-off of ≥ 2.0 as SUV_{ratio} has a very high predictive value for PVE (100% sensitivity, 91% specificity) after proper standardization of the scanner (European Association of Nuclear Medicine Research Ltd–EARL, accreditation program).[132]

Several physiological variants and pathological conditions that enter the differential diagnosis with IE/CIED infection should be recognized to prevent misinterpretation of a positive scan such as lipomatous hypertrophy of the interatrial septum,[133] active thrombi,[134] soft atherosclerotic plaques,[135] primary cardiac tumors,[136] cardiac metastasis,[48] and in case of Libman-Sacks endocarditis.[51]

One of the major findings that should be recognized is the presence of faint and homogeneous [^{18}F]FDG uptake strictly limited to the valve annulus,[137] most likely as the result of the persistent host reaction against the biomaterial coating the sewing ring of the prosthetic valve. A recent experience by Pizzi and colleagues[138] suggests that the metabolic and anatomic patterns might help distinguish between inflammation and infection in these patients. In particular, a postoperative

inflammatory response may result in nonspecific [^{18}F]FDG uptake immediately after surgery.[139] However, Mathieu and colleagues[140] have recently shown that the mean amount of [^{18}F]FDG uptake did not significantly differ in patients scanned within 3 months. This has been confirmed in a recent multicenter study on a large cohort of patients, where recent valve implantation was not a significant predictor of false positive interpretation.[132]

As already discussed, antimicrobial therapy and/or vegetation size could account for false negative results on [^{18}F]FDG-PET/CT.

CLINICS CARE POINTS

- In patients who present with fever and positive blood culture, [18F]FDG-PET/CT and imaging with labeled leukocytes (WBC) may be useful in identifying foci of infection, both cardiac and extracardiac.

- These imaging techniques have a greater role in the evaluation of prosthetic valve endocarditis, where echocardiography may be limited; in native valve endocarditis they should be considered to detect distant embolic events.

- Diagnostic criteria should be included in the report of [18F]FDG-PET/CT.

- WBC imaging is particularly useful in the evaluation of infection with pyogenic bacteria.

- WBC imaging and [18F]FDG-PET/CT are useful in patients with implantable electronic device infections (CIEDs) as a guide for choosing the most appropriate treatment, differentiating superficial incisional infection from isolated pocket infection and pocket infections associated with lead infection and systemic infection and/or infectious endocarditis of CIEDs.

- In patients with congenital heart disease, [18F]FDG-PET/CT maintains the same diagnostic accuracy as in adult patients.

REFERENCES

1. Hoen B, Alla F, Selton-Suty C, et al. Changing profile of infective endocarditis: results of a 1-year survey in France. JAMA 2002;288(1):75–81.
2. Selton-Suty C, Célard M, Le Moing V, et al. Preeminence of Staphylococcus aureus in infective endocarditis: a 1-year population-based survey. Clin Infect Dis 2012;54(9):1230–9.
3. Habib G, Erba PA, Iung B, et al. Clinical presentation, aetiology and outcome of infective

endocarditis. Results of the ESC-EORP EURO-ENDO (European infective endocarditis) registry: a prospective cohort study. Eur Heart J 2019;40: 3222–32.

4. Kollef MH, Sharpless L, Vlasnik J, et al. The impact of nosocomial infections on patient outcomes following cardiac surgery. Chest 1997;112(3):666–75.

5. Brown PP, Kugelmass AD, Cohen DJ, et al. The frequency and cost of complications associated with coronary artery bypass grafting surgery: results from the United States Medicare program. Ann Thorac Surg 2008;85(6):1980–6.

6. Edwards JR, Peterson KD, Mu Y, et al. National healthcare safety network (NHSN) report: data summary for 2006 through 2008, issued december 2009. Am J Infect Control 2009;37(10):783–805.

7. Dudeck MA, Weiner LM, Allen-Bridson K, et al. National healthcare safety network (NHSN) report, data summary for 2012, device-associated module. Am J Infect Control 2013;41(12):1148–66.

8. Gelijns AC, Moskowitz AJ, Acker MA, et al. Management practices and major infections after cardiac surgery. J Am Coll Cardiol 2014;64(4):372–81.

9. Pérez de Isla L, Zamorano J, Lennie V, et al. Negative blood culture infective endocarditis in the elderly: long-term follow-up. Gerontology 2007; 53(5):245–9.

10. Habib G, Lancellotti P, Antunes MJ, et al. 2015 ESC guidelines for the management of infective endocarditis: the task force for the management of infective endocarditis of the European society of Cardiology (ESC). Endorsed by: European association for cardio-thoracic surgery (EACTS), the European association of nuclear medicine (EANM). Eur Heart J 2015;36(44):3075–128.

11. Otto CM, Nishimura RA, Bonow RO, et al. 2020 ACC/AHA guideline for the management of patients with valvular heart disease: a report of the American College of Cardiology/American heart association joint committee on clinical practice guidelines. Circulation 2021;143(5):e72–227.

12. Habib G, Hoen B, Tornos P, et al. Guidelines on the prevention, diagnosis, and treatment of infective endocarditis (new version 2009): the task force on the prevention, diagnosis, and treatment of infective endocarditis of the European society of Cardiology (ESC). Endorsed by the European society of clinical microbiology and infectious diseases (ESCMID) and the international society of chemotherapy (ISC) for infection and cancer. Eur Heart J 2009;30(19):2369–413.

13. Erba PA, Pizzi MN, Roque A, et al. Multimodality imaging in infective endocarditis: an imaging Team within the endocarditis Team. Circulation 2019; 140(21):1753–65.

14. Habib G, Badano L, Tribouilloy C, et al. Recommendations for the practice of echocardiography

in infective endocarditis. Eur J Echocardiogr 2010;11(2):202–19.

15. Roe MT, Abramson MA, Li J, et al. Clinical information determines the impact of transesophageal echocardiography on the diagnosis of infective endocarditis by the duke criteria. Am Heart J 2000; 139(6):945–51.

16. Jacob S, Tong AT. Role of echocardiography in the diagnosis and management of infective endocarditis. Curr Opin Cardiol 2002;17(5):478–85.

17. Hill EE, Herijgers P, Claus P, et al. Abscess in infective endocarditis: the value of transesophageal echocardiography and outcome: a 5-year study. Am Heart J 2007;154(5):923–8.

18. Ren Z, Zhang J, Chen H, et al. Preoperative false-negative transthoracic echocardiographic results in native valve infective endocarditis patients: a retrospective study from 2001 to 2018. Cardiovasc Ultrasound 2021;19(1):2.

19. Habib G. Management of infective endocarditis. Heart 2006;92(1):124–30.

20. Saby L, Laas O, Habib G, et al. Positron emission tomography/computed tomography for diagnosis of prosthetic valve endocarditis: increased valvular 18F-fluorodeoxyglucose uptake as a novel major criterion. J Am Coll Cardiol 2013;61(23):2374–82.

21. Bruun NE, Habib G, Thuny F, et al. Cardiac imaging in infectious endocarditis. Eur Heart J 2014;35(10): 624–32.

22. Erba PA, Conti U, Lazzeri E, et al. Added value of 99mTc-HMPAO-labeled leukocyte SPECT/CT in the characterization and management of patients with infectious endocarditis. J Nucl Med 2012; 53(8):1235–43.

23. Erba PA, Lancellotti P, Vilacosta I, et al. Recommendations on nuclear and multimodality imaging in IE and CIED infections. Eur J Nucl Med Mol Imaging 2018;45(10):1795–815.

24. Sollini M, Berchiolli R, Delgado Bolton RC, et al. The "3M" approach to cardiovascular infections: multimodality, multitracers, and multidisciplinary. Semin Nucl Med 2018;48(3):199–224.

25. Rasmussen RV, Høst U, Arpi M, et al. Prevalence of infective endocarditis in patients with Staphylococcus aureus bacteraemia: the value of screening with echocardiography. Eur J Echocardiogr 2011; 12(6):414–20.

26. Østergaard L, Bruun NE, Voldstedlund M, et al. Prevalence of infective endocarditis in patients with positive blood cultures: a Danish nationwide study. Eur Heart J 2019;40(39):3237–44.

27. van der Vaart TW, Prins JM, Soetekouw R, et al. Prediction rules for ruling out endocarditis in patients with staphylococcus aureus bacteremia. Clin Infect Dis 2022;74(8):1442–9.

28. Showler A, Burry L, Bai AD, et al. Use of transthoracic echocardiography in the management of

low-risk staphylococcus aureus bacteremia: results from a retrospective multicenter cohort study. JACC Cardiovasc Imaging 2015;8(8):924–31.

29. Diekema DJ, Hsueh PR, Mendes RE, et al. The microbiology of bloodstream infection: 20-year trends from the SENTRY antimicrobial surveillance program, Antimicrobial Agents Chemother, 63(7), 2019, 00355-19.

30. Dahl A, Hernandez-Meneses M, Perissinotti A, et al. Echocardiography and FDG-PET/CT scan in Gram-negative bacteremia and cardiovascular infections. Curr Opin Infect Dis 2021;34(6):728–36.

31. Grob A, Thuny F, Villacampa C, et al. Cardiac multidetector computed tomography in infective endocarditis: a pictorial essay. Insights Imaging 2014; 5(5):559–70.

32. Feuchtner GM, Stolzmann P, Dichtl W, et al. Multi-slice computed tomography in infective endocarditis: comparison with transesophageal echocardiography and intraoperative findings. J Am Coll Cardiol 2009;53(5):436–44.

33. Fagman E, Perrotta S, Bech-Hanssen O, et al. ECG-gated computed tomography: a new role for patients with suspected aortic prosthetic valve endocarditis. Eur Radiol 2012;22(11):2407–14.

34. Sifaoui I, Oliver L, Tacher V, et al. Diagnostic performance of transesophageal echocardiography and cardiac computed tomography in infective endocarditis. J Am Soc Echocardiogr 2020;33(12): 1442–53.

35. Kestler M, Muñoz P, Rodríguez-Créixems M, et al. Role of (18)F-FDG PET in patients with infectious endocarditis. J Nucl Med 2014;55(7):1093–8.

36. Kouijzer IJ, Vos FJ, Janssen MJ, et al. The value of 18F-FDG PET/CT in diagnosing infectious endocarditis. Eur J Nucl Med Mol Imaging 2013;40(7): 1102–7.

37. Granados U, Fuster D, Pericas JM, et al. Diagnostic accuracy of 18F-FDG PET/CT in infective endocarditis and implantable cardiac electronic device infection: a cross-sectional study. J Nucl Med 2016;57(11):1726–32.

38. Gomes A, Glaudemans AWJM, Touw DJ, et al. Diagnostic value of imaging in infective endocarditis: a systematic review. Lancet Infect Dis 2017; 17(1):e1–14.

39. Rouzet F, Chequer R, Benali K, et al. Respective performance of 18F-FDG PET and radiolabeled leukocyte scintigraphy for the diagnosis of prosthetic valve endocarditis. J Nucl Med 2014; 55(12):1980–5.

40. Ricciardi A, Sordillo P, Ceccarelli L, et al. 18-Fluoro-2-deoxyglucose positron emission tomography-computed tomography: an additional tool in the diagnosis of prosthetic valve endocarditis. Int J Infect Dis 2014;28:219–24.

41. Bartoletti M, Tumietto F, Fasulo G, et al. Combined computed tomography and fluorodeoxyglucose positron emission tomography in the diagnosis of prosthetic valve endocarditis: a case series. BMC Res Notes 2014;7:32.

42. Pizzi MN, Roque A, Fernández-Hidalgo N, et al. Improving the diagnosis of infective endocarditis in prosthetic valves and intracardiac devices with 18F-Fluorodeoxyglucose positron emission tomography/computed tomography angiography: initial results at an infective endocarditis referral center. Circulation 2015;132(12):1113–26.

43. Fagman E, van Essen M, Fredén Lindqvist J, et al. 18F-FDG PET/CT in the diagnosis of prosthetic valve endocarditis. Int J Cardiovasc Imaging 2016;32(4):679–86.

44. Salomäki SP, Saraste A, Kemppainen J, et al. F-FDG positron emission tomography/computed tomography in infective endocarditis. J Nucl Cardiol 2017;24(1):195–206.

45. Pizzi MN, Dos-Subirà L, Roque A, et al. F-FDG-PET/CT angiography in the diagnosis of infective endocarditis and cardiac device infection in adult patients with congenital heart disease and prosthetic material. Int J Cardiol 2017;248:396–402.

46. Philip M, Tessonier L, Mancini J, et al. Comparison between ESC and duke criteria for the diagnosis of prosthetic valve infective endocarditis. JACC Cardiovasc Imaging 2020;13(12):2605–15.

47. Hyafil F, Rouzet F, Lepage L, et al. Role of radiolabelled leucocyte scintigraphy in patients with a suspicion of prosthetic valve endocarditis and inconclusive echocardiography. Eur Heart J Cardiovasc Imaging 2013;14(6):586–94.

48. San Román JA, Vilacosta I, López J, et al. Role of transthoracic and transesophageal echocardiography in right-sided endocarditis: one echocardiographic modality does not fit all. J Am Soc Echocardiogr 2012;25(8):807–14.

49. Morokuma H, Minato N, Kamohara K, et al. Three surgical cases of isolated tricuspid valve infective endocarditis. Ann Thorac Cardiovasc Surg 2010; 16(2):134–8.

50. Winslow TM, Redberg RF, Foster E, et al. Transesophageal echocardiographic detection of abnormalities of the tricuspid valve in adults associated with spontaneous closure of perimembranous ventricular septal defect. Am J Cardiol 1992;70(9): 967–9.

51. San Román JA, Vilacosta I. Role of transesophageal echocardiography in right-sided endocarditis. Echocardiography 1995;12(6):669–72.

52. Vilacosta I, Sarriá C, San Román JA, et al. Usefulness of transesophageal echocardiography for diagnosis of infected transvenous permanent pacemakers. Circulation 1994;89(6):2684–7.

53. Sohail MR, Uslan DZ, Khan AH, et al. Infective endocarditis complicating permanent pacemaker and implantable cardioverter-defibrillator infection. Mayo Clin Proc 2008;83(1):46–53.

54. Di Filippo S. Clinical outcomes for congenital heart disease patients presenting with infective endocarditis. Expert Rev Cardiovasc Ther 2020;18(6): 331–42.

55. Kuijpers JM, Koolbergen DR, Groenink M, et al. Incidence, risk factors, and predictors of infective endocarditis in adult congenital heart disease: focus on the use of prosthetic material. Eur Heart J 2017;38(26):2048–56.

56. Moore B, Cao J, Kotchetkova I, et al. Incidence, predictors and outcomes of infective endocarditis in a contemporary adult congenital heart disease population. Int J Cardiol 2017;249:161–5.

57. Fatima S, Dao B, Jameel A, et al. Epidemiology of infective endocarditis in rural upstate New York, 2011 - 2016. J Clin Med Res 2017;9(9):754–8.

58. Yener N, Oktar GL, Erer D, et al. Bicuspid aortic valve. Ann Thorac Cardiovasc Surg 2002;8(5): 264–7.

59. Berglund E, Johansson B, Dellborg M, et al. High incidence of infective endocarditis in adults with congenital ventricular septal defect. Heart 2016; 102(22):1835–9.

60. Ishiwada N, Niwa K, Tateno S, et al. Causative organism influences clinical profile and outcome of infective endocarditis in pediatric patients and adults with congenital heart disease. Circ J 2005; 69(10):1266–70.

61. Verheugt CL, Uiterwaal CS, van der Velde ET, et al. Turning 18 with congenital heart disease: prediction of infective endocarditis based on a large population. Eur Heart J 2011;32(15):1926–34.

62. Chau A, Renella P, Arrieta A. Multimodality cardiovascular imaging in the diagnosis and management of prosthetic valve infective endocarditis in children report of two cases and brief review of the literature. Cardiol Young 2019;29(12):1526–9.

63. Miranda WR, Connolly HM, Bonnichsen CR, et al. Prosthetic pulmonary valve and pulmonary conduit endocarditis: clinical, microbiological and echocardiographic features in adults. Eur Heart J Cardiovasc Imaging 2016;17(8):936–43.

64. Niwa K, Nakazawa M, Tateno S, et al. Infective endocarditis in congenital heart disease: Japanese national collaboration study. Heart 2005;91(6): 795–800.

65. Habets J, Tanis W, Reitsma JB, et al. Are novel noninvasive imaging techniques needed in patients with suspected prosthetic heart valve endocarditis? A systematic review and meta-analysis. Eur Radiol 2015;25(7):2125–33.

66. Ishikita A, Sakamoto I, Yamamura K, et al. Usefulness of. Circ J 2021;85(9):1505–13.

67. Venet M, Jalal Z, Ly R, et al. Diagnostic value of 18F-Fluorodeoxyglucose positron emission tomography computed tomography in prosthetic pulmonary valve infective endocarditis. JACC Cardiovasc Imaging 2022;15(2):299–308.

68. Managing cardiovascular implantable electronic devices (CIEDs) during perioperative care. The Anesthesia Patient Safety Foundation. J Patient Saf 2013;28(2):29–48.

69. Podoleanu C, Deharo JC. Management of cardiac implantable electronic device infection. Arrhythm Electrophysiol Rev 2014;3(3):184–9.

70. Thuny F, Grisoli D, Collart F, et al. Management of infective endocarditis: challenges and perspectives. Lancet 2012;379(9819):965–75.

71. Baddour LM, Epstein AE, Erickson CC, et al. Update on cardiovascular implantable electronic device infections and their management: a scientific statement from the American Heart Association. Circulation 2010;121(3):458–77.

72. Voigt A, Shalaby A, Saba S. Rising rates of cardiac rhythm management device infections in the United States: 1996 through 2003. J Am Coll Cardiol 2006;48(3):590–1.

73. Margey R, McCann H, Blake G, et al. Contemporary management of and outcomes from cardiac device related infections. Europace 2010;12(1):64–70.

74. Baman TS, Gupta SK, Valle JA, et al. Risk factors for mortality in patients with cardiac device-related infection. Circ Arrhythm Electrophysiol 2009;2(2): 129–34.

75. Cacoub P, Leprince P, Nataf P, et al. Pacemaker infective endocarditis. Am J Cardiol 1998;82(4): 480–4.

76. Klug D, Lacroix D, Savoye C, et al. Systemic infection related to endocarditis on pacemaker leads: clinical presentation and management. Circulation 1997;95(8):2098–107.

77. Murdoch DR, Corey GR, Hoen B, et al. Clinical presentation, etiology, and outcome of infective endocarditis in the 21st century: the International Collaboration on Endocarditis-Prospective Cohort Study. Arch Intern Med 2009;169(5):463–73.

78. Peacock JE, Stafford JM, Le K, et al. Attempted salvage of infected cardiovascular implantable electronic devices: are there clinical factors that predict success? Pacing Clin Electrophysiol 2018; 41(5):524–31.

79. Lebeaux D, Fernández-Hidalgo N, Chauhan A, et al. Management of infections related to totally implantable venous-access ports: challenges and perspectives. Lancet Infect Dis 2014;14(2):146–59.

80. Kusumoto FM, Schoenfeld MH, Wilkoff BL, et al. 2017 HRS expert consensus statement on cardiovascular implantable electronic device lead management and extraction. Heart Rhythm 2017; 14(12):e503–51.

81. Li JS, Sexton DJ, Mick N, et al. Proposed modifications to the Duke criteria for the diagnosis of infective endocarditis. Clin Infect Dis 2000;30(4): 633–8.

82. Blomström-Lundqvist C, Traykov V, Erba PA, et al. European heart rhythm association (EHRA) international consensus document on how to prevent, diagnose, and treat cardiac implantable electronic device infections-endorsed by the heart rhythm society (HRS), the asia pacific heart rhythm society (APHRS), the Latin American heart rhythm society (LAHRS), international society for cardiovascular infectious diseases (ISCVID) and the European society of clinical microbiology and infectious diseases (ESCMID) in collaboration with the European association for cardio-thoracic surgery (EACTS). Europace 2020;22(4):515–49.

83. Golzio PG, Errigo D, Peyracchia M, et al. Prevalence and prognosis of lead masses in patients with cardiac implantable electronic devices without infection. J Cardiovasc Med 2019;20(6):372–8.

84. Downey BC, Juselius WE, Pandian NG, et al. Incidence and significance of pacemaker and implantable cardioverter-defibrillator lead masses discovered during transesophageal echocardiography. Pacing Clin Electrophysiol 2011;34(6): 679–83.

85. Diemberger I, Biffi M, Lorenzetti S, et al. Predictors of long-term survival free from relapses after extraction of infected CIED. Europace 2018;20(6): 1018–27.

86. Bongiorni MG, Di Cori A, Soldati E, et al. Intracardiac echocardiography in patients with pacing and defibrillating leads: a feasibility study. Echocardiography 2008;25(6):632–8.

87. Narducci ML, Pelargonio G, Russo E, et al. Usefulness of intracardiac echocardiography for the diagnosis of cardiovascular implantable electronic device-related endocarditis. J Am Coll Cardiol 2013;61(13):1398–405.

88. Chang D, Gabriels J, Laighold S, et al. A novel diagnostic approach to a mass on a device lead. HeartRhythm Case Rep 2019;5(6):306–9.

89. Goodman LR, Almassi GH, Troup PJ, et al. Complications of automatic implantable cardioverter defibrillators: radiographic, CT, and echocardiographic evaluation. Radiology 1989;170(2):447–52.

90. Diemberger I, Bonfiglioli R, Martignani C, et al. Contribution of PET imaging to mortality risk stratification in candidates to lead extraction for pacemaker or defibrillator infection: a prospective single center study. Eur J Nucl Med Mol Imaging 2019;46(1):194–205.

91. Litzler PY, Manrique A, Etienne M, et al. Leukocyte SPECT/CT for detecting infection of left-ventricular-assist devices: preliminary results. J Nucl Med 2010;51(7):1044–8.

92. Ploux S, Riviere A, Amraoui S, et al. Positron emission tomography in patients with suspected pacing system infections may play a critical role in difficult cases. Heart Rhythm 2011;8(9):1478–81.

93. Vos FJ, Bleeker-Rovers CP, Sturm PD, et al. 18F-FDG PET/CT for detection of metastatic infection in gram-positive bacteremia. J Nucl Med 2010; 51(8):1234–40.

94. Abikhzer G, Turpin S, Bigras JL. Infected pacemaker causing septic lung emboli detected on FDG PET/CT. J Nucl Cardiol 2010;17(3):514–5.

95. Costo S, Hourna E, Massetti M, et al. Impact of F-18 FDG PET-CT for the diagnosis and management of infection in JARVIK 2000 device. Clin Nucl Med 2011;36(12):e188–91.

96. Bensimhon L, Lavergne T, Hugonnet F, et al. Whole body [(18) F]fluorodeoxyglucose positron emission tomography imaging for the diagnosis of pacemaker or implantable cardioverter defibrillator infection: a preliminary prospective study. Clin Microbiol Infect 2011;17(6):836–44.

97. Sarrazin JF, Philippon F, Tessier M, et al. Usefulness of fluorine-18 positron emission tomography/computed tomography for identification of cardiovascular implantable electronic device infections. J Am Coll Cardiol 2012;59(18):1616–25.

98. Juneau D, Golfam M, Hazra S, et al. Positron emission tomography and single-photon emission computed tomography imaging in the diagnosis of cardiac implantable electronic device infection: a systematic review and meta-analysis. Circ Cardiovasc Imaging 2017;10(4):e005772.

99. Matsushita K, Tsuboi N, Nanasato M, et al. Intravenous vegetation of methicillin-resistant Staphylococcus aureus induced by central venous catheter in a patient with implantable cardioverter-defibrillator: a case report. J Cardiol 2002;40(1):31–5.

100. Memmott MJ, James J, Armstrong IS, et al. The performance of quantitation methods in the evaluation of cardiac implantable electronic device (CIED) infection: a technical review. J Nucl Cardiol 2016;23(6):1457–66.

101. Erba PA, Sollini M, Conti U, et al. Radiolabeled WBC scintigraphy in the diagnostic workup of patients with suspected device-related infections. JACC Cardiovasc Imaging 2013;6(10):1075–86.

102. Ahmed FZ, James J, Cunnington C, et al. Early diagnosis of cardiac implantable electronic device generator pocket infection using 18F-FDG-PET/CT. Eur Heart J Cardiovasc Imaging 2015;16(5):521–30.

103. Amraoui S, Tlili G, Sohal M, et al. Contribution of PET imaging to the diagnosis of septic embolism in patients with pacing lead endocarditis. JACC Cardiovasc Imaging 2016;9(3):283–90.

104. Paparoupa M, Spineli L, Framke T, et al. Pulmonary embolism in pneumonia: still a diagnostic

challenge? results of a case-control study in 100 patients. Dis Markers 2016;2016:8682506.

105. Holman WL, Naftel DC, Eckert CE, et al. Durability of left ventricular assist devices: interagency registry for mechanically assisted circulatory support (INTERMACS) 2006 to 2011. J Thorac Cardiovasc Surg 2013;146(2):437–41.e1.

106. Köhler AK, Körperich H, Morshuis M, et al. Pre-operative risk factors for driveline infection in left ventricular-assist device patients. ESC Heart Fail 2022.

107. Xie A, Phan K, Yan TD. Durability of continuous-flow left ventricular assist devices: a systematic review. Ann Cardiothorac Surg 2014;3(6):547–56.

108. Wickline SA, Fischer KC. Can infections be imaged in implanted devices? ASAIO J 2000;46(6):S80–1.

109. Siméon S, Flécher E, Revest M, et al. Left ventricular assist device-related infections: a multicentric study. Clin Microbiol Infect 2017;23(10):748–51.

110. Koval CE, Rakita R, Practice AIDCo. Ventricular assist device related infections and solid organ transplantation. Am J Transplant 2013;13(Suppl 4):348–54.

111. Dell'Aquila AM, Mastrobuoni S, Alles S, et al. Contributory role of fluorine 18-fluorodeoxyglucose positron emission tomography/computed tomography in the diagnosis and clinical management of infections in patients supported with a continuous-flow left ventricular assist device. Ann Thorac Surg 2016;101(1):87–94 [discussion].

112. Tam MC, Patel VN, Weinberg RL, et al. Diagnostic Accuracy of FDG PET/CT in Suspected LVAD Infections: a case series, systematic review, and meta-analysis. JACC Cardiovasc Imaging 2020; 13(5):1191–202.

113. Friedman SN, Mahmood M, Geske JR, et al. Positron emission tomography objective parameters for assessment of left ventricular assist device infection using. Am J Nucl Med Mol Imaging 2020;10(6):301–11.

114. Avramovic N, Dell'Aquila AM, Weckesser M, et al. Metabolic volume performs better than SUVmax in the detection of left ventricular assist device driveline infection. Eur J Nucl Med Mol Imaging 2017;44(11):1870–7.

115. Duval X, Delahaye F, Alla F, et al. Temporal trends in infective endocarditis in the context of prophylaxis guideline modifications: three successive population-based surveys. J Am Coll Cardiol 2012;59(22):1968–76.

116. Vilacosta I, Graupner C, San Román JA, et al. Risk of embolization after institution of antibiotic therapy for infective endocarditis. J Am Coll Cardiol 2002; 39(9):1489–95.

117. Baddour LM, Wilson WR, Bayer AS, et al. Infective endocarditis in adults: diagnosis, antimicrobial therapy, and management of complications: a scientific statement for healthcare professionals from the american heart association. Circulation 2015; 132(15):1435–86.

118. Habib G. Embolic risk in subacute bacterial endocarditis: determinants and role of transesophageal echocardiography. Curr Cardiol Rep 2003;5(2): 129–36.

119. Hubert S, Thuny F, Resseguier N, et al. Prediction of symptomatic embolism in infective endocarditis: construction and validation of a risk calculator in a multicenter cohort. J Am Coll Cardiol 2013;62(15): 1384–92.

120. Thuny F, Di Salvo G, Disalvo G, et al. Risk of embolism and death in infective endocarditis: prognostic value of echocardiography: a prospective multicenter study. Circulation 2005;112(1):69–75.

121. Di Salvo G, Habib G, Pergola V, et al. Echocardiography predicts embolic events in infective endocarditis. J Am Coll Cardiol 2001;37(4):1069–76.

122. Steckelberg JM, Murphy JG, Ballard D, et al. Emboli in infective endocarditis: the prognostic value of echocardiography. Ann Intern Med 1991; 114(8):635–40.

123. García-Cabrera E, Fernández-Hidalgo N, Almirante B, et al. Neurological complications of infective endocarditis: risk factors, outcome, and impact of cardiac surgery: a multicenter observational study. Circulation 2013;127(23):2272–84.

124. Erba PA, Leo G, Sollini M, et al. Radiolabelled leucocyte scintigraphy versus conventional radiological imaging for the management of late, low-grade vascular prosthesis infections. Eur J Nucl Med Mol Imaging 2014;41(2):357–68.

125. Osborne MT, Hulten EA, Murthy VL, et al. Patient preparation for cardiac fluorine-18 fluorodeoxyglucose positron emission tomography imaging of inflammation. J Nucl Cardiol 2017;24(1):86–99.

126. Jamar F, Buscombe J, Chiti A, et al. EANM/SNMMI guideline for 18F-FDG use in inflammation and infection. J Nucl Med 2013;54(4):647–58.

127. Rabkin Z, Israel O, Keidar Z. Do hyperglycemia and diabetes affect the incidence of false-negative 18F-FDG PET/CT studies in patients evaluated for infection or inflammation and cancer? A Comparative analysis. J Nucl Med 2010;51(7): 1015–20.

128. Scholtens AM, van Aarnhem EE, Budde RP. Effect of antibiotics on FDG-PET/CT imaging of prosthetic heart valve endocarditis. Eur Heart J Cardiovasc Imaging 2015;16(11):1223.

129. Raplinger K, Chandler K, Hunt C, et al. Effect of steroid use during chemotherapy on SUV levels in PET/CT. J Nucl Med 2012;53(supplement 1): 2718.

130. Mikail N, Benali K, Ou P, et al. Detection of mycotic aneurysms of lower limbs by whole-body (18)F-FDG-PET. JACC Cardiovasc Imaging 2015;8(7): 859–62.

131. Bucerius J, Mani V, Moncrieff C, et al. Optimizing 18F-FDG PET/CT imaging of vessel wall inflammation: the impact of 18F-FDG circulation time, injected dose, uptake parameters, and fasting blood glucose levels. Eur J Nucl Med Mol Imaging 2014;41(2):369–83.·

132. Swart LE, Gomes A, Scholtens AM, et al. Improving the diagnostic performance of circulation. Circulation 2018;138(14):1412–27.

133. Fan CM, Fischman AJ, Kwek BH, et al. Lipomatous hypertrophy of the interatrial septum: increased uptake on FDG PET. AJR Am J Roentgenol 2005; 184(1):339–42.

134. Sochowski RA, Chan KL. Implication of negative results on a monoplane transesophageal echocardiographic study in patients with suspected infective endocarditis. J Am Coll Cardiol 1993; 21(1):216–21.

135. Salaun E, Aldebert P, Jaussaud N, et al. Early endocarditis and delayed left ventricular pseudoaneurysm complicating a transapical transcatheter mitral valve-in-valve implantation: percutaneous closure under local anesthesia and echocardiographic guidance. Circ Cardiovasc Interv 2016; 9(10):e003886.

136. Baddour LM, Wilson WR, Bayer AS, et al. Infective endocarditis: diagnosis, antimicrobial therapy, and management of complications: a statement for healthcare professionals from the committee on rheumatic fever, endocarditis, and kawasaki disease, council on cardiovascular disease in the young, and the councils on clinical Cardiology, stroke, and cardiovascular surgery and anesthesia, American heart association: endorsed by the infectious diseases society of America. Circulation 2005;111(23):e394–434.

137. Keidar Z, Pirmisashvili N, Leiderman M, et al. 18F-FDG uptake in noninfected prosthetic vascular grafts: incidence, patterns, and changes over time. J Nucl Med 2014;55(3):392–5.

138. Pizzi MN, Roque A, Cuéllar-Calabria H, et al. F-FDG-PET/CTA of prosthetic cardiac valves and valve-tube grafts: infective versus inflammatory patterns. JACC Cardiovasc Imaging 2016;9(10): 1224–7.

139. Schouten LR, Verberne HJ, Bouma BJ, et al. Surgical glue for repair of the aortic root as a possible explanation for increased F-18 FDG uptake. J Nucl Cardiol 2008;15(1):146–7.

140. Mathieu C, Mikaïl N, Benali K, et al. Characterization of 18F-fluorodeoxyglucose uptake pattern in noninfected prosthetic heart valves. Circ Cardiovasc Imaging 2017;10(3):e005585.

Positron Emission Tomography Imaging in Vasculitis

Kornelis S.M. van der Geest, MD, PhD[a], Berend G.C. Slijkhuis, MD[b],
Alessandro Tomelleri, MD[c], Olivier Gheysens, MD, PhD[d],
William F. Jiemy, PhD[a], Costanza Piccolo, BSc[c], Pieter Nienhuis, BSc[e],
Maria Sandovici, MD, PhD[a], Elisabeth Brouwer, MD, PhD[a],
Andor W.J.M. Glaudemans, MD, PhD[e], Douwe J. Mulder, MD, PhD[b],
Riemer H.J.A. Slart, MD, PhD[e,f],*

KEYWORDS

• Vasculitis • Heart • FDG-PET/CT • Novel tracers

KEY POINTS

• Systemic vasculitides can affect any type of blood vessel, including the coronary arteries and aorta.
• [18F]-fluoro-2-deoxy-D-glucose positron emission tomography/computed tomography aids in the diagnosis and therapeutic monitoring of large-sized and medium-sized vessel vasculitides.
• Innovations, such as newer generations of PET scanners and development of immune cell-specific tracers, may further improve the assessment and monitoring of disease extent in patients with vasculitis.

INTRODUCTION

General Introduction

Systemic vasculitides are autoimmune diseases characterized by inflammation of blood vessels. Their categorization is based on the size of the preferentially affected blood vessels: large-vessel, medium-vessel, and small-vessel vasculitides.[1] Demographic, serologic, and pathologic findings further define the specific forms of vasculitis.

The diagnosis of vasculitis requires a comprehensive clinical and laboratory evaluation. Laboratory testing typically reveals an elevation of nonspecific inflammation markers in the blood.

Serologic testing for antineutrophil cytoplasmic antibodies and cryoglobulines may aid in the diagnosis of small-vessel vasculitis. A biopsy of affected organs can provide direct evidence for vascular inflammation. However, a biopsy is invasive and not every vessel and tissue can be sampled. Imaging may provide alternative evidence for vascular inflammation in the large and medium vasculitides. Furthermore, imaging can reveal vascular complications of these vasculitides: aneurysm formation, stenosis, and occlusion.

The management of systemic vasculitides requires substantial immunosuppressive treatment. Glucocorticoid treatment has a key role in the

[a] Department of Rheumatology and Clinical Immunology, University Medical Center Groningen, University of Groningen, the Netherlands; [b] Division of Vascular Medicine, Department of Internal Medicine, University of Groningen, University Medical Center Groningen, the Netherlands; [c] Unit of Immunology, Rheumatology, Allergy and Rare Diseases (UnIRAR), IRCCS San Raffaele Hospital, Vita-Salute San Raffaele University, Milan, Italy; [d] Department of Nuclear Medicine, Cliniques Universitaires Saint-Luc and Institute of Clinical and Experimental Research (IREC), Université Catholique de Louvain (UCLouvain), Brussels, Belgium; [e] Department of Nuclear Medicine and Molecular Imaging, Medical Imaging Center, University Medical Center Groningen, University of Groningen, the Netherlands; [f] Biomedical Photonic Imaging Group, Faculty of Science and Technology, University of Twente, Enschede, the Netherlands
* Corresponding author.
E-mail address: r.h.j.a.slart@umcg.nl

Cardiol Clin 41 (2023) 251–265
https://doi.org/10.1016/j.ccl.2023.01.012
0733-8651/23/© 2023 Elsevier Inc. All rights reserved.

induction phase of treatment. Other immunosuppressive treatments are typically required for the maintenance of remission and can also play a role in the induction phase of treatment. A correct diagnosis of vasculitis is important in order to prevent irreversible damage while precluding unnecessary exposure to potentially toxic treatments in patients without vasculitis. Ascertaining the specific type of systemic vasculitis is critical to select the correct immunosuppressive treatment regimen. The role of imaging in the diagnosis of vasculitis, as well as the assessment of disease activity and damage during treatment, is currently emerging, especially in the large-vessel vasculitides (LVVs).

Vasculitis and the Heart

The heart can be involved in systemic vasculitis.[2] Coronary artery vasculitis can result into aneurysm formation, stenosis, and thrombosis. Coronary artery involvement is most commonly seen in Kawasaki disease (KD). Takayasu arteritis (TAK) is the most common large-vessel vasculitis to involve the heart and can result in myocardial infarction and aortic incompetence.[3] In addition, inflammation of the ascending aorta in the LVVs can be associated with aortic regurgitation, which is incidentally also observed in IgG4-related disease (IgG4-RD). Myocarditis and pericarditis are described in varying frequencies across the entire vasculitis spectrum. Cardiac manifestations of giant cell arteritis (GCA) are very rare. Isolated reports exist of pericardial effusion and coronary arteritis in the context of GCA.[4] Cardiac involvement has been described in 4% to 18% of patients with polyarteritis nodosa (PAN).[5] Involvement of the heart in Behçet disease (BD) is usually in the form of intracardiac masses, thrombosis, or endomyocardial fibrosis.[6]

Premature atherosclerosis may occur secondary to systemic vasculitis.[7] Furthermore, past and current glucocorticoid use increases the risk of cardiovascular events. A greater risk is conferred by higher dose of glucocorticoid use partly related to incidental hypertension and steroid-induced diabetes. Patients on current glucocorticoid therapy have a 2-to-3-fold greater risk of developing heart failure and a 1-to-2-fold greater risk of developing ischemic heart disease.[8] There is a reasonable pool of evidence to suggest favorable modulation of this cardiovascular risk by using other glucocorticoid-sparing, immunosuppressive agents.[9,10]

IMAGING IN VASCULITIS

Depending on the caliber and location of the vessels affected,[11] different imaging modalities can be applied to diagnose vasculitis: ultrasonography (US), magnetic resonance angiography (MRA), computed tomography angiography (CTA), and [18F]-fluoro-2-deoxy-D-glucose positron emission tomography/computed tomography (FDG-PET/CT). These imaging tools can provide complementary information regarding the state of the vessels (**Table 1**). Conventional angiography has been largely replaced by MRA and CTA.[11] However, conventional angiography is sometimes required in patients with PAN to detect the classic microaneurysms.[11]

US allows for the assessment of large-sized and medium-sized arteries. Vasculitis lesions are identified by an increased intima-media thickness that is concentric and homogenous, and mostly explained by intima hyperplasia.[12,13] The thickened vessel wall is hypoechoic early in the disease, probably due to inflammation-induced edema. The intima-media complex can be readily identified in grayscale mode in large arteries, such as the axillary, carotid, and subclavian arteries. With high-frequency probes ($\geq$22 MHz), the intima-media complex of smaller and more superficial arteries, such as the temporal arteries, can also be measured directly.[14] However, the assessment of temporal arteries with lower frequency transducers requires color Doppler signal in order to detect the "halo sign" (ie, dark hypoechoic area surrounding the luminal flow) in case of arteritic lesions.[15] Doppler spectral analysis allows to determine the degree of stenosis and occlusion. US has limited use for deeply located arteries, such as the aortic arch.

CTA and MRA may aid in the detection of inflammation of large arteries in the neck, chest, abdomen, and pelvic area.[11] CTA can also be applied to investigate coronary artery involvement in vasculitis. MRA may also identify inflammation of the medium-sized, temporal arteries.[16] Both imaging tools may reveal concentric vessel wall thickening (cuffing) and mural enhancement of affected arteries. Disease complications such as stenosis and aneurysms can also be detected. CTA is typically more readily available than MRA, but comes with a substantial radiation burden. MRA provides better insight into the soft tissues surrounding the vessels and can be combined with protocols that assess the function and morphology of the heart.

[18F]-fluoro-2-deoxy-D-Glucose Positron Emission Tomography/Computed Tomography

FDG-PET/CT is a widely used, whole-body imaging modality. FDG is a radiolabeled glucose analogue in which the C-2 hydroxyl group is

Table 1
Pros and cons for imaging techniques in vasculitis

Technique	Arterial Regions—Examination for Vasculitis	Pro	Con
Ultrasound	• Head: superficial arteries • Neck: carotid, vertebral arteries • Upper and lower extremities: for example, axillary and femoral arteries • Chest: subclavian arteries, proximal ascending aorta • Abdomen: abdominal aorta (especially perivascular inflammation)	• Cheap • No radiation • Doppler (flow measurement, stenosis, obstruction) • High spatial resolution for superficial arteries • Combine with echocardiography • Rapid access (if expertise available in center) • Assessment of stenosis and dilatation	• Unable to scan deep arteries; or, if possible, with poor resolution • Operator dependent and time consuming • No whole body imaging possible
CTA	• Neck, chest, and abdomen: all large and medium arteries • Coronary arteries	• High spatial resolution • Short scanning time needed • Rapid access • Assessment of stenosis and dilatation	• Radiation • Risk of contrast nephrotoxicity
MRA	• Neck, chest, and abdomen: all large and medium arteries • Head: superficial and deep arteries, including cerebral arteries	• No radiation • Combine with cardiac function studies • Examination of tissues surrounding the arteries • Assessment of stenosis and dilatation	• Long scanning time needed • Resolution decreases when scanning larger areas • Not compatible with body devices (eg, pacemaker) • Claustrophobia • Risk of gadolinium toxicity/interactions with certain drugs
FDG-PET/CT	• Neck, chest, and abdomen: all large and medium arteries • Head: superficial and deep arteries, excluding cerebral arteries • Upper and lower extremities: all large and medium arteries	• Standard whole body imaging • Measures metabolic activity in arterial wall • Detection of other pathologic conditions (eg, cancer, infection, PMR in patients with GCA, lymphadenopathy in IgG4) • Cardiac evaluation possible with low carb diet • EARL PET procedural standardization	• Radiation • Expensive • Reduced sensitivity in patients with hyperglycemia

replaced by the positron emitting fluorine-18 atom. After intravenous administration, FDG is transported across the cell membrane through facilitative glucose transporters and phosphorylated intracellularly by the hexokinase enzyme to FDG-6-phosphate. In contrast to glucose-6-phosphate, FDG-6-phosphate is not further metabolized in the glycolytic pathway and gets accumulated intracellularly. The main mechanism of FDG uptake in inflammatory diseases is linked to the high expression levels of glucose transporters and hexokinase activity of cells involved in the inflammatory response, especially neutrophils and the monocytes/macrophages.[17,18] The introduction of hybrid PET-CT cameras that allow a more accurate anatomic localization and semiquantification of pathologic FDG uptake, together with the widespread availability from the early 2000s and recent technological advances in hardware have made PET/CT an indispensable tool for imaging of inflammatory disorders. Large vessel vasculitides were one of the first major indications for FDG-PET/CT in inflammatory disorders.[19]

THE ROLE OF [18F]-FLUORO-2-DEOXY-D-GLUCOSE POSITRON EMISSION TOMOGRAPHY/COMPUTED TOMOGRAPHY IN THE DIAGNOSIS OF DIFFERENT TYPES OF VASCULITIS
Large-Vessel Vasculitides

Giant cell arteritis
GCA is a systemic vasculitis of the large and medium arteries with unknown cause, affecting almost exclusively people aged older than 50 years. The peak incidence is between 70 and 79 years of age. GCA is more common in women than in men. The incidence of GCA is 10.0 per 100,000 in people aged 50 years or older. Vascular inflammation in GCA is characterized by a transmural infiltrate composed of lymphocytes, macrophages, and giant cells. Intimal hyperplasia may occur and is associated with the occurrence of ischemic visual loss.[13] Cranial (C)-GCA predominantly affects the branches of the external carotid artery (eg, temporal artery) and causes "classic" symptoms such as headache and jaw claudication.[20] Large-vessel (LV)-GCA involves the aorta and its primary branches (eg, the subclavian and axillary arteries) and initially presents with constitutional symptoms such as fever, weight loss, and fatigue. Two-thirds of patients have overlapping C-GCA and LV-GCA.[21] GCA shows a strong overlap with polymyalgia rheumatica (PMR), which is an inflammatory syndrome of the shoulder and hip girdle. The incidence of heart involvement by GCA is low (<5%). Cardiac manifestations of GCA encompass pericarditis, myocarditis, coronary vasculitis, and aortic regurgitation secondary to aortic root aneurysm involving the aortic valve.[2]

US and MRA are used to detect C-GCA, whereas CTA, MRA, and FDG-PET/CT are useful for detecting LV-GCA in patients presenting with general symptoms (**Fig. 1**A).[22] With the new-generation PET/CT scanners also GCA of the cranial arteries can be visualized by FDG-PET/CT (**Fig. 1**B).[23,24] FDG-PET/CT can also show inflammation of periarticular and articular synovial structures in overlapping PMR (see **Fig. 1**A).[25]

In a prospective study of PET imaging in patients with GCA, vascular FDG uptake was noted in 83% of patients, particularly at the subclavian arteries (74%) but also in the thoracic and abdominal aorta (>50%) and the femoral arteries (37%).[26] A meta-analysis of 6 studies evaluating PET for the diagnosis of GCA reported an overall sensitivity of 80% and specificity of 89%. Moreover, the negative predictive value of a PET scan for GCA was excellent (88%).[27] Glucocorticoid therapy may decrease the sensitivity of the FDG-PET scan particularly when longer than 3 days.[28]

Takayasu arteritis
TAK also affects large and medium vessels, including the aorta and its primary branches.[29] Women are affected in up to 90% of cases and the age of onset is usually between 10 and 40 years. TAK has a worldwide distribution, with the highest prevalence in Asian populations.[30,31] A variable inflammatory infiltrate is observed in the adventitia and media layers of the arterial wall, with hyperplasia and neovascularization in the intima.[32] Any tract of the aorta and all its main branches can be involved in TAK, usually with a symmetric pattern.[33] Stenoses and aneurysms frequently occur (>90% and 25%, respectively).[29] The most affected vessels are the subclavian and carotid arteries; the thoracic tract of the aorta is involved more frequently than the abdominal tract.[34] Patients present with nonspecific constitutional symptoms,[35] in addition to symptoms reflecting individual artery involvement: limb claudication and blood pressure difference between arms (femoral and subclavian arteries), carotidynia, abdominal angina (mesenteric artery), and renovascular hypertension.[36] Coronary artery involvement can be disclosed in up to 10% of patients; hence, TAK should always be suspected in young female patients experiencing acute coronary syndrome.[37] In most patients with TAK, the disease course follows a 2-stage process, in which a "prepulseless" phase characterized by constitutional symptoms is followed by a chronic phase where typical vascular symptoms prevail.[38] In most severe cases, patients experience acute and potentially fatal ischemic events, such as acute coronary syndrome or stroke.[39]

A presumptive diagnosis of TAK can be made starting from demographic, laboratory, and clinical features but imaging confirmation is mandatory.[22] CTA and MRA are the modalities of choice in clinical practice to evaluate both early signs of inflammation within the arterial wall and late complications correlated to longstanding disease.[40] US can represent a viable alternative in case of subclavian or carotid artery involvement.[41] FDG-PET/CT is widely used for the diagnosis of TAK (**Fig. 1**C).[42] One meta-analysis,[43] including patients with TAK and LV-GCA, reported a sensitivity of 76% and specificity of 93% for FDG-PET/CT.

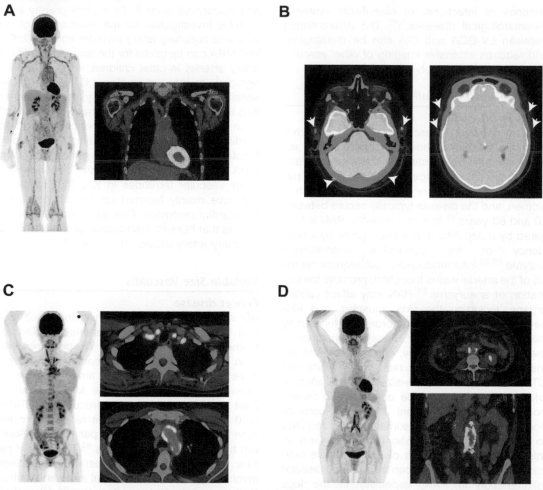

Fig. 1. Large-vessel vasculitis on FDG-PET/CT. For the assessment of large-vessel vasculitis, the arterial wall FDG uptake is visually compared with FDG uptake by the liver[110]: arterial wall FDG uptake similar to the liver possibly indicates active vasculitis, whereas uptake higher than the liver is considered positive for active vasculitis. (*A*) Large-vessel giant cell arteritis in a patient with constitutional symptoms. FDG-PET/CT shows inflammation of the thoracic aorta and its major branches, as well as uptake around shoulders, hips, and knees indicates PMR. (*B*) Cranial giant cell arteritis. Left panel: FDG-PET/CT showing inflammation of superficial temporal arteries (*arrows*) and occipital arteries (*arrow heads*). Right panel: Inflammation of the frontal and parietal branches arising from the superficial temporal arteries (*arrows*). (*C*) Large-vessel involvement in TAK. FDG-PET/CT shows inflammation of the aorta, proximal subclavian arteries, and both carotid arteries. (*D*) Isolated aortitis in a patient presenting with pain in the back and upper legs. FDG-PET/CT shows intense and heterogeneous FDG uptake in the distal part of the abdominal aorta extending to the proximal parts of both iliac arteries. The diagnosis of isolated aortitis was made in the absence of other affected organs/arteries.

Clinically isolated aortitis

Aortitis is an all-encompassing term ascribed to inflammation of the aorta.[44] It includes "true" aortitis limited to the vascular wall and periaortitis involving the adventitial layer and potentially surrounding fat and other soft tissues. Periaortitis may also present as inflammatory aneuryms and/or retroperitoneal fibrosis. FDG-PET/CT allows distinction between these conditions, which is important for identifying the underlying cause (eg, infectious and noninfectious conditions).

Notably, mild and heterogeneous metabolic activity of the aortic wall is frequently seen in the absence of vasculitis, especially in atherosclerotic aneurysms.[45] Periaortitis is uniquely characterized by a periaortic soft tissue mass surrounding the aorta visible on radiographical imaging and ultrasound excentric to the calcifications of the media. FDG-uptake is an important indicator of active disease, potentially allowing follow-up.[46] Clinically isolated aortitis (CIA; **Fig. 1**D) is a diagnosis made per exclusionem because it requires the absence of infections, or classifiable systemic rheumatological diseases.[1,47] The differentiation between LV-GCA and CIA can be challenging, and requires extensive imaging of other vascular territories typically involved in GCA.

Medium-Vessel Vasculitides

Polyarteritis nodosa

PAN is mostly a vasculitis of medium-sized, muscular arteries, although small and large arteries can also be affected. PAN is a rare disease with an annual incidence rate of less than 10 per million.[48] Men are more frequently affected than women, and the disease typically occurs between 40 and 60 years.[48] In some patients, PAN is triggered by a hepatitis B viral infection or by a deficiency of the adenosine deaminase-2 enzyme.[49,50] Inflammation and subsequent necrosis of the arterial wall is thought to promote the formation of aneurysms.[51] PAN may affect various organs, including the skin, muscles, and kidneys.[52] Involvement of the coronary arteries may lead to cardiac ischemia.[2] Biopsy, for instance of the skin, muscle or kidney, can help to establish the diagnosis.[52] Imaging tests for PAN include CTA and MRA of medium-sized visceral arteries, whereas CTA can also be performed to assess coronary artery involvement.[11] However, conventional angiography may sometimes be required to detect the characteristic microaneurysms in this disease. Small series of patients have indicated that FDG-PET/CT can also reveal vascular inflammation in PAN, especially in the legs (**Fig. 2**). Enhanced FDG uptake can be found in the muscles, as well as in medium-sized and large-sized arteries of the legs.[53–55]

Kawasaki disease

KD is a systemic vasculitis predominantly affecting medium-sized, muscular arteries. This condition more frequently affects men than women.[56] Most patients are aged younger than 5 years, and the disease affects 20 per 100.000 children in this age category.[56] Patients present with systemic inflammation, conjunctivitis, mucositis, erythema of the palms and soles and cervical lymphadenopathy. These disease features are usually self-limiting within several weeks. Coronary artery involvement and abnormalities occur in almost 25% of nontreated patients.[57] Abnormalities include coronary artery dilation, aneurysm formation, and stenosis. Coronary artery abnormalities typically progress during the first 4 to 6 weeks of the disease. Mild abnormalities may recover, whereas severe changes such as giant aneurysms usually persist. Aneurysms may occur in peripheral arteries, most often the brachial and iliac arteries

and abdominal aorta.[58] Echocardiography is the first-line investigation for the assessment of cardiac and coronary artery involvement in KD. CTA and MRA can be useful for the assessment of coronary arteries in older children, when echocardiography might not suffice. CTA has higher sensitivity for detecting coronary artery abnormalities than MRA but it comes at the expense of radiation exposure. MRA can be combined with cardiac MRI protocols evaluating the anatomy, function, and perfusion of the heart. CTA and MRA can be used to identify the involvement of other vascular territories in KD. PET studies in KD have mainly focused on the assessment of myocardial perfusion. One case report has suggested that FDG-PET/MRI could potentially detect coronary artery inflammation in KD.[59]

Variable Size Vasculitis

Behçet disease

BD is a systemic vasculitis involving small-sized and large-sized veins and arteries.[60] Men and women are affected equally.[61] The peak incidence is in the third and fourth decades, and disease severity often decreases over time.[61] The highest prevalence is reported in the Middle East and East Asia (the Silk route), particularly in Türkiye (370 per 100,000), whereas it ranges from less than 1 (United Kingdom) to 16 per 100,000 (Southern Italy) in Western countries.[60] The clinical picture of BD is heterogeneous. Mucocutaneous involvement with recurrent oral and genital ulcers is the most typical manifestation.[62] Ulcerations can also affect the gastrointestinal system, thereby mimicking Crohn disease.[63] Eye involvement ranges from mild conjunctivitis or episcleritis to sight-threatening uveitis and retinal vasculitis.[64] BD-associated vasculitis is an early manifestation, can affect both the veins and the arteries, and is the main predictor of mortality.[65] Vein inflammation can lead to thrombophlebitis or deep vein thrombosis, sometimes involving the central nervous system or causing the Budd-Chiari syndrome.[66] Intracardiac thrombus formation can occur mainly in the right chambers but this complication is exceedingly rare.[67] Arterial involvement can affect the pulmonary arteries, the aorta, and, in fewer cases, peripheral and visceral arteries (mainly, subclavian and femoral arteries).[68] The most common vascular complication of BD is aneurysm formation.[69] Stenosis, occlusion, and pseudoaneurysm of coronary arteries have been described.[65] MRA and, especially, CTA play a pivotal role in the diagnosis and characterization of vascular involvement in patients with BD. The latter can also identify intraluminal thrombosis.

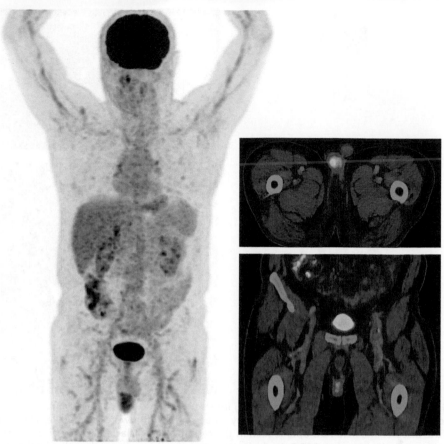

Fig. 2. PAN on FDG-PET/CT. FDG-PET/CT shows inflammation of the brachial, iliac, and femoral arteries. In addition, FDG uptake is seen at the smaller branches arising from the femoral arteries.

Peripheral veins and the heart can also be investigated by ultrasound; however, not all intracardiac thrombi can be detected by transthoracic echocardiography. The role of FDG-PET/CT in diagnosing BD is poorly understood. Some reports have described radiotracer uptake in vascular lesions, both arteries and veins,[70] and, of note, also in a patient with intracardiac thrombosis.[71] However, it is unclear whether FDG-PET/CT provides adjunctive information to MRA and CTA.

Cogan syndrome
Cogan syndrome is characterized by the presence of ocular inflammation, inner ear disease leading to vestibuloauditory dysfunction, and systemic vasculitis. Cogan syndrome is a rare condition typically occurring around the age of 30 years without a strong gender predilection. Vasculitis in Cogan syndrome can manifest as an aortitis with aortic valve insufficiency, as a TAK-like vasculitis, and less commonly as a vasculitis of small vessels (eg, glomerulonephritis, cutaneous vasculitis).[72,73] Little is known about the role of imaging in

detecting vascular inflammation in Cogan syndrome, although imaging techniques similar to those in other vasculitides are typically applied.

Other Forms of Vasculitis

IgG4-related disease
IgG4-RD is a fibroinflammatory, multisystem disease. It is histopathologically recognized by a lymphoplasmacytic infiltrate enriched with IgG4-positive plasma cells, storiform fibrosis, and obliterative phlebitis.[74] Serum IgG4 concentrations are elevated in 40% to 50% of patients. Cardiovascular manifestations are common in IgG4-RD. Vascular manifestations include perivascular infiltration of the aorta and branching arteries that may lead to aneurysms, dissections, and retroperitoneal fibrosis. Cardiac involvement includes coronary artery stenosis, pericardial disease, cardiac masses, and valvular heart disease. Although CT, MRI, and sometimes US can detect and raise the suspicion of IgG4-RD (eg, characteristic perivascular cuffing of the aorta), a distinction between active and

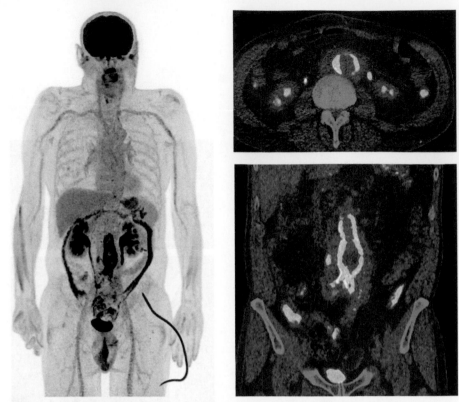

Fig. 3. IgG4-RD on FDG-PET/CT. FDG-PET/CT showing intense FDG uptake of the abdominal aorta and proximal iliac arteries. The abdominal aorta is surrounded by tissue mass with lower FDG uptake, likely reflecting the fibrosis of the disease. The mild FDG uptake seen in the carotid and subclavian/axillary arteries was still considered normal because the intensity of FDG uptake by the arterial walls was lower than that by the liver.[110] Intense FDG uptake in the colon was not associated with symptoms suggestive of colitis.

quiescent disease is difficult to make.[69] Case series have demonstrated the added value of FDG-PET/CT in diagnosis and assessment of systemic involvement of IgG4-RD.[75] Multiorgan involvement is demonstrated in 70% to 80% of patients using FDG-PET/CT,[76] of which large vascular involvement was present in approximately 40%, most prominently in the iliac arteries, followed by the infrarenal abdominal aorta (**Fig. 3**).[77] Furthermore, subclinical vascular inflammation is frequently detected in patients with IgG4-RD, of which the clinical relevance has yet to be determined.[78] Moreover, FDG-PET/CT may aid the detection of rare cardiac manifestations such as myocardial and sinoatrial node involvement.[79]

Relapsing polychondritis

Relapsing polychondritis (RP) is a systemic inflammatory disease affecting cartilaginous structures.[80,81] RP equally affects men and women, with an incidence of 0.7 to 3.5 per million persons.[82,83] Age of onset is typically between 40 and 60 years.[84] Auricular and nasal chondritis are the most typical manifestations but eye inflammation (mostly, scleritis or episcleritis), costochondritis, laryngotracheal chondritis, arthritis, and cardiovascular involvement may occur.[80] The entire aorta can be affected but the most common site is the aortic root, where the inflammatory process can lead to dilation, often accompanied by aortic valve regurgitation.[85] Less frequently, the main aortic branches (eg, coronary, epiaortic, renal, and iliac arteries) can be involved, leading to features resembling those typically seen in TAK.[86] Echocardiography has a central role in the early assessment of aortic valve and aortic root disease and should be routinely performed in patients with RP.[87] Conversely, there is still debate regarding the best way to investigate the remaining tracts of the aorta and its large branches. CTA and MRA allow an accurate morphologic evaluation of these vessels, whereas CTA is the technique of choice to detect coronary involvement.[86] FDG-PET/CT can be useful in displaying the presence of active vascular inflammation even before it becomes clinically relevant (ie, symptomatic). This can have prognostic implications because cardiovascular involvement is the

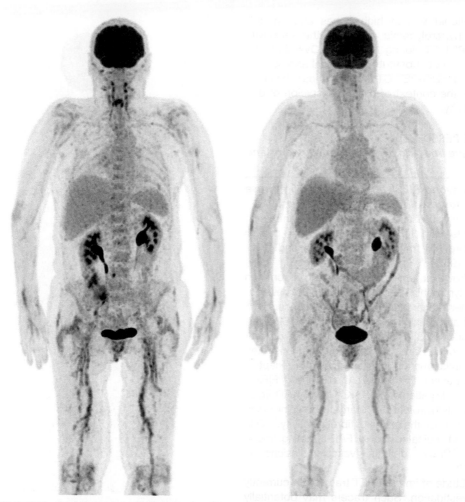

Fig. 4. GCA/PMR before and after treatment. A 70-year-old-female with complaints of headache and fever. Maximum intensity projection FDG-PET scan at baseline (*left*) shows increased uptake in the vertebral arteries and the arteries in the upper leg with concomitant findings compatible with PMR. Maximum intensity projection FDG-PET scan during treatment with interleukin-6 (*right*) shows a clear reduction of FDG uptake at the affected sites.

second most common cause of death in patients with RP and it is often silent in the first phase.[87] In addition, FDG-PET/CT allows to visualize cartilaginous inflammation at the nose, ears, and costochondral junctions.[88]

THE ROLE OF [18F]-FLUORO-2-DEOXY-D-GLUCOSE POSITRON EMISSION TOMOGRAPHY/COMPUTED TOMOGRAPHY FOR THERAPY MONITORING

Because the assessment of disease activity during treatment can be challenging, FDG-PET/CT is gaining increasing interest as a tool for therapeutic monitoring in patients with vasculitis.[89] Studies have primarily focused on large-vessel vasculitides. FDG uptake by large-sized and medium-sized arteries in patients with GCA, and TAK

seems to decrease during treatment-induced remission, although complete resolution does not necessarily occur (**Fig. 4**).[90,91] A meta-analysis suggested that FDG-PET/CT provides an overall sensitivity of 77% and specificity of 71% for discriminating between remission and relapsing/refractory disease in patients receiving treatment of GCA/TAK.[90] Whether FDG-PET/CT can predict clinical relapse is still a matter of debate.[92] Less is known about the role of FDG-PET/CT for monitoring disease activity in other types of vasculitis, although this could be of interest. Radiation exposure by FDG-PET/CT can be an issue in younger patients, where repetitive imaging by other techniques such as MRA and color Doppler US might be more appropriate. Nevertheless, the radiation burden of FDG-PET/CT continues to decrease with newer generation of scanners. Additionally, glucocorticoid use at high doses and steroid-induced hyperglycemia may limit the sensitivity of FDG-PET/CT during treatment. Overall, FDG-PET/CT cannot substitute the clinical assessment of patients. FDG-PET/CT findings should be interpreted in the context of clinical suspicion of disease activity.

FUTURE PERSPECTIVES
Innovative Imaging: New Camera Systems and Tracers

Tracers beyond [18F]-fluoro-2-deoxy-D-glucose in imaging vasculitides

Successful visualization of vessel-wall inflammation in patients with LVV using translocator protein (TSPO)-targeted tracers, [11C]PK11195 and [11C]-(R)-PK11195,[93,94] have been reported. These tracers, however, are unable to bind to a common TSPO polymorphism, which prompted the development of new-generation TSPO-targeted tracers.[95,96] A recent study using a new-generation TSPO-targeted tracer, [11C]PBR28, failed to detect vascular inflammation.[97] One case report demonstrated vascular inflammation with somatostatin receptor-targeted tracers, [68Ga]DOTATATE and [18F]FET-βAG-TOCA, in patients with TAK.[98] In IgG4-RD, fibroblast activation protein (FAP)-targeted imaging could allow to visualize the extent of fibrotic activity.[99] One case report indicated that a FAP-targeting tracer, [68Ga]FAPI-04, detects vascular lesions in GCA.[100,101]

A multitude of immunoPET tracers are currently underinvestigation. Such tracers may potentially bind to specific molecules on immune cells infiltrating the vessel wall of patients with vasculitis.[102] For instance, tracers targeting CD206 and folate receptor β on macrophages, CD20 on B cells and CD8 on cytotoxic T cells could be of interest in GCA because these immune cells are abundantly present in the temporal arteries and the aorta of patients with this disease.[103,104] As shown in rheumatoid arthritis,[105] novel immunoPET tracers may also potentially stratify patients for precision medicine. Overall, these studies warrant further investigation into the utility of novel radiotracers for imaging vasculitides.

Total Body Positron Emission Tomography: Heart–Vascular Axis

An important new development in nuclear medicine is the introduction of a long axial field of view (LAFOV) or total body (TB) PET. This substantially increases the sensitivity (a factor of 10–40 depending on of the number of detectors, ie, the actual length of the FOV compared with a conventional PET scanner (**Fig. 5**).[106,107] This new PET

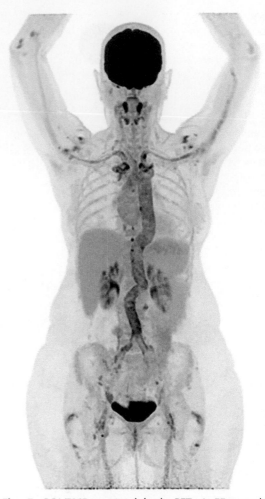

Fig. 5. GCA/PMR on total body PET. A 55-year-old woman with pathologic FDG uptake in the large arteries; the abdominal and thoracic aorta, the subclavian, axillary, carotid, iliac, and femoral arteries, indicating large-vessel vasculitis, or GCA. FDG uptake is also observed in the proximal articular joints and periarticular structures, indicating synovitis, due to PMR.

modality allows cardiovascular researchers to establish multiorgan dynamic PET analyses. Acquisition of dynamic uptake images delineating the large-sized and medium-sized arteries of the whole body can be done with the LAFOV and the TB PET scanner, expanding on the ability to understand the pathophysiological mechanisms of various cardiovascular disorders such as vasculitis. Combing LAFOV or TB PET with novel immunoPET tracers for vasculitis would allow a more thorough insight of how each specific cell is involved in the pathogenesis of specific types of vasculitis and how these cells behave. Moreover, the multiorgan changes regarding kinetic uptake of immunoPET tracer after appropriate treatment of vasculitis could be assessed with the LAFOV and the TB PET scanner, something that was not possible before the development of this type of scanner.[108] Pugliese and colleagues proved already with a standard PET scanner using dynamic tracing with [11C]-PK11195 that inflammation is more prominent in symptomatic patients with vasculitis.[93]

Further, the main differential with systemic vasculitis is the presence of systemic atherosclerosis because inflammation plays an important role in the pathogenesis of atherosclerotic plaques. PET usually excels at differentiating one from the other because vasculitis lesions usually have a higher and a more homogenous uptake than atherosclerotic lesions but a TB PET could further characterize differences in these 2 cardiovascular entities using dynamic PET evaluations.[109]

SUMMARY

FDG-PET/CT is an important diagnostic tool for detecting inflammation of large-sized and medium-sized vessels in patients with systemic vasculitides. FDG-PET/CT can also provide complementary information to other vascular imaging techniques such as US, CTA, and MRA. Furthermore, FDG-PET/CT has an emerging role for therapeutic monitoring of patients with vasculitis. A new generation of long axial FOV/TB PET scanners can limit radiation exposure while providing excellent sensitivity. The introduction of novel immune-cell targeted radiotracers will potentially allow to directly visualize inflammatory cell infiltrates in the vasculature of patients with vasculitis.

CLINICS CARE POINTS

- FDG-PET/CT is an important diagnostic tool for detecting inflammation of large-sized and medium-sized vessels in patients with systemic vasculitides.
- FDG-PET/CT can also provide complementary information to other vascular imaging techniques such as US, CTA, and MRA-FDG-PET/CT has an emerging role for therapeutic monitoring of patients with vasculitis.
- A new generation of long axial FOV/TB PET scanners can limit radiation exposure while providing excellent sensitivity.
- The introduction of novel immune-cell targeted radiotracers will potentially allow to directly visualize inflammatory cell infiltrates in the vasculature of patients with vasculitis.

DECLARATION OF INTERESTS

K.S.M. van der Geest: received a speaker fee from Roche paid to the UMCG. A. Tomelleri: received a speaker fee from MS. A.W.J.M. Glaudemans: received unrestricted research grants from Siemens Healthineers, The Netherlands. R.H.J.A. Slart: received unrestricted research grants from Siemens Healthineers, The Netherlands. Remaining authors have nothing to disclose.

REFERENCES

1. Jennette JC, Falk RJ, Bacon PA, et al. 2012 Revised international chapel hill consensus conference nomenclature of vasculitides. Arthritis Rheum 2013;65(1):1–11.
2. Miloslavsky E, Unizony S. The heart in vasculitis. Rheum Dis Clin N Am 2014;40(1):11–26.
3. Kim H, Barra L. Ischemic complications in Takayasu's arteritis: a meta-analysis. Semin Arthritis Rheum 2018;47(6):900–6.
4. Misra DP, Shenoy SN. Cardiac involvement in primary systemic vasculitis and potential drug therapies to reduce cardiovascular risk. Rheumatol Int 2017;37(1):151–67.
5. Deok Bae Y, Jin Choi H, Chan Lee J, et al. Clinical features of polyarteritis nodosa in Korea. J Korean Med Sci 2006;21:591–6.
6. Chuang KW, Chang HC. Risk of ischaemic heart diseases and stroke in behçet disease: a systematic review and meta-analysis. Eur J Clin Invest 2022;52(8):e13778.
7. Cohen Tervaert JW. Cardiovascular disease due to accelerated atherosclerosis in systemic vasculitides. Best Pract Res Clin Rheumatol 2013;27(1):33–44.
8. Souverein PC, Berard A, van Staa TP, et al. Use of oral glucocorticoids and risk of cardiovascular and cerebrovascular disease in a population based case-control study. Heart 2004;90(8):859–65.
9. Hsue PY, Scherzer R, Grunfeld C, et al. Depletion of B-cells with rituximab improves endothelial function and reduces inflammation among individuals with rheumatoid arthritis. J Am Heart Assoc 2014;3(5). https://doi.org/10.1161/JAHA.114.001267.
10. Micha R, Imamura F, Wyler Von Ballmoos M, et al. Systematic review and meta-analysis of methotrexate use and risk of cardiovascular disease. Am J Cardiol 2011;108(9):1362–70.
11. Aghayev A, Steigner ML, Azene EM, et al. ACR appropriateness Criteria® noncerebral vasculitis. J Am Coll Radiol 2021;18(11):S380–93.
12. Chrysidis S, Duftner C, Dejaco C, et al. Definitions and reliability assessment of elementary ultrasound lesions in giant cell arteritis: a study from the OMERACT large vessel vasculitis ultrasound

working group. RMD Open 2018;4(1). https://doi.org/10.1136/rmdopen-2017-000598.

13. van der Geest KSM, Wolfe K, Borg F, et al. Ultrasonographic Halo Score in giant cell arteritis: association with intimal hyperplasia and ischaemic sight loss. Rheumatology 2021;60(9):4361–6.

14. Schäfer VS, Jin L, Schmidt WA. Imaging for diagnosis, monitoring, and outcome prediction of large vessel vasculitides. Curr Rheumatol Rep 2020;22(11). https://doi.org/10.1007/s11926-020-00955-y.

15. van der Geest KSM, Borg F, Kayani A, et al. Novel ultrasonographic Halo Score for giant cell arteritis: assessment of diagnostic accuracy and association with ocular ischaemia. Ann Rheum Dis 2019;79(3):393–9.

16. Rhéaume M, Rebello R, Pagnoux C, et al. High-resolution magnetic resonance imaging of scalp arteries for the diagnosis of giant cell arteritis: results of a prospective cohort study. Arthritis Rheumatol 2017;69(1):161–8.

17. Yamada S, Kubota K, Kubota R, et al. High accumulation of fluorine-18-fluorodeoxyglucose in turpentine-induced inflammatory tissue. J Nucl Med 1995;36(7):1301–6. Available at: http://www.ncbi.nlm.nih.gov/pubmed/7790960.

18. Mochizuki T, Tsukamoto E, Kuge Y, et al. FDG uptake and glucose transporter subtype expressions in experimental tumor and inflammation models. J Nucl Med 2001;42(10):1551–5. Available at: http://www.ncbi.nlm.nih.gov/pubmed/11585872.

19. Jamar F, Buscombe J, Chiti A, et al. EANM/SNMMI guideline for 18F-FDG use in inflammation and infection. J Nucl Med 2013;54(4):647–58.

20. van der Geest KSM, Sandovici M, Brouwer E, et al. Diagnostic accuracy of symptoms, physical signs, and laboratory tests for giant cell arteritis. JAMA Intern Med 2020;180(10):1295.

21. van Sleen Y, Graver JC, Abdulahad WH, et al. Leukocyte dynamics reveal a persistent myeloid dominance in giant cell arteritis and polymyalgia rheumatica. Front Immunol 2019;1. https://doi.org/10.3389/fimmu.2019.01981. Available at: www.frontiersin.org.

22. Dejaco C, Ramiro S, Duftner C, et al. EULAR recommendations for the use of imaging in large vessel vasculitis in clinical practice. Ann Rheum Dis 2018;77(5):636–43.

23. Nienhuis PH, Sandovici M, Glaudemans AW, et al. Visual and semiquantitative assessment of cranial artery inflammation with FDG-PET/CT in giant cell arteritis. Semin Arthritis Rheum 2020;50(4):616–23.

24. Nielsen BD, Hansen IT, Kramer S, et al. Simple dichotomous assessment of cranial artery inflammation by conventional 18F-FDG PET/CT shows high accuracy for the diagnosis of giant cell arteritis: a case-control study. Eur J Nucl Med Mol Imag 2019;46(1):184–93.

25. van der Geest KSM, van Sleen Y, Nienhuis P, et al. Comparison and validation of FDG-PET/CT scores for polymyalgia rheumatica. Rheumatology 2022;61(3):1072–82.

26. Blockmans D, Bley T, Schmidt W. Imaging for large-vessel vasculitis. Curr Opin Rheumatol 2009;21(1):19–28.

27. Besson FL, Parienti JJ, Bienvenu B, et al. Diagnostic performance of 18F-fluorodeoxyglucose positron emission tomography in giant cell arteritis: a systematic review and meta-analysis. Eur J Nucl Med Mol Imag 2011;38(9):1764–72.

28. Nielsen BD, Gormsen LC, Hansen IT, et al. Three days of high-dose glucocorticoid treatment attenuates large-vessel 18F-FDG uptake in large-vessel giant cell arteritis but with a limited impact on diagnostic accuracy. Eur J Nucl Med Mol Imag 2018;45(7):1119–28.

29. Saadoun D, Vautier M, Cacoub P. Medium- and large-vessel vasculitis. Circulation 2021;143(3):267–82.

30. Sanchez-Alvarez C, Crowson CS, Koster MJ, et al. Prevalence of Takayasu arteritis: a population-based study. J Rheumatol 2021;48(6):952.

31. Watts RA, Hatemi G, Burns JC, et al. Global epidemiology of vasculitis. Nat Rev Rheumatol 2022;18(1):22–34.

32. Stone JR, Bruneval P, Angelini A, et al. Consensus statement on surgical pathology of the aorta from the society for cardiovascular pathology and the association for European cardiovascular pathology: I. Inflammatory diseases. Cardiovasc Pathol 2015;24(5):267–78.

33. Goel R, Bates Gribbons K, Carette S, et al. Derivation of an angiographically based classification system in Takayasu's arteritis: an observational study from India and North America Rheumatology key messages. Rheumatology 2020;59:1118–27.

34. Chung JW, Kim HC, Choi YH, et al. Patterns of aortic involvement in Takayasu arteritis and its clinical implications: evaluation with spiral computed tomography angiography. J Vasc Surg 2007;45(5):906–14.

35. Serra R, Butrico L, Fugetto F, et al. Updates in pathophysiology, diagnosis and management of Takayasu arteritis. Ann Vasc Surg 2016;35:210–25.

36. de Souza AWS, de Carvalho JF. Diagnostic and classification criteria of Takayasu arteritis. J Autoimmun 2014;48-49:79–83.

37. Cavalli G, Tomelleri A, di Napoli D, et al. Prevalence of Takayasu arteritis in young women with acute ischemic heart disease. Int J Cardiol 2018;252:21–3.

38. Johnston SL, Lock RJ, Gompels MM. Takayasu arteritis: a review. J Clin Pathol 2002;55(7):481–6.

39. Yu RY, AlSolimani R, Khalidi N, et al. Characteristics of Takayasu arteritis patients with severe ischemic events. J Rheumatol 2020;47(8):1224–8.

40. Sarma K, Handique A, Phukan P, et al. Magnetic resonance angiography and multidetector CT angiography in the diagnosis of takayasu's arteritis: assessment of disease extent and correlation with disease activity. Current Medical Imaging Formerly Current Medical Imaging Reviews 2021;18(1):51–60.

41. Svensson C, Eriksson P, Zachrisson H. Vascular ultrasound for monitoring of inflammatory activity in Takayasu arteritis. Clin Physiol Funct Imag 2020; 40(1):37–45.

42. Danve A, O'Dell J. The role of 18F fluorodeoxyglucose positron emission tomography scanning in the diagnosis and management of systemic vasculitis. International Journal of Rheumatic Diseases 2015;18(7):714–24.

43. Lee YH, Choi SJ, Ji JD, et al. Diagnostic accuracy of 18F-FDG PET or PET/CT for large vessel vasculitis. Z Rheumatol 2016;75(9):924–31.

44. Gornik HL, Creager MA. Aortitis. Circulation 2008; 117(23):3039–51.

45. Barwick TD, OTA Lyons, Mikhaeel NG, et al. 18F-FDG PET-CT uptake is a feature of both normal diameter and aneurysmal aortic wall and is not related to aneurysm size. Eur J Nucl Med Mol Imag 2014;41(12):2310–8.

46. Treglia G, Stefanelli A, Mattoli MV, et al. Usefulness of 18F-FDG PET/CT in evaluating disease activity at different times in a patient with chronic periaortitis. Nuclear Medicine and Molecular Imaging 2013; 47(1):69–71.

47. Cinar I, Wang H, Stone JR. Clinically isolated aortitis: pitfalls, progress, and possibilities. Cardiovasc Pathol 2017;29:23–32.

48. Watts RA, Lane SE, Scott DGI. Epidemiology of vasculitis in europe. Ann Rheum Dis 2001;60(12): 1156a–11157a.

49. Lee PY, Aksentijevich I, Zhou Q. Mechanisms of vascular inflammation in deficiency of adenosine deaminase 2 (DADA2). Semin Immunopathol 2022;44(3):269–80.

50. Guillevin L, Lhote F, Cohen P, et al. Polyarteritis nodosa related to hepatitis B virus A prospective study with long-term observation of 41 patients. Medicine 1995;74(5):238–53.

51. Matsumoto T, Kobayashi S, Ogishima D, et al. Isolated necrotizing arteritis (localized polyarteritis nodosa): examination of the histological process and disease entity based on the histological classification of stage and histological differences from polyarteritis nodosa. Cardiovasc Pathol 2007;16(2): 92–7.

52. Hernández-Rodríguez J, Alba MA, Prieto-González S, et al. Diagnosis and classification of polyarteritis nodosa. J Autoimmun 2014;48-49:84–9.

53. Chen Z, Zhao Y, Wang Q, et al. Imaging features of 18F-FDG PET/CT in different types of systemic vasculitis. Clin Rheumatol 2022;41(5):1499–509.

54. Bleeker-Rovers CP, Bredie SJH, van der Meer JWM, et al. F-18-fluorodeoxyglucose positron emission tomography in diagnosis and follow-up of patients with different types of vasculitis. Neth J Med 2003;61(10):323–9. Available at: http://www. ncbi.nlm.nih.gov/pubmed/14708910.

55. Fagart A, MacHet T, Collet G, et al. Fluorodeoxyglucose positron emission tomography-computed tomography findings in a first series of 10 patients with polyarteritis nodosa. Rheumatology 2022; 61(4):1663–8.

56. Holman RC, Belay ED, Christensen KY, et al. Hospitalizations for Kawasaki syndrome among children in the United States, 1997-2007. Pediatr Infect Dis J 2010;29(6):483–8.

57. McCrindle BW, Rowley AH, Newburger JW, et al. Diagnosis, treatment, and long-term management of Kawasaki disease: a scientific statement for health professionals from the American heart association. Circulation 2017;135(17). https://doi.org/10.1161/CIR.0000000000000484.

58. Hoshino S, Tsuda E, Yamada O. Characteristics and fate of systemic artery aneurysm after Kawasaki disease. J Pediatr 2015;167(1):108–12. e2.

59. Danchin MH, Abo Y, Akikusa J, et al. FDG-PET imaging in a child with Kawasaki disease: systemic and coronary artery inflammation without dilatation. Arch Dis Child 2022;107(6):619.

60. Yazici Y, Hatemi G, Bodaghi B, et al. Behçet syndrome. Nat Rev Dis Prim 2021;7(1):67.

61. Yazici H, Seyahi E, Hatemi G, et al. Behçet syndrome: a contemporary view. Nature Publishing Group; 2018. p. 14. https://doi.org/10.1038/nrrheum.2017.208.

62. Oh SH, Han EC, Lee JH, et al. Comparison of the clinical features of recurrent aphthous stomatitis and Behçet's disease. Clin Exp Dermatol 2009; 34(6):e208–12.

63. Bayraktar Y, Ozaslan E, van Thiel DH. Gastrointestinal manifestations of Behçet's disease. J Clin Gastroenterol 2000;30(2):144–54.

64. Tugal-Tutkun I, Onal S, Altan-Yaycioglu R, et al. Uveitis in Behçet disease: an analysis of 880 patients. Am J Ophthalmol 2004;138(3):373–80.

65. Toledo-Samaniego N, Oblitas CM, Peñaloza-Martínez E, et al. Arterial and venous involvement in Behçet's syndrome: a narrative review. J Thromb Thrombolysis 2022;54(1):162–71.

66. Tascilar K, Melikoglu M, Ugurlu S, et al. Vascular involvement in Behçet's syndrome: a retrospective analysis of associations and the time course. Rheumatology 2014;53(11):2018–22.

67. Aksu T, Tufekcioglu O. Intracardiac thrombus in Behçet's disease: four new cases and a comprehensive literature review. Rheumatol Int 2015; 35(7):1269–79.

68. Saadoun D, Asli B, Wechsler B, et al. Long-term outcome of arterial lesions in Behçet disease: a

series of 101 patients. Medicine 2012;91(1): 18–24.

69. Zhou J, Shi J, Liu J, et al. The clinical features, risk factors, and outcome of aneurysmal lesions in behcet's disease. Journal of Immunology Research 2019;2019:1–8.

70. Cho S bin, Yun M, Lee JH, et al. Detection of cardiovascular system involvement in behçet's disease using fluorodeoxyglucose positron emission tomography. Semin Arthritis Rheum 2011;40(5): 461–6.

71. Xi XY, Gao W, Guo XJ, et al. Multiple cardiovascular involvements in Behçet's disease: unique utility of 18F-FDG PET/CT in diagnosis and follow-up. Eur J Nucl Med Mol Imag 2019;46(10):2210–1.

72. Gluth MB, Baratz KH, Matteson EL, et al. Cogan syndrome: a retrospective review of 60 patients throughout a half century. Mayo Clin Proc 2006; 81(4):483–8.

73. Grasland A, Pouchot J, Hachulla E, et al. Typical and atypical Cogan's syndrome: 32 cases and review of the literature. Rheumatology 2004;43: 1007–15.

74. Stone JH, Zen Y, Deshpande V. IgG4-Related disease. N Engl J Med 2012;366(6):539–51.

75. Pucar D, Hinchcliff M. FDG PET vascular imaging in IgG4-RD: potential and challenges. J Nucl Cardiol 2021;29(6):2934–7.

76. Zhang J, Chen H, Ma Y, et al. Characterizing IgG4-related disease with 18F-FDG PET/CT: a prospective cohort study. Eur J Nucl Med Mol Imag 2014; 41(8):1624–34.

77. Yabusaki S, Oyama-Manabe N, Manabe O, et al. Characteristics of immunoglobulin G4-related aortitis/periaortitis and periarteritis on fluorodeoxyglucose positron emission tomography/computed tomography co-registered with contrast-enhanced computed tomography. EJNMMI Res 2017;7(1):20.

78. Imai S, Tahara N, Igata S, et al. Vascular/perivascular inflammation in IgG4-related disease. J Nucl Cardiol 2021;29(6):2920–33.

79. Carbajal H, Waters L, Popovich J, et al. IgG4 related cardiac disease. Methodist DeBakey Cardiovascular Journal 2013;9(4):230.

80. Kingdon J, Roscamp J, Sangle S, et al. Relapsing polychondritis: a clinical review for rheumatologists. Rheumatology 2018;57(9):1525–32.

81. Foidart JM, Abe S, Martin GR, et al. Antibodies to type II collagen in relapsing polychondritis. N Engl J Med 1978;299(22):1203–7.

82. Hazra N, Dregan A, Charlton J, et al. Incidence and mortality of relapsing polychondritis in the UK: a population-based cohort study. Rheumatology 2015;54(12):2181–7.

83. Horvath A, Pall N, Molnar K, et al. A nationwide study of the epidemiology of relapsing polychondritis. Clin Epidemiol 2016;8:211–30.

84. Alqanatish JT, Alshanwani JR. Relapsing polychondritis in children: a review. Mod Rheumatol 2020; 30(5):788–98.

85. Erdogan M, Esatoglu SN, Hatemi G, et al. Aortic involvement in relapsing polychondritis: case-based review. Rheumatol Int 2021;41(4):827–37.

86. Tomelleri A, Campochiaro C, Sartorelli S, et al. Large-vessel vasculitis affecting the aorta and its branches in relapsing polychondritis: case series and systematic review of the literature. J Rheumatol 2020;47(12):1780–4.

87. Erdogan M, Sinem ·, Esatoglu N, et al. CASE BASED REVIEW Aortic involvement in relapsing polychondritis: case-based review. Rheumatol Int 2021;41:827–37.

88. Okuda S, Hirooka Y, Itami T, et al. FDG-PET/CT and auricular cartilage biopsy are useful for diagnosing with relapsing polychondritis in patients without auricular symptoms. Life 2021;11(9):956.

89. Slart RHJA, Glaudemans AWJM, Brouwer E, et al. Therapy response evaluation in large-vessel vasculitis: a new role for [18F]FDG-PET/CT? Rheumatology 2021;60(8):3494–5.

90. van der Geest KSM, Treglia & G, Glaudemans AWJM, et al. Diagnostic value of [18F]FDG-PET/CT for treatment monitoring in large vessel vasculitis: a systematic review and meta-analysis. Eur J Nucl Med Mol Imag 2021;48:3886–902.

91. Schönau V, Roth J, Tascilar K, et al. Resolution of vascular inflammation in patients with new-onset giant cell arteritis: data from the RIGA study. Rheumatology 2021;60(8):3851–61.

92. Grayson PC, Alehashemi S, Bagheri AA, et al. 18F-Fluorodeoxyglucose-Positron emission tomography as an imaging biomarker in a prospective, longitudinal cohort of patients with large vessel vasculitis. Arthritis Rheumatol 2018;70(3):439–49.

93. Pugliese F, Gaemperli O, Kinderlerer AR, et al. Imaging of vascular inflammation with [11C]-PK11195 and positron emission tomography/computed tomography angiography. J Am Coll Cardiol 2010; 56(8):653–61.

94. Lamare F, Hinz R, Gaemperli O, et al. Detection and quantification of large-vessel inflammation with 11C-(R)-PK11195 PET/CT. J Nucl Med 2011; 52(1):33–9.

95. Owen DR, Yeo AJ, Gunn RN, et al. An 18-kDa translocator protein (TSPO) polymorphism explains differences in binding affinity of the PET radioligand PBR28. J Cereb Blood Flow Metabol 2012;32(1):1–5.

96. Owen DRJ, Gunn RN, Rabiner EA, et al. Mixed-affinity binding in humans with 18-kDa translocator protein ligands. J Nucl Med 2011;52(1):24–32.

97. Schollhammer R, Lepreux S, Barthe N, et al. In vitro and pilot in vivo imaging of 18 kDa translocator protein (TSPO) in inflammatory vascular disease. EJNMMI Res 2021;11:45.

98. Tarkin JM, Wall C, Gopalan D, et al. Novel approach to imaging active Takayasu arteritis using somatostatin receptor positron emission tomography/magnetic resonance imaging circulation: cardiovascular imaging. Circ Cardiovasc Imaging 2020;13:10389.

99. Schmidkonz C, Rauber S, Atzinger A, et al. Disentangling inflammatory from fibrotic disease activity by fibroblast activation protein imaging. Ann Rheum Dis 2020;79(11):1485–91.

100. Hicks RJ, Roselt PJ, Kallur KG, et al. Fapi PET/CT: will it end the hegemony of 18F-FDG in oncology? J Nucl Med 2021;62(3):296–302.

101. Luo Y, Pan Q, Yang H, et al. Fibroblast activation protein–targeted PET/CT with 68Ga-FAPI for imaging IgG4-related disease: comparison to 18F-FDG PET/CT. J Nucl Med 2021;62(2):266–71.

102. van der Geest KSM, Sandovici M, Nienhuis PH, et al. Novel PET imaging of inflammatory targets and cells for the diagnosis and monitoring of giant cell arteritis and polymyalgia rheumatica. Front Med 2022;9. https://doi.org/10.3389/fmed.2022.902155.

103. van Sleen Y, Jiemy WF, Pringle S, et al. A distinct macrophage subset mediating tissue destruction and neovascularization in giant cell arteritis: implication of the YKL-40/interleukin-13 receptor α2 Axis. Arthritis Rheumatol 2021;73(12):2327–37.

104. Jiemy WF, Sleen Y, Geest KS, et al. Distinct macrophage phenotypes skewed by local granulocyte macrophage colony-stimulating factor (GM-CSF) and macrophage colony-stimulating factor (M-CSF) are associated with tissue destruction and intimal hyperplasia in giant cell arteritis. Clinical &

Translational Immunology 2020;9(9). https://doi.org/10.1002/cti2.1164.

105. Bruijnen S, Tsang-A-Sjoe M, Raterman H, et al. B-cell imaging with zirconium-89 labelled rituximab PET-CT at baseline is associated with therapeutic response 24 weeks after initiation of rituximab treatment in rheumatoid arthritis patients. Arthritis Res Ther 2016;18(1):266.

106. Slart RHJA, Tsoumpas C, Glaudemans AWJM, et al. Long axial field of view PET scanners: a road map to implementation and new possibilities. Eur J Nucl Med Mol Imag 2021;48(13):4236–45.

107. Alberts I, Hünermund JN, Prenosil G, et al. Clinical performance of long axial field of view PET/CT: a head-to-head intra-individual comparison of the Biograph Vision Quadra with the Biograph Vision PET/CT. Eur J Nucl Med Mol Imaging 2021;48(8):2395–404.

108. Rodriguez JA, Selvaraj S, Bravo PE. Potential cardiovascular applications of total-body PET imaging. Pet Clin 2021;16(1):129–36.

109. Nienhuis PH, van Praagh GD, Glaudemans AWJM, et al. A review on the value of imaging in differentiating between large vessel vasculitis and atherosclerosis. J Pers Med 2021;11(3):236. Published online.

110. Slart RHJA, Glaudemans AWJM, Chareonthaitawee P, et al. FDG-PET/CT(A) imaging in large vessel vasculitis and polymyalgia rheumatica: joint procedural recommendation of the EANM, SNMMI, and the PET Interest Group (PIG), and endorsed by the ASNC. Eur J Nucl Med Mol Imag 2018;45(7):1250–69.

Radionuclide Imaging of Heart-Brain Connections

Shady Abohashem, MD[a,b], Simran S. Grewal, DO[b,c], Ahmed Tawakol, MD[b,c], Michael T. Osborne, MD[b,c],*

KEYWORDS

- Molecular imaging • Heart-brain • Inflammation • Radionuclides • Positron emission tomography
- Psychosocial stress

KEY POINTS

- Growing evidence supports a complex pathologic interplay between the heart and brain that has been challenging to clarify and has important differences between sexes.
- Molecular imaging is uniquely equipped to provide novel insights into the heart-brain connection through its ability to simultaneously evaluate biological processes in disparate tissues.
- Radiotracers targeting processes, such as inflammation, autonomic nervous and neurohormonal system activity, metabolism, and perfusion, have elucidated important aspects of the relationship between the heart and brain.
- An enhanced understanding of the underlying mechanisms may lead to greater clinical attention and improved patient care.

INTRODUCTION

Recent scientific advances have led to greater attention on the heart-brain connection in disease processes involving both organs. Epidemiologic studies have identified links between maladies of the 2 systems in diverse populations. The stress response that occurs through autonomic and neurohormonal mechanisms has historically played a central role in this interplay. In addition, growing evidence supports an intimate and complex relationship between the heart and brain that involves significant crosstalk, changes in neural networks, and immune modulation to contribute to pathologic condition in both organs.[1,2] Furthermore, there appears to be variation in these mechanisms between sexes.[3]

Although investigating the heart-brain connection has remained challenging, molecular imaging using positron emission tomography (PET) and single-photon emission tomography (SPECT) is well-positioned to provide insights into the multi-system mechanisms underlying this relationship. These techniques allow simultaneous assessment of both organ systems using a variety of radiotracers that probe tissue metabolism, perfusion, innervation, and inflammation among other processes.[2,4] Furthermore, findings can be linked to imaging indices from other modalities and serologic biomarkers to generate novel observations.[1] This review focuses on describing the currently available radiotracers that facilitate the evaluation of the heart-brain connection and the mechanistic insights they provide.

DISCUSSION

Clinical Associations

Acute or chronic cardiac or neurologic disease increases the risk for concurrent disease of both organs. The most common pathologic condition that impacts both organs is atherosclerosis, which manifests clinically as myocardial infarction (MI)

a Department of Radiology, Massachusetts General Hospital, 55 Fruit Street, Boston, MA 02114, USA;
b Massachusetts General Hospital, Cardiovascular Imaging Research Center, 165 Cambridge Street, Suite 400, Boston, MA 02114, USA; c Division of Cardiology, Department of Medicine, Massachusetts General Hospital, 55 Fruit Street, Boston, MA 02114, USA
* Corresponding author. 55 Fruit Street, Yawkey 5B, Boston, MA 02114.
E-mail address: mosborne@mgh.harvard.edu

Cardiol Clin 41 (2023) 267–275
https://doi.org/10.1016/j.ccl.2023.01.013
0733-8651/23/© 2023 Elsevier Inc. All rights reserved.

or cerebrovascular accident, and typically stems from cardiovascular disease (CVD) risk factors, such as hypertension, diabetes, dyslipidemia, and smoking. MI associates with chronic heart failure, and both MI and heart failure are associated with impaired cognition owing to vascular and nonvascular causes.[5-7] Similarly, a cerebrovascular accident enhances the risk for cognitive impairment, MI, and heart failure (even without myocardial ischemia).[8,9] These relationships imply that additional connections beyond atherosclerosis contribute to disease in both organs.

In addition, the association between psychosocial stress and psychiatric disorders with adverse cardiovascular and neurologic outcomes has been increasingly recognized. People with severe psychiatric illnesses, including schizophrenia, bipolar disorder, and major depressive disorder, have 2 to 3 times higher rates of cardiovascular morbidity and mortality than the general population.[10,11] Similarly, individuals under acute and chronic stress have a greater risk for cognitive dysfunction as well as adverse cardiovascular outcomes, including atherosclerotic events and Takotsubo syndrome.[12-15] Accordingly, an enhanced understanding of this heart-brain interplay beyond atherosclerosis is needed to optimize patient care and develop novel therapeutic and preventative strategies.

Importantly, there is substantial evidence of variation in the heart-brain connection in men and women.[3] Generally, women have a profile of a lower burden of coronary artery disease (CAD) but worse clinical outcomes compared with men. Furthermore, women more commonly suffer from a type of Takotsubo syndrome, described as broken heart syndrome, that is often triggered by negative emotions.[16] Alternatively, recent findings have identified a rare type of Takotsubo syndrome, referred to as happy heart syndrome, that is more prevalent in men and is consequent to positive emotions.[17] These differences suggest additional complexity in the heart-brain connection related to sex that may explain dimorphisms in disease presentation and outcomes.

Mechanisms

Multiple pathophysiologic mechanisms contribute to the complex crosstalk underlying heart-brain connections (**Fig. 1**). The autonomic nervous system, renin-aldosterone system, and hypothalamic-pituitary-adrenal (HPA) axis all play integral roles in governing the response to both physiologic injury and psychosocial stress.[1-3] Activation of these systems culminates in increased inflammation and leukopoiesis that

have a systemic impact through cellular migration and cytokine release.[1,2] This enhanced systemic inflammatory state is closely coupled with neuroinflammation. Neuroinflammation is caused by the activation of microglia and may result from either local injury or an insult to another organ, such as the heart, through its intimate link to the peripheral immune system.[1] Over time, neuroinflammation results in neurodegeneration, whereas peripheral inflammation contributes to the progression of CVD risk factors, such as diabetes, hypertension, and hyperlipidemia, as well as CVDs, such as atherosclerosis and heart failure.[1,2] This feedforward loop between the heart and brain manifests as a potentially bidirectional and cyclical neuroimmune process that propagates itself once an initial injury occurs to either organ and contributes to disease in both.[1]

Psychosocial stress activates stress-responsive neural networks (that include fear-responsive brain regions, such as the amygdala, as well as regulatory cortical regions) and modulates the autonomic nervous system and HPA axis to culminate in changes in blood pressure and heart rate as well as heightened inflammation.[2] In addition, there are important sex variations in the stress response. Women with CAD are more likely to have mental stress-induced (but not exercise-induced) ischemia than their male counterparts.[18,19] As a consequence of stress hormones, men have higher baseline sympathetic tone, whereas women have greater baseline parasympathetic tone.[20] Despite these differences, women appear to be more susceptible to the adverse consequences of sympathetic hyperactivity.[21] Furthermore, there are important sex differences in inflammation, as women have a greater inflammatory response to stress and higher baseline C-reactive protein levels.[22,23] Accordingly, stress may act variably through these neuroimmune mechanisms to result in the development of CVD risk factors, atherosclerosis, Takotsubo syndrome, sudden cardiac death, and cognitive impairment in both sexes and provide another avenue to activate this complex heart-brain relationship.[2,14,24,25]

The importance of these relationships in linking the heart and brain was strengthened by a recent study that provided novel insights into the neuroimmune cardiovascular interfaces contributing to atherosclerosis in both mice and humans. The findings provide further supportive evidence of a biological link involving the central nervous system, including the amygdala, and the peripheral nervous system that drives atherosclerosis and can be attenuated by ligation of the splenic nerve, resulting in decreased autonomic input, inflammation, and atherosclerotic disease.[24,26]

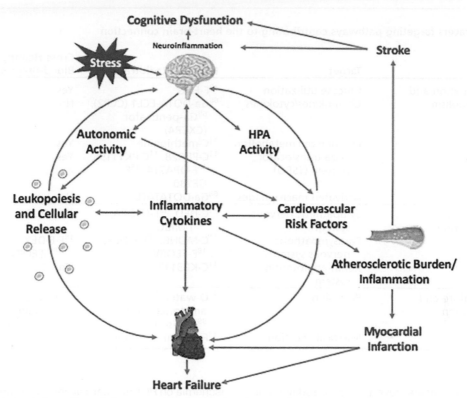

Fig. 1. Mechanistic outline of the potentially bidirectional cross talk between the heart and brain.

Radiotracers

Radiotracers targeting heart-brain connections continue to emerge (**Table 1**). Many of these radiotracers can provide an evaluation of both organs; however, the blood-brain barrier precludes the implementation of several for brain imaging. Nevertheless, some of the radiotracers that cannot penetrate the central nervous system still provide mechanistic insights through the evaluation of their peripheral uptake.

^{18}F-fluorodeoxyglucose (FDG) -PET has been extensively leveraged by systems-based approaches. ^{18}F-FDG provides an assessment of glucose metabolism throughout the body and is taken up with high avidity in tissues with high metabolic rates, such as the brain, myocardium, inflammatory cells, and malignant tumors. Furthermore, uptake of ^{18}F-FDG within the arterial wall is a validated measure that correlates with the degree of inflammatory cell infiltration and associates with downstream CVD risk.[2] In several recent studies, the relationships between arterial ^{18}F-FDG uptake and that of other organs have been explored. These studies have shown that increased resting metabolic activity in stress-associated neural networks (ie, the ratio of amygdalar to regulatory cortical uptake) and in leukopoietic tissues (ie, the bone marrow and spleen) associates with heightened inflammation in the arterial wall in individuals without CVD as well as those with acute MI.[24,27] Furthermore, this neural network activity associates with perceived stress scores as well as common psychosocial stressors, such as neighborhood income and transportation noise exposure.[24,28,29] Moreover, these neural changes may have a greater impact on inflammation and CVD in women.[22,30] Interestingly, increased uptake in the same neural networks has also been associated with the onset and timing of Takotsubo syndrome.[14] On the other hand, a recent study showed that heightened cardiovascular risk scores and carotid plaque burden associate with lower global cerebral metabolic activity on ^{18}F-FDG-PET, providing further evidence of systemic crosstalk and complex interplay between the brain and heart.[31] Although ^{18}F-FDG provides useful insights into inflammatory atherosclerosis, other radiotracers, such as ^{18}F-sodium fluoride and ^{68}Ga-tetraazacyclododecane tetraacetic acid octreotate (DOTATATE), that detect microcalcifications and somatostatin receptors, respectively, provide additional information about plaque biology and CVD risk.[32,33]

Table 1
Radiotracers targeting pathways contributing to the heart-brain connection

System	Target	Example Radiotracers	Cross Healthy Blood-Brain Barrier?
Inflammation and metabolism	Glucose utilization	^{18}F-FDG	Yes
	Chemokines/cytokines	^{68}Ga-DOTA-ECL1 (CCR2), ^{68}Ga-pentixafor (CXCR4)	No
	Immune cell metabolism	^{11}C-methionine	Yes
	18-kDa translocator protein (TSPO)	^{11}C-PBR28, ^{11}C-PK11195, ^{18}F-DPA714, ^{18}F-GE180	Yes
	Activated macrophages	^{68}Ga-DOTATATE	No
Autonomic regulation	Sympathetic nervous system	^{11}C-HED, ^{18}F-FDOPA, ^{123}I-MIBG	^{18}F-FDOPA
	Parasympathetic nervous system	^{11}C-MQNB, ^{18}F-F-DEX, ^{18}F-FEOBV	^{18}F-F-DEX, ^{18}F-FEOBV
	Renin-angiotensin system	^{11}C-KR31173	No
Vasculature and perfusion	Perfusion	^{15}O-water, ^{13}N-ammonia, ^{82}Rb, ^{99m}Tc-sestamibi	^{15}O-water, ^{13}N-ammonia
	Microcalcification	^{18}F-sodium fluoride	No

Perfusion tracers have provided additional insights into the heart-brain connection by clarifying how each organ responds to stimuli and therapies. Perfusion of both organs can be measured with PET imaging; however, the short half-lives of the commonly implemented radiotracers often require multiple imaging positions (and therefore multiple injections) to accurately evaluate first-pass imaging. Even still, increased perfusion measured in stress-responsive brain regions under conditions of mental stress using ^{15}O-water PET has been associated with shortened telomeres, a marker of aging, in white blood cells in patients with known CAD.[34] Furthermore, mental stress has long been known to provoke ischemia on SPECT myocardial perfusion imaging.[35] Further evaluation with SPECT myocardial perfusion imaging has compared the prognostic impact of mental stress-induced and conventional stress-induced ischemia.[36,37] Interestingly, those with conventional stress-induced myocardial ischemia are more likely to have obstructive epicardial CAD, whereas those with mental stress-induced ischemia without ischemia induced by conventional stress are more likely to have endothelial and microvascular dysfunction.[35] Moreover, those with both mental stress and conventional stress-induced ischemia had the greatest risk for CVD death or nonfatal MI followed by those with mental stress-induced ischemia alone.[37] Similarly, among patients with CAD, mental stress-induced

ischemia on PET myocardial perfusion imaging using ^{13}N-ammonia associates with a worse prognosis than ischemia induced by conventional methods.[37] These findings suggest that the pathologic links involve both epicardial atherosclerotic lesions and coronary microvascular dysfunction.

Several other radionuclides have become available to facilitate imaging of neurohormonal pathways that participate in the heart-brain connection. The renin-aldosterone system contributes to the response to tissue injury and can be imaged in both the heart and the brain via ^{11}C-KR31173, a PET radiotracer that binds to the angiotensin II type I receptor.[38]

The autonomic nervous system can also be interrogated by several tracers that are specific to either the sympathetic or the parasympathetic nervous system. These systems directly connect the brain and heart and act through leukopoietic tissues to contribute to changes in hemodynamics, cardiac rhythm, myocardial contractility, and systemic inflammation.[1,39] Sympathetic activity is chronically upregulated in heart failure as well as in cerebral and myocardial ischemia, and it contributes to increased inflammation, leukopoiesis, and HPA axis activity.[1,2,39] Radiotracers that allow the assessment of myocardial sympathetic innervation include ^{123}I-meta-iodobenzylguanidine (MIBG) for SPECT imaging and ^{11}C-hydroxyephedrine (HED) and ^{18}F-fluorodopa (FDOPA) for PET imaging.[40–42] Notably, FDOPA has also been

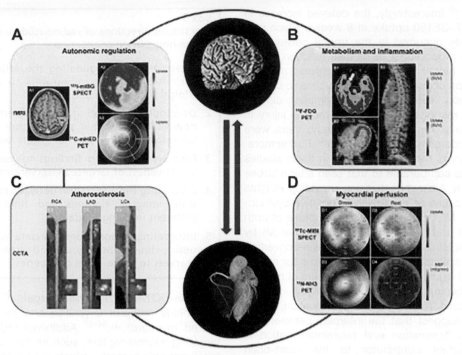

Fig. 2. Application of various imaging modalities to visualize mechanisms underlying the heart-brain relationship. (*A*) Visualizing autonomic regulation using functional MRI (*A1*), ^{123}I-mIBG-SPECT (*A2*), and ^{11}C-mHED-PET (*A3*). (*B*) ^{18}F-FDG-PET images of metabolism and inflammation with increased ^{18}F-FDG uptake in the right amygdala (*B1; white arrow*), myocardium (*B2*), and bone marrow (*B3*). (*C*) CCTA imaging of calcified and noncalcified atherosclerotic plaques shows mid-RCA-positive remodeling (*C1*), mid-LAD calcified plaque (*C2*), and mid-LCx spotty calcification (*C3*). Red boxes show the cross-sectional view at the level of the corresponding plaque for each vessel. (*D*) Myocardial perfusion images show a reversible myocardial perfusion defect of the inferior wall of the left ventricle during stress (*D1*) versus rest (*D2*). Low MBF (mL/g/min) in the myocardial territory supplied by the LAD (*D3*) did not increase during stress (*D3*) as compared with rest (*D4*). ^{11}C-mHED, ^{11}C-meta-hydroxyephedrine; ^{123}I-mIBG, ^{123}I-metaiodobenzylguanidine; ^{13}N-NH3, ^{13}N-ammonia; ^{99}Tc-MIBI, [99]Technetium-methoxyisobutyl isonitrile; CCTA, coronary computed tomography angiography; fMRI, functional magnetic resonance imaging; LAD, left anterior descending coronary artery; LCx, left circumflex coronary artery; MBF, myocardial blood flow; MR, magnetic resonance; RCA, right coronary artery; SUV, standard uptake value. (*From* Rossi A, Mikail N, Bengs S, et al. Heart-brain interactions in cardiac and brain diseases: why sex matters. Eur Heart J. 2022;43(39):3971-3980.)

applied to assess autonomic dysfunction in primary neurologic diseases (eg, Parkinson disease).[41] Alternatively, several other radiotracers target the parasympathetic nervous system, which counteracts the sympathetic nervous system, through their affinity to targets in cholinergic neurons. Examples include ^{11}C-methylquinuclidinyl benzilate (MQNB), ^{18}F-fluorobenzyl dexetimide (F-DEX), and ^{18}F-fluoroethoxy-benzovesamicol (FEOBV).[43–45]

Beyond ^{18}F-FDG, which is nonspecific for inflammation, many other radionuclide tracers have been developed to target this critical process and have provided important insights into the role of inflammation in the heart-brain connection. These tracers exhibit different patterns of uptake in different leukocyte populations, allowing them

to differentially characterize the actions of the immune system in different tissues.[46]

Tracers targeting the 18-kDa translocator protein (TSPO) have been particularly informative. These tracers bind to a protein expressed by the mitochondria of activated immune cells and can cross the blood-brain barrier. Therefore, they localize to both activated peripheral macrophages and microglia to provide information about systemic and neuroinflammation. Following MI, TSPO tracers concentrate in the bone marrow and spleen for an extended period of time, indicating increased leukopoietic activity.[46,47] In a murine study of MI, ^{18}F-GE180 localized to CD68-positive macrophages in the region of MI as well as CD68-positive microglia within 1 week before declining at 4 weeks and again increasing at

8 weeks.[48] Interestingly, the delayed increase in neural ^{18}F-GE180 uptake at 8 weeks, which predominately occurred in the frontal cortex, was inversely proportional to cardiac function, which provides further argument that chronic neuroinflammation occurs consequent to chronic cardiac dysfunction. Notably, neuroinflammation did not occur in response to a skeletal muscle injury in the same study. In a human study, there were similar findings with ^{11}C-PK11195.[48] Furthermore, the observed neuroinflammation in these studies of MI was comparable to that seen after a stroke or in early Alzheimer disease, providing insights into the cause of progressive cognitive dysfunction after MI.[49,50] Importantly, the uptake of both the heart and brain was decreased after MI by the administration of an angiotensin-converting enzyme inhibitor, indicating a key role for neurohormonal signaling in the development of multiorgan inflammation.[47] Although these precise mechanisms require further clarification, these findings suggest that the interplay between peripheral inflammation and neuroinflammation is an important contributor to the heart-brain connection following injury to either the heart or the brain.

A recent investigation explored the impact of the SARS-CoV-2 pandemic on neuroinflammation in individuals without viral infection using a TSPO tracer. It compared healthy individuals imaged before and after the lockdown using ^{11}C-PBR28 PET and showed heightened brain levels of TSPO activity after the lockdown compared with before. Furthermore, the individuals demonstrated nonsignificant trends toward increased interleukin-16 and monocyte chemoattractant protein-1, which both associate with greater atherosclerotic disease, after the lockdown.[51] These findings suggest that neuroinflammation may also be a consequence of psychosocial stress that contributes to downstream pathologic conditions of the heart and brain.

Several other radiotracers facilitate evaluation of the role of inflammation in the heart-brain connection. ^{11}C-methionine further characterizes the role of the immune system in the heart-brain relationship by targeting leukocyte amino acid metabolism, a process initiated at the onset of immune activation. After MI, uptake of ^{11}C-methionine in the injured myocardium rises rapidly before subsequent proportionally increased brain uptake that localizes to astroglia.[52,53] In addition, radiotracers targeting cytokines and chemokines localize to inflammatory cell infiltration. These include ^{68}Ga-pentixafor, which targets C-X-C motif chemokine receptor 4 (CXCR4) and localizes to atherosclerotic plaques, MI, and stroke, as well

as ^{68}Ga-DOTA-ECL1, which targets C-C motif chemokine receptor 2 (CCR2) and localizes to injured myocardium.[54–57] Additional radiotracers targeting neuroreceptors, such as the fast inhibitory ionotropic gamma-aminobutyric acid receptor (^{18}F-flumazenil), have facilitated research into the emotional response to stress.[58]

Other Imaging Modalities

Imaging modalities aside from nuclear techniques have been leveraged to evaluate the link between the heart and brain (**Fig. 2**). Several insights have arisen from findings on ^{18}F-FDG-PET imaging and concurrently acquired attenuation correction computed tomography (CT) imaging. For example, 1 such study identified a relationship between an increased ratio of ^{18}F-FDG uptake in the amygdala relative to cortical tissue and increased visceral adiposity, an important CVD risk factor.[59] In a study of patients with psoriasis, heightened ^{18}F-FDG uptake in the amygdala relative to cortical tissue associated with greater coronary plaque burden on CT-angiography.[60] Other studies have implemented structural and functional MRI to evaluate the heart-brain connection. Studies of patients with prior Takotsubo syndrome demonstrated altered regional brain volumes and connectivity relative to controls.[61–63] Accordingly, several other imaging tools offer complementary insights that further the understanding of this relationship beyond those derived from molecular imaging.

SUMMARY

Greater recognition of the neuroimmune axis and its component mechanisms that underlie the

---

Box 1
Key future directions of radionuclide imaging of the heart-brain connection

1. Establishing and validating the efficacy of currently available radiotracers to expand clinical recognition and access

2. Developing, validating, and implementing new radiotracers that allow further characterization of complex multisystem biology

3. Leveraging imaging findings to assess the effectiveness of targeted interventions

4. Evaluating the association between radionuclide imaging findings and findings on different imaging modalities

5. Integrating imaging-derived data with genetics, clinical phenotypes, and systemic biomarkers to make novel discoveries

heart-brain connection will result in greater clinical recognition and attention to factors that contribute to heightened crosstalk between these organs. Molecular imaging is uniquely positioned to study the heart-brain connection through its capacity to perform targeted whole-body imaging with a variety of tracers that characterize biological processes, such as perfusion, metabolism, autonomic nervous system and neurohormonal activity, and inflammation. Although additional research is needed (**Box 1**), these tracers can be leveraged in conjunction with other imaging modalities and serologic biomarkers to further refine the understanding of the underlying biology and how it varies between sexes. Furthermore, these same techniques can then be used to identify potential therapies as well as evaluate their impact on disparate tissues and biological intermediaries with the goal of reducing the consequent disease in both the heart and the brain.

CLINICS CARE POINTS

- Increasing evidence supports the presence of an important link between the heart and brain that contributes to pathologic condition in both organs.

- Nevertheless, this relationship is often overlooked clinically because the biological pathways linking the 2 organs are complex and have been challenging to disentangle.

- Molecular nuclear imaging provides a significant opportunity to evaluate a variety of contributory mechanisms simultaneously in disparate tissues, including inflammation, autonomic nervous and neurohormonal system activity, metabolism, and perfusion.

- Although many of these molecular imaging approaches are not yet available clinically, the insights generated from ongoing research will increase clinical awareness of the heart-brain connection and may yield novel insights into potential therapeutic approaches.

DISCLOSURE

Dr M.T. Osborne is supported in part by the United States National Institutes of Health K23HL151909 and receives consulting fees from WCG Intrinsic Imaging, LLC for unrelated work. Dr A. Tawakol is supported in part by the United States National Institutes of Health (NIH R01AR077187, R01HL152957, R01HL137913, P01HL131478, R01HL149516), International Atomic Energy Agency, and Lung Biotechnology, Inc for unrelated work. Drs S. Abohashem and S.S. Grewal have no disclosures.

REFERENCES

1. Bengel FM, Hermanns N, Thackeray JT. Radionuclide imaging of the molecular mechanisms linking heart and brain in ischemic syndromes. Circulation Cardiovascular imaging 2020;13(8):e011303.

2. Osborne MT, Abohashem S, Zureigat H, et al. Multimodality molecular imaging: gaining insights into the mechanisms linking chronic stress to cardiovascular disease. J Nucl Cardiol 2021;28(3):955–66.

3. Rossi A, Mikail N, Bengs S, et al. Heart-brain interactions in cardiac and brain diseases: why sex matters. Eur Heart J 2022. https://doi.org/10.1093/eurheartj/ehac061.

4. Thackeray JT. Imaging the molecular footprints of the heart-brain axis in cardiovascular disease. J Nucl Med. Jun 2019;60(6):728–9.

5. Breteler MM, Claus JJ, Grobbee DE, et al. Cardiovascular disease and distribution of cognitive function in elderly people: the Rotterdam Study. BMJ 1994;308(6944):1604–8.

6. Xie W, Zheng F, Yan L, et al. Cognitive decline before and after incident coronary events. J Am Coll Cardiol 2019;73(24):3041–50.

7. Qiu C, Winblad B, Marengoni A, et al. Heart failure and risk of dementia and Alzheimer disease: a population-based cohort study. Arch Intern Med 2006;166(9):1003–8.

8. Gunnoo T, Hasan N, Khan MS, et al. Quantifying the risk of heart disease following acute ischaemic stroke: a meta-analysis of over 50,000 participants. BMJ Open 2016;6(1):e009535.

9. Laowattana S, Zeger SL, Lima JA, et al. Left insular stroke is associated with adverse cardiac outcome. Neurology 2006;66(4):477–83 [discussion: 463].

10. Brown S, Kim M, Mitchell C, et al. Twenty-five year mortality of a community cohort with schizophrenia. Br J Psychiatry 2010;196(2):116–21.

11. Dar T, Radfar A, Abohashem S, et al. Psychosocial stress and cardiovascular disease. Curr Treat Options Cardiovasc Med 2019;21(5):23.

12. Leor J, Poole WK, Kloner RA. Sudden cardiac death triggered by an earthquake. N Engl J Med 1996;334(7):413–9.

13. Rosengren A, Hawken S, Ôunpuu S, et al. Association of psychosocial risk factors with risk of acute myocardial infarction in 11 119 cases and 13 648 controls from 52 countries (the INTERHEART study): case-control study. Lancet 2004;364(9438):953–62.

14. Radfar A, Abohashem S, Osborne MT, et al. Stress-associated neurobiological activity associates with

the risk for and timing of subsequent Takotsubo syndrome. Eur Heart J 2021;42(19):1898–908.

15. McEwen BS, Sapolsky RM. Stress and cognitive function. Curr Opin Neurobiol 1995;5(2):205–16.

16. Arcari L, Nunez Gil IJ, Stiermaier T, et al. Gender differences in Takotsubo syndrome. J Am Coll Cardiol 2022;79(21):2085–93.

17. Stiermaier T, Walliser A, El-Battrawy I, et al. Happy heart syndrome. JACC (J Am Coll Cardiol): Heart Fail 2022;10(7):459–66.

18. Truong QA, Rinehart S, Abbara S, et al. Coronary computed tomographic imaging in women: an expert consensus statement from the Society of Cardiovascular Computed Tomography. Journal of Cardiovascular Computed Tomography 2018;12(6):451–66.

19. Vaccarino V, Shah AJ, Rooks C, et al. Sex differences in mental stress-induced myocardial ischemia in young survivors of an acute myocardial infarction. Psychosom Med 2014;76(3):171–80.

20. Dart AM, Du XJ, Kingwell BA. Gender, sex hormones and autonomic nervous control of the cardiovascular system. Cardiovasc Res Feb 15 2002;53(3):678–87.

21. Gebhard CE, Maredziak M, Portmann A, et al. Heart rate reserve is a long-term risk predictor in women undergoing myocardial perfusion imaging. Eur J Nucl Med Mol Imaging 2019;46(10):2032–41.

22. Fiechter M, Haider A, Bengs S, et al. Sex-dependent association between inflammation, neural stress responses, and impaired myocardial function. Eur J Nucl Med Mol Imaging 2019. https://doi.org/10.1007/s00259-019-04537-8.

23. Khera A, McGuire DK, Murphy SA, et al. Race and gender differences in C-reactive protein levels. J Am Coll Cardiol 2005;46(3):464–9.

24. Tawakol A, Ishai A, Takx RA, et al. Relation between resting amygdalar activity and cardiovascular events: a longitudinal and cohort study. Lancet 2017;389(10071):834–45.

25. Osborne MT, Ishai A, Hammad B, et al. Amygdalar activity predicts future incident diabetes independently of adiposity. Psychoneuroendocrinology 2018;100:32–40.

26. Mohanta SK, Peng L, Li Y, et al. Neuroimmune cardiovascular interfaces control atherosclerosis. Nature 2022;605(7908):152–9.

27. Kang DO, Eo JS, Park EJ, et al. Stress-associated neurobiological activity is linked with acute plaque instability via enhanced macrophage activity: a prospective serial 18F-FDG-PET/CT imaging assessment. Eur Heart J 2021;42(19):1883–95.

28. Osborne MT, Radfar A, Hassan MZO, et al. A neurobiological mechanism linking transportation noise to cardiovascular disease in humans. Eur Heart J 2020;41(6):772–82.

29. Tawakol A, Osborne MT, Wang Y, et al. Stress-associated neurobiological pathway linking socioeconomic disparities to cardiovascular disease. J Am Coll Cardiol 2019;73(25):3243–55.

30. Fiechter M, Roggo A, Burger IA, et al. Association between resting amygdalar activity and abnormal cardiac function in women and men: a retrospective cohort study. European Heart Journal Cardiovascular Imaging 2019;20(6):625–32.

31. Cortes-Canteli M, Gispert JD, Salvado G, et al. Subclinical atherosclerosis and brain metabolism in middle-aged individuals: the PESA study. J Am Coll Cardiol 2021;77(7):888–98.

32. Kwiecinski J, Tzolos E, Adamson PD, et al. Coronary (18)F-sodium fluoride uptake predicts outcomes in patients with coronary artery disease. J Am Coll Cardiol 2020;75(24):3061–74.

33. Tarkin JM, Joshi FR, Evans NR, et al. Detection of atherosclerotic inflammation by (68)Ga-DOTATATE PET compared to [(18)F]FDG PET imaging. J Am Coll Cardiol 2017;69(14):1774–91.

34. Almuwaqqat Z, Wittbrodt MT, Moazzami K, et al. Neural correlates of stress and leucocyte telomere length in patients with coronary artery disease. J Psychosom Res 2022;155:110760.

35. Hammadah M, Al Mheid I, Wilmot K, et al. The mental stress ischemia prognosis study: objectives, study design, and prevalence of inducible ischemia. Psychosom Med 2017;79(3):311–7.

36. Vaccarino V, Sullivan S, Hammadah M, et al. Mental stress-induced-myocardial ischemia in young patients with recent myocardial infarction: sex differences and mechanisms. Circulation 2018;137(8):794–805.

37. Vaccarino V, Almuwaqqat Z, Kim JH, et al. Association of mental stress-induced myocardial ischemia with cardiovascular events in patients with coronary heart disease. JAMA 2021;326(18):1818–28.

38. Higuchi T, Fukushima K, Xia J, et al. Radionuclide imaging of angiotensin II type 1 receptor upregulation after myocardial ischemia-reperfusion injury. J Nucl Med 2010;51(12):1956–61.

39. Dutta P, Courties G, Wei Y, et al. Myocardial infarction accelerates atherosclerosis. Nature 2012;487(7407):325–9.

40. Henderson EB, Kahn JK, Corbett JR, et al. Abnormal I-123 metaiodobenzylguanidine myocardial washout and distribution may reflect myocardial adrenergic derangement in patients with congestive cardiomyopathy. Circulation 1988;78(5 Pt 1):1192–9.

41. Kuten J, Linevitz A, Lerman H, et al. [18F] FDOPA PET may confirm the clinical diagnosis of Parkinson's disease by imaging the nigro-striatal pathway and the sympathetic cardiac innervation: proof-of-concept study. J Integr Neurosci 2020;19(3):489–94.

42. Allman KC, Wieland DM, Muzik O, et al. Carbon-11 hydroxyephedrine with positron emission tomography for serial assessment of cardiac adrenergic

neuronal function after acute myocardial infarction in humans. J Am Coll Cardiol 1993;22(2):368–75.

43. Delforge J, Le Guludec D, Syrota A, et al. Quantification of myocardial muscarinic receptors with PET in humans. J Nucl Med 1993;34(6):981–91.

44. Pain CD, O'Keefe GJ, Ackermann U, et al. Human biodistribution and internal dosimetry of 4-[(18)F]fluorobenzyl-dexetimide: a PET radiopharmaceutical for imaging muscarinic acetylcholine receptors in the brain and heart. EJNMMI Res 2020;10(1):61.

45. Saint-Georges Z, Zayed VK, Dinelle K, et al. First-in-human imaging and kinetic analysis of vesicular acetylcholine transporter density in the heart using [(18)F]FEOBV PET. J Nucl Cardiol 2021;28(1):50–4.

46. Borchert T, Beitar L, Langer LBN, et al. Dissecting the target leukocyte subpopulations of clinically relevant inflammation radiopharmaceuticals. J Nucl Cardiol 2021;28(4):1636–45.

47. Borchert T, Hess A, Lukacevic M, et al. Angiotensin-converting enzyme inhibitor treatment early after myocardial infarction attenuates acute cardiac and neuroinflammation without effect on chronic neuroinflammation. Eur J Nucl Med Mol Imaging 2020; 47(7):1757–68.

48. Thackeray JT, Hupe HC, Wang Y, et al. Myocardial inflammation predicts remodeling and neuroinflammation after myocardial infarction. J Am Coll Cardiol 2018;71(3):263–75.

49. Heiss WD. The ischemic penumbra: how does tissue injury evolve? Ann N Y Acad Sci 2012;1268:26–34.

50. Long JM, Holtzman DM. Alzheimer disease: an update on pathobiology and treatment strategies. Cell 2019;179(2):312–39.

51. Brusaferri L, Alshelh Z, Martins D, et al. The pandemic brain: neuroinflammation in non-infected individuals during the COVID-19 pandemic. Brain Behav Immun 2022;102:89–97.

52. Thackeray JT, Bankstahl JP, Wang Y, et al. Targeting amino acid metabolism for molecular imaging of inflammation early after myocardial infarction. Theranostics 2016;6(11):1768–79.

53. Bascunana P, Hess A, Borchert T, et al. 11)C-Methionine PET identifies astroglia involvement in heart-brain inflammation networking after acute myocardial infarction. J Nucl Med 2020;61(7):977–80.

54. Hyafil F, Pelisek J, Laitinen I, et al. Imaging the cytokine receptor CXCR4 in atherosclerotic plaques with the radiotracer (68)Ga-pentixafor for PET. J Nucl Med 2017;58(3):499–506.

55. Reiter T, Kircher M, Schirbel A, et al. Imaging of C-X-C Motif Chemokine Receptor CXCR4 expression after myocardial infarction with [(68)Ga]Pentixafor-PET/CT in correlation with cardiac MRI. JACC Cardiovasc Imaging 2018;11(10):1541–3.

56. Schmid JS, Schirbel A, Buck AK, et al. [68Ga]Pentixafor-positron emission tomography/computed tomography detects chemokine receptor CXCR4 expression after ischemic stroke. Circulation Cardiovascular Imaging 2016;9(9):e005217.

57. Heo GS, Kopecky B, Sultan D, et al. Molecular imaging visualizes recruitment of inflammatory monocytes and macrophages to the injured heart. Circ Res 2019;124(6):881–90.

58. Geuze E, van Berckel BN, Lammertsma AA, et al. Reduced GABAA benzodiazepine receptor binding in veterans with post-traumatic stress disorder. Mol Psychiatr 2008;13(1):74–83, 3.

59. Ishai A, Osborne MT, Tung B, et al. Amygdalar metabolic activity independently associates with progression of visceral adiposity. J Clin Endocrinol Metab 2019;104(4):1029–38.

60. Goyal A, Dey AK, Chaturvedi A, et al. Chronic stress-related neural activity associates with subclinical cardiovascular disease in psoriasis: a prospective cohort study. JACC Cardiovasc Imaging 2020;13(2 Pt 1):465–77.

61. Silva AR, Magalhaes R, Arantes C, et al. Brain functional connectivity is altered in patients with Takotsubo syndrome. Sci Rep 2019;9(1):4187.

62. Templin C, Hanggi J, Klein C, et al. Altered limbic and autonomic processing supports brain-heart axis in Takotsubo syndrome. Eur Heart J 2019; 40(15):1183–7.

63. Hiestand T, Hanggi J, Klein C, et al. Takotsubo syndrome associated with structural brain alterations of the limbic system. J Am Coll Cardiol 20 2018;71(7): 809–11.

Moving?

Make sure your subscription moves with you!

To notify us of your new address, find your **Clinics Account Number** (located on your mailing label above your name), and contact customer service at:

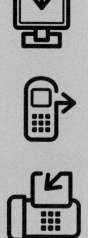

Email: journalscustomerservice-usa@elsevier.com

800-654-2452 (subscribers in the U.S. & Canada)
314-447-8871 (subscribers outside of the U.S. & Canada)

Fax number: 314-447-8029

Elsevier Health Sciences Division
Subscription Customer Service
3251 Riverport Lane
Maryland Heights, MO 63043

*To ensure uninterrupted delivery of your subscription, please notify us at least 4 weeks in advance of move.

Printed and bound by CPI Group (UK) Ltd, Croydon, CR0 4YY

03/10/2024

01040367-0015